Post registration qualifications for dental care professionals

Questions and answers

Post registration qualifications for dental care professionals

Questions and answers

Nicola Rogers RDN, NEBDN National Certificate in Dental Nursing, NEBDN Certificate in Dental Sedation Nursing, NEBDN Certificate in Dental Radiography, NEBDN Certificate in Oral Health Education

Tutor of the Year 2010 (DDU Educational Awards)
Author of *Basic Guide to Dental Sedation Nursing*
Dental Nurse Tutor, Pre and Post Registration Training
Bristol Dental Hospital
Bristol, UK

Rebecca Davies BChD (Hons), MFDSRCS (Eng), MSc, DDRRCR

Consultant and Honorary Senior Lecturer in Dental and Maxillofacial Radiology
University Hospitals Bristol NHS Foundation Trust
Bristol Dental Hospital
Bristol, UK

Wendy Lee Dip Orth Ther (Edin)

DCP Tutor
Bristol Dental Hospital
Bristol, UK

Dominic O'Sullivan BDS, FDSRCS (Eng), PhD, FDS (Rest Dent) RCS, FHEA

Professor in Restorative Dentistry
Programme Director for MSc in Dental Implantology
Graduate Director for School of Oral and Dental Sciences
Bristol Dental Hospital
Bristol, UK

Frances Marriott RDH MRSPH Cert Ed, Diploma in Dental Hygiene

Royal Society of Public Health–Diploma in Nutrition and Diet
Stonebridge Associated Colleges–Diploma in Post Traumatic Stress Disorder
Certificate in Education (University of Plymouth)
Company Director–Focus Oral Health CIC
Plymouth, UK

WILEY Blackwell

Library of Congress Cataloging-in-Publication Data

Rogers, Nicola, 1962- , author.
   Post registration qualifications for dental care professionals : questions and answers / Nicola Rogers, Rebecca Davies, Wendy Lee, Dominic O'Sullivan, Frances Marriott.
      p. ; cm.
   ISBN 978-1-118-71116-3 (pbk.)
   I. Davies, Rebecca, 1972- , author. II. Lee, Wendy, 1963- , author. III. O'Sullivan, Dominic, 1968- , author. IV. Marriott, Frances, 1958- , author. V. Title.
   [DNLM: 1. Dental Assistants–Examination Questions. 2. Dental Care–Examination Questions. WU 18.2]
   RK57
   617.60076–dc23

                            2015022533

A catalogue record for this book is available from the British Library.

Set in 9/11.5pt TimesLTStd by SPi Global, Chennai, India
Printed and bound in Malaysia by Vivar Printing Sdn Bhd

1   2016

Contents

How to use this book

This book is a revision resource tool which has been written with dental nurses in mind to assist them in establishing any gaps in their personal knowledge, enabling them to prepare for any final assessment/examination. However, it could be used by other members of the dental team preparing for forthcoming examinations. It is split into subject areas, assigning a chapter to each topic to reflect the current ones where dental nurses can access courses and qualifications, being designed to aid preparation for final examinations. It has been written in a user-friendly manner covering all aspects relevant to the National Examining Board for Dental Nurses' examinations.

Although subjects are stand-alone, additional questions relating to common topics such as law and ethics, medical emergencies, cross-infection control, health and safety, and patient care may be found in other chapters.

There is no intention of instructing/criticising clinicians, or any professionals on their role in the clinical environment, which has only been explained to further the knowledge of dental nurses through this revision resource book. Any offence is entirely unintended and apologies are tendered for any perceived affront.

Dental nurses are subsequently reminded/warned that on no account should they under-take any duty that is solely the province of any other General Dental Council or Health Care Professional.

Acknowledgements

Nicola Rogers

To my husband David and son Sean, both of whom I am very proud for their own personal achievements, for the love, perseverance and continual support they have shown while I have been writing this chapter.

To my parents Nigel and Valerie for always being there for me, encouraging and supporting me in everything I do, especially my Father who has constantly given his time to reading and helping me correct the sedation chapter.

To the other authors for agreeing to write their chapters within this book and Wiley Blackwell for publishing it, thereby making my vision possible to provide DCPs with a valuable revision resource.

Rebecca Davies

I have endeavoured to write a selection of questions primarily to test dental nurses, hygienists and therapists on dental radiography and radiology. I give no excuses for some of the difficult questions that lie ahead. For those of you who will take dental radiographs you have a responsibility to your patients, your colleagues, members of the public and yourselves to have a good knowledge and respect for ionising radiation.

Many people have helped me along this journey, and to all of them I am extremely grateful.

To my friend Nikki Rogers, thank you for asking me to join your collaboration and for your continual support.

To my departmental colleagues Jos Sewell, Stuart Grange, Lynn Wilcox, Tracey Cunningham, Jane Luker, and Louise Denning, thank you for all you have done.

To John Rout and Eric Whaites, I am truly grateful for the time you have given in providing your feedback and expert advice on the content of this chapter. Both of you have inspired me with your teaching and knowledge over the years.

To my mum, Margaret, heartfelt thanks for reading my work and correcting the grammar. Some things never change.

Finally, special thanks to my husband Scott and my beautiful children Esme and Harry for their help, love, encouragement and understanding at all times.

Wendy Lee

Dedicated to all the dental nurses who have shown, and will continue to show, enormous commitment and effort to improve their professional skills and understanding of Orthodontics to the benefit of their patients.

Special thanks must go to Clare McNamara, Consultant Orthodontist, whose inspirational leadership and enthusiasm ensures a high standard is taught within our courses.

Dominic O'Sullivan

To Nikki and Wiley Blackwell for inviting me to take part in this book. To my parents and family for encouraging me and supporting me throughout my education and career and for always being there for me. Especially my father for his incredibly wise words of advice over the years.

Frances Marriott

First of all, a huge thank you to my dear husband Steve and sons Bryn and Dean for all of their support. Steve has been at my side for practically the whole of my dental career (we met very soon after I had qualified as a Dental Hygienist). He continues to provide unwavering support through all of the very personal and professional challenges I am still working through to this very day. Indeed, my lovely family can state the key dental public health messages with 100% accuracy too!

Over the years, other family members and good friends have been a real source of support too. Through their continued positivity, kindness and generous goodwill, the vision of having a totally 'non-clinical' community based Oral Health Education and Information service (Focus Oral Health CIC) has been achieved – special thanks go to my colleague Lorraine and her family for signing up to our 'journey'.

Without a doubt, I also thank all of the patients I have cared for throughout my years in Special Care Dentistry. It has been a true privilege to meet such a diverse community of people who, in all honesty, have both enriched my clinical practice and actually taught me my 'job'. It is intentional, therefore, that some details within my chapters on Special Care Dentistry and Oral Health Education is indeed based on personal learning and authentic experience.

About the companion website

This book is accompanied by a companion website:

www.wiley.com/go/rogers/post-registration-dental-care-questions

The website includes:

Example questions reflecting different methods of assessment.

CHAPTER 1

Special care dental nursing

Post Registration Qualifications for Dental Care Professionals: Questions and Answers, First Edition.
Nicola Rogers, Rebecca Davies, Wendy Lee, Dominic O'Sullivan and Frances Marriott.
© 2016 John Wiley & Sons, Ltd. Published 2016 by John Wiley & Sons, Ltd.
Companion Website: www.wiley.com/go/rogers/post-registration-dental-care-questions

SECTION I Questions: Disability awareness

LEARNING OUTCOMES

At the end of this section, you should be able to identify any gaps in knowledge associated with the following:

- Impairment and disability
- Related legislation and guidelines – consent
- Barriers to access

Impairment and disability

1. Define the term 'Impairment'.

2. Define the term 'Disability'.

3. Disability can be listed under four main classifications. What are these?

4. Give an example of an impairment for each of the four classifications of disability.

5. What is meant by the Social Model of Disability?

6. What is meant by the Medical Model of Disability?

Related legislation and guidelines – consent

1. State three key legislative Acts which help inform the delivery of Special Care Dentistry.

2. In 2011, the 'Public Sector Equality Duty' became part of the Equality Act. State one action the amendment required that public organisations need to take.

3. State three 'dentally related' documents which help inform delivery of oral health care for people with disabilities.

4. In relation to Health and Social Care, a new Act was introduced in 2012 – what was it called?

5. When determining a new way of working or a new policy in healthcare provision, what is an EIA?

6. From date of diagnosis, progressive conditions such as HIV, Cancer and Multiple Sclerosis are covered by which key disability related legislation?

7. In relation to obtaining consent in England and Wales, what do the letters MCA stand for?

8. When did the MCA come into force?

9. In relation to obtaining consent in Scotland, which Act is involved?

10. When did this Act come into force?

11. A person who supports another person (who lacks capacity and has no appropriate family or friends to consult) to make decisions is called an IMCA? What does this stand for?

12. State two types of situation when the services of an IMCA may be necessary.

13. Another form of advocacy support is via an IMHA – what do these letters stand for?

14. To protect a vulnerable person from harm, DoLS may be implemented – what is this?

15. State three ways in which the 'principles' of informed consent can be implemented.

Barriers to access

1. State two ways patient general anxiety may be triggered/increased in the dental waiting room.

2. State three 'physical' environmental barriers to access dental care.

3. State three 'organisational' barriers to access dental care.

4. State three 'social' barriers to access dental care.

5. State two 'cultural' barriers to access dental care.

6. State three 'medical' barriers in relation to patient care and management.

7. State three 'communication' barriers in relation to patient care and management.

SECTION II Questions: Facilitating access

> **LEARNING OUTCOMES**
>
> At the end of this section, you should be able to identify any gaps in knowledge associated with the following:
> - Providing special care dentistry
> - Reasonable adjustments
> - Oral health screening

Providing special care dentistry

1. What is Special Care Dentistry?

2. Describe three 'community' providers of Special Care Dentistry.

3. State three dental specialties that may be found in the Hospital setting.

4. Describe the purpose of a mobile dental unit.

5. State four ways that provision of a dental service in a mobile dental unit may differ from working in a fixed clinic?

Reasonable adjustments

1. Describe four examples of environmental 'reasonable adjustments' for gaining access to the dental clinical setting.

2. Describe four examples of environmental 'reasonable adjustments' upon entering the dental clinical setting.

3. State three considerations in relation to seating arrangements in the waiting room.

4. Give an example of a 'reasonable adjustment' in relation to information provision.

5. How can a patient who needs help to complete their medical history be supported?

6. Give an example of 'inclusive' language to replace the statement 'disabled toilet'.

7. 'Disability etiquette' is important. Give an example of steps to take when meeting a person who is a wheelchair user.

8. Give an example of considerations to take when meeting a person who requires help with navigation.

Oral health screening

1. Oral health screenings are carried out by Community Dental Services. What is the correct name for this work?

2. Give two advantages of carrying out oral health screenings.

3. Give three disadvantages of carrying out oral health screenings.

4. State five considerations during the initial planning of an oral health screening.

5. State three considerations required on arriving at the venue on day of oral health screening.

6. State six items required for carrying out an oral health screening.

7. State three considerations required for after an oral health screening has been carried out.

SECTION III Questions: Communication

LEARNING OUTCOMES

At the end of this section, you should be able to identify any gaps in knowledge associated with:

- Pre-visit information – supporting patient and carer
- Sensory impairment
- Alternative communication

Pre-visit information – supporting patient and carer

1. When scheduling an initial dental visit, state at least three considerations to be made.

2. State two pieces of information a Dental Nurse could provide to the patient/carer prior to attending the dental clinic.

3. State two pieces of information a Dental Nurse could provide to the patient/carer prior to attending for actual dental treatment.

4. 'Personal preference' information helps in determining successful outcomes for patients – give four examples of what this could include.

5. What communication and interpersonal skills are required to enhance support for individuals with diverse needs?

6. State two health-related conditions that may impair communication.

7. What are the four modalities of language?

8. What does the term Dysarthria mean?

9. What is an inability to understand spoken or written work known as?

10. State three 'environmental' barriers to effective communication in the clinical setting.

Sensory impairment

1. What is meant by the term sight loss?

2. Partial sight is categorised by different levels – what are they?

3. Define the term blindness.

4. What are the leading causes of sight loss?

5. What are the leading causes of blindness?

6. Define visual impairment.

7. What is meant by visual acuity?

8. Myopia is the clinical term for which eye condition?

9. What is the role of an Optometrist?

10. What is the role of an Ophthalmologist?

11. What is the role of an Orthoptist?

12. How can hearing impairment occur?

13. What is tinnitus?

14. State three ways in which effective communication for people with hearing impairment may be facilitated.

15. What is a hearing loop system?

16. What is a Cochlear implant?

17. State three ways in which effective communication for someone with visual impairment may be facilitated.

18. State three ways information may be effectively provided for someone with visual impairment.

19. State three ways effective communication for people with a cognitive disability may be facilitated.

20. When providing information for a person with Learning Disability – what is meant by the term 'sequencing'?

21. State three ways in which effective communication for people with speech impairment may be facilitated.

22. State three ways in which effective communication for people with mobility impairment may be facilitated.

23. A person with Autism may have several 'sensory' challenges – name four.

Alternative communication

1. BSL is a communication method used predominately by members of the Deaf community – what is it?

2. Lip reading is what type of communication?

3. The Total Communication approach uses a combination of communication methods – state five methods that may be included.

4. What is Makaton?

5. Give the name of two commonly used picture symbol sets.

6. What is Braille?

7. What is Moon?

8. What is the deaf-blind manual alphabet?

9. How does the 'block alphabet' differ from the deaf-blind manual alphabet?

10. Name two non-verbal methods of communication that are based purely on physical movement.

11. State an alternative method for verbal communication to occur via use of technology.

12. What is a picture board?

13. When could an Alternative and Augmentative Communication (AAC) system be used?

14. State one way in which an Alternative and Augmentative Communication (AAC) system may be operated.

15. How can telecommunications items be adapted to support effective communication?

16. Interpreters can be employed to assist with communication – name two types of interpreters.

17. Describe the three common steps used during the teaching of a new skill.

18. What is the purpose of a palatal lift (training) device?

SECTION IV Questions: Diversity of need

LEARNING OUTCOMES

At the end of this section, you should be able to identify any gaps in knowledge associated with provision of dental care for patients of all ages who may have:
- Medically compromising conditions
- Cancer and palliative care
- Learning and physical disabilities

Medically compromising conditions

1. What is the difference between a sign and a symptom?

2. In relation to 'cardiac' complications, what is a VSD?

3. What is meant by the term cardiovascular disease (CVD)?

4. Mention two types of CVD.

5. In relation to CVD, there are two main reasons for a 'reduced' blood flow – what are they?

6. In relation to respiratory complications, what do the letters COPD stand for?

7. When trying to ascertain how far a patient may be able to lie back in dental chair, what useful, simple questions may be asked?

8. What is Asthma?

9. Application of topical fluoride varnish is contraindicated in some patients with Asthma – state the exclusion criteria.

10. What is a tracheotomy (or tracheostomy)?

11. What is Anaemia?

12. State three common orofacial signs/symptoms of Anaemia.

13. Define what is meant by a 'bleeding disorder'.

14. What is Haemophilia?

15. Factor VIII is used in the treatment of which coagulation disorder?

16. What is Christmas disease?

17. What intraoral signs may be seen in relation to von Willebrand's disease?

18. What do the letters INR stand for?

19. Which is the commonly prescribed drug monitored by carrying out INR checks?

20. Diabetes can occur in all ages – what are the two main types?

21. Give the name of a drug commonly prescribed in relation to Diabetes controlled by diet.

22. What is Liver Cirrhosis?

23. How may Liver Cirrhosis be caused?

24. State an oral presentation affecting 'hard' dental tissue that may present in a patient with Liver Cirrhosis.

25. State an oral presentation affecting 'soft' oral tissue that may present in a patient with Liver Cirrhosis.

26. What is Hepatitis?

27. Hepatitis viruses are referred to as 'types' – state two of the five main ones.

28. Which types of Hepatitis are of particular interest in the dental setting?

29. For which Hepatitis a vaccination can be given as part of 'Personal Protective Equipment'?

30. What do the letters HIV stand for?

31. State three oral lesions/conditions strongly associated with HIV infection.

32. Advanced stage HIV may progress to AIDS – what do these letters AIDS stand for?

33. The CD4 count for a person with AIDS is likely to be below which level?

34. Define the term Kidney Disease.

35. How does End Stage Renal Disease (ERSD) differ from chronic Kidney Disease?

36. What is the difference between Peritoneal Dialysis and Haemodialysis?

37. Define the term Gastrointestinal Disease.

38. What is Crohn's Disease?

39. State two orofacial signs of Crohn's Disease.

40. What do the letters GERD (or GORD) stand for?

41. What is Rheumatoid Arthritis?

42. How can Rheumatoid Arthritis impact on oral health?

43. What is Sjogren's Syndrome?

44. How can Sjogren's Syndrome impact on oral health?

45. What is Scleroderma?

46. How can Scleroderma affect oral care?

47. What is meant by Neurodisability?

48. State three types of difficulty that may occur due to Neurodisability.

49. Give an example of a 'progressive' neurological disease.

50. State two reasons why acquired brain injury may occur.

51. What is the correct term to describe a 'lack of oxygen' to the brain or other tissues?

52. Give an example of a neurological 'acquired' disability.

53. What is the correct medical term for a Stroke and why may a Stroke occur?

54. In relation to the risk of Stroke – what is a TIA?

55. What is Dementia?

56. State two types of Dementia.

57. What is Multiple Sclerosis?

58. Multiple Sclerosis may present in three different stages – what are these?

59. Epilepsy is a symptom of an underlying neurological disorder – what is a seizure?

60. What sort of physical presentations may precede a seizure?

61. What does the term 'absence' mean in relation to seizures?

62. Describe what may be seen in relation to Tonic and Clonic seizures.

63. What is the name of the condition involving a neural tube defect of the spinal cord at birth?

64. What is Huntington's Disease?

65. What is Cystic Fibrosis?

Cancer and palliative care

1. Define Chemotherapy.

2. Define Radiotherapy.

3. In relation to treatment of cancer, what is Oral Mucositis?

4. State two signs/symptoms of Oral Mucositis.

5. What is trismus?

6. Define the terms benign and malignant.

7. Define the term lesion.

8. Define the term histopathology.

9. Define the term sedative filling.

10. What does the term therapeutic mean?

11. What does the term palliative care mean?

12. Pain control can also be influenced by use of an appropriate bed and bedding – state two types of mattress that may enhance patient comfort.

13. A palliative care team could include a variety of members from the multidisciplinary team – state two disciplines that may be included.

Learning and physical disabilities

1. What is meant by 'Learning Disability, Learning Difficulty and Intellectual Disability' within adult Health and Social Care.

2. Define 'Learning Difficulty' within education services.

3. In UK education services, what do the letters SEN stand for?

4. What type of need/s may a person with Profound and Multiple Learning Disability (PMLD) have?

5. What do the letters 'IQ' stand for?

6. What is Dyslexia?

7. What is Fragile X Syndrome?

8. What is Duchenne Muscular Dystrophy?

9. What is Down's Syndrome and how does it occur?

10. State five physical features that may present in a patient with Down's Syndrome.

11. When treating a patient with Down's Syndrome, care must be taken with positioning in relation to neck region – why?

12. Drinking alcohol during pregnancy may result in the baby being born with which syndrome?

13. Autism is a lifelong developmental disability. When does it tend to appear?

14. Which 'umbrella term' covers the range of disorders that includes Autism?

15. In relation to Autistic Spectrum Disorder (ASD) – what is the 'Triad of Impairment'?

16. What is Asperger's Syndrome?

17. What does ADHD stand for?

18. Name a bone disorder commonly found in older women.

19. What is Paget's Disease?

20. What is Scoliosis?

21. Spinal Cord Injury may result in Monoplegia, Paraplegia or Quadriplegia – how do they differ from each other?

22. In what other ways can Spinal Cord Injury affect the limbs and the body?

23. What does the term 'gait' relate to?

24. Give an example of 'fine' and 'gross' motor movements.

25. Which part of the brain controls balance and muscle tone?

26. What is Dyskinesia?

27. What is Dyspraxia or Apraxia?

28. What is the difference between Hypertonia and Hypotonia?

29. Describe the term Dystonia.

30. What is the name of the toxin used to treat patients who have Dystonia?

31. Define Cerebral Palsy.

32. What are the main causes of Cerebral Palsy?

33. State two factors that may increase the risk of Cerebral Palsy.

34. State two main types of Cerebral Palsy.

35. What common orofacial presentations may be seen in Cerebral Palsy?

SECTION V Questions: Preparing for patient visit

LEARNING OUTCOMES

At the end of this section, you should be able to identify any gaps in knowledge associated with caring for patients in clinical and domiciliary settings:

- Patient assessment
- Organising patient transport
- Domiciliary care

Patient assessment

1. The term 'vulnerable/disadvantaged' groups commonly refer to which key 'age' groups?

2. The term 'vulnerable/disadvantaged' groups include which 'income-related' groups?

3. The term 'vulnerable/disadvantaged' groups may include groups who experience 'discrimination or other social disadvantage' – State three examples.

4. What sort of 'population areas' could the term 'vulnerable/disadvantaged' be applied to?

5. What key information needs to be collated prior to the patient attending for treatment? State four considerations.

6. State three considerations to be taken when caring specifically for people who are wheelchair users.

7. Give three ways how the dental nurse can ensure that an appropriate 'treatment setting' is available for patient.

8. State three patient criteria likely to be included in a Special Care 'case mix' model.

9. State five steps that can be taken to help reduce the risk of medical emergencies.

10. What does the abbreviation ASA stand for?

11. What is the name of an assessment scale commonly used to measure dental anxiety?

12. What is meant by the term Dysphagia?

13. What are the factors involved in Dysphagia?

14. State three signs or symptoms of Dysphagia.

15. What is the main purpose of carrying out a 'videofluoroscopy'?

16. Why are IV bisphonates of interest to the dental team?

Organising patient transport

1. State three considerations around 'patient assistance' that can help inform arrangement of patient transport.

2. State two considerations around 'patient treatment' that can help inform arrangement of patient transport.

3. State two factors that may influence the type of transport organised.

4. State two factors to take into account if the patient requires ambulance transport.

5. State two considerations around 'patient treatment' that can help inform arrangement of transport to take the patient home.

6. State some ways to minimise the risk of difficulties with 'organised' transport.

Domiciliary care

1. State two types of patients who may require domiciliary dental care.

2. Give two 'pros' for carrying out domiciliary dental care.

3. Give two 'cons' for carrying out domiciliary dental care.

4. Risk assessments are required for provision of domiciliary dental care – state five topic areas that these could/should cover.

5. State four planning considerations required for a domiciliary visit in relation to safety of **dental team**.

6. State four planning considerations required for a domiciliary visit in relation to **patient safety**.

7. On arrival at venue, what measures can be implemented to support delivery of safe and effective dental care?

8. State two types of treatment that may be carried out in the domiciliary setting.

9. State two ways **how** treatment may be modified especially if working in the 'non-clinical' setting.

10. Give three reasons **why** treatment may need to be modified especially if working in the 'non-clinical' setting.

11. When working on a domiciliary basis, list ten items that may be found in the 'dental treatment kit'.

12. When working on a domiciliary basis, list five items that may be found in the 'administration kit'.

SECTION VI Questions: Patient care during treatment

LEARNING OUTCOMES

At the end of this section, you should be able to identify any gaps in knowledge associated with the care of patients with diverse needs during treatment:

- Role of the dental nurse
- Ongoing risk assessment
- Treatment modification

Role of the dental nurse

1. State two ways in which a patient with diverse needs may be supported during treatment.

2. What are the main four ways in which the dental nurse can provide support for a patient?

3. How can dental team ensure that patient is kept as fully informed as possible throughout treatment?

4. For a patient with dental phobia, state two 'management' techniques that could be used.

5. Suggest three ways in which a patient with Autism may be supported during dental treatment.

6. Describe what is meant by a 'physical' intervention.

7. State three ways of supporting patients with an extreme gag reflex to cope with treatment.

8. State two reasons how oral function and/or structure may prevent access to the mouth.

9. What is the correct term for a very small lower jaw?

10. What is the correct term for a very large tongue?

11. In what ways a very large tongue can impact on delivery of dental treatment?

12. What is a 'frenum'?

13. How can a 'frenum' or 'frena' impact on delivery of oral care?

14. What is Ankyloglossia?

15. State one way in which safe access to the oral cavity during treatment may be achieved.

16. State how the Dental Nurse can provide ongoing support for patients during treatment.

Ongoing risk assessment

1. State three key areas of training very pertinent to Special Care Dentistry.

2. State three factors in relation to the safe moving and handling of a patient.

3. What is the purpose of a 'wheelchair platform'?

4. What additional factor needs to be considered if a patient has no sensation in his or her legs?

5. Describe two items that may be used to assist a patient to 'transfer' to the dental chair.

6. The letters FAST assist as a 'check list' for early recognition of a Stroke – what do the letters stand for?

7. How can the risk of medical emergencies be reduced?

8. Some medical conditions can be aggravated by stress. – Give one example.

9. Some conditions can affect patient ability to co-operate. Give one example

10. State one long-term condition that can impact on actual dental treatment.

11. When providing dental care for people with Special Care Needs, what medical/health barriers may need to be considered? State two examples.

Treatment modification

1. Give three reasons <u>why</u> treatment may need to be modified.

2. State two ways in which the delivery 'timeframe' for treatment can be modified.

3. State three ways in which the delivery of treatment can be modified.

SECTION VII Questions: Pain and anxiety management

LEARNING OUTCOMES

At the end of this section, you should be able to identify any gaps in knowledge associated with the identification of pain in people, particularly those with cognitive impairment:

• Different types of pain
• Non-pharmacological pain and behavioural management
• Mental health

Different types of pain

1. In relation to dental pain, what signs may be noted in people who are unable to verbally express their need?

2. People with Special Care Needs will experience dental pain both on an acute and chronic basis. State two reasons for dental pain.

3. What is the difference between the clenching of the teeth and bruxism?

4. What does the term 'extra-oral' mean?

5. Describe the term 'mucous membrane'.

6. Mention two different types of pain.

7. What is Acupuncture?

8. What is Acupressure?

9. Thinking about unpredictable patient responses, what is the term for an exaggerated response to pain?

10. What is Allodynia?

Non-pharmacological pain and behavioural management

1. What is meant by the term 'non-pharmacological' interventions?

2. What factors need to be taken into account in relation to a non-pharmacologic approach?

3. What is meant by the term 'behavioural management'?

4. Give an example of behavioural management technique.

5. What is a papoose board used for?

6. Distraction may be used to support pain management. How is the technique thought to work?

7. Providing information for a patient may help to alleviate their stress. What factors need considering prior to offering this?

8. A patient may have his or her own techniques for controlling pain. What might these be?

9. Application of either heat or cold can help with pain relief. Describe how both may work.

10. Appropriate 'patient positioning' contributes to both pain relief and comfort. How can this be achieved?

11. Young children can be supported by using the 'knee to knee' approach. What is this?

12. What is Cognitive Behavioural Therapy?

13. What do the letters NLP stand for?

14. State four simple steps that can be taken to help acclimatise a person with Special Care Needs to the dental clinical environment.

Mental health

1. Define the term 'Mental Health Impairment'.

2. What are Affective Disorders?

3. How may a patient with 'depression' present in the dental setting?

4. What is Manic Depression also known as?

5. Sometimes a person may hear voices or have periods where they see things that other people may not. What is the name of this disorder?

6. How may Mental Health and related treatments affect oral health and dental care?

7. If a patient had a personality disorder, how may this affect his or her behaviour?

8. What sort of feelings a person who self-harms may have?

9. What is Agoraphobia?

10. What is a Phobia?

11. A patient who is anxious may have several physical symptoms. State two of them.

12. What signs and symptoms may be seen during a panic attack?

13. What is meant by the term 'Neurosis'?

14. Obsessive Compulsive Disorder has two main parts – what are they?

15. What is the name of the appetite disorder that involves compulsive eating?

16. What is Pica?

17. Name two commonly known Eating Disorders.

18. Orthorexia is classed as a similar condition to an Eating Disorder. What does it mean?

19. What is the S.C.O.F.F questionnaire?

20. What is the layer of fine body hair that can develop on a person with an Eating Disorder called?

21. State three physical signs that a dental professional may notice in a person with an Eating Disorder.

22. State some orofacial signs of Recreational Drug use.

23. State some other ways in which alcohol abuse may impact on health.

SECTION VIII Questions: Promoting good oral health

> **LEARNING OUTCOMES**
>
> At the end of this section, you should be able to identify any gaps in knowledge associated with early development and shared care with the wider interdisciplinary team:
>
> - Whole life spectrum
> - Interdisciplinary and multi-agency working
> - Facilitating good oral health

Whole life spectrum

1. What are the age ranges in relation to the terms Infant, Child and Adolescent?

2. The 'perinatal' period covers which time period?

3. What does the term 'congenital' mean?

4. What is meant by the term 'birth defect'?

5. State one type of defect that comes under the classification of 'birth defect'?

6. Define the term cleft palate.

7. What is an 'acquired' disability?

8. Give an example of a 'physical' acquired disability.

9. What is the age range for a 'developmental disability' to occur?

10. What is meant by the term 'developmental delay'?

11. State two domains (types) of developmental delay that may be found in children.

12. What is meant by the term 'global' developmental delay?

13. State three reasons why 'developmental disability' may occur.

14. What is 'intellectual' disability?

15. In relation to the ageing process, what terms may help indicate the potential level of support that may be needed?

16. What term is used to describe dental care provision specifically for children?

17. What term is used to describe dental care specifically provided towards an 'older' population group?

18. During growth and development of facial structures, an orthognathic opinion may be required – what would this assessment primarily involve?

19. What is meant by the term 'prosthesis'?

20. What is an obturator?

Interdisciplinary and multi-agency working

1. In relation to holistic care, what is meant by the letters 'MDT'?

2. Delivering Better Oral Health, 3rd edition, contains a letter template for a GDP to communicate with a GMP – what is the purpose of the template?

3. Health Care colleagues work in many different patient care areas. Which care areas are identified by the letters SALT, CPN and OT ?

4. State the name of the main nutritional screening tool used in care settings.

5. What is the difference between Enteral and Parenteral Nutrition?

6. State three methods of Enteral Nutrition.

7. A patient is receiving Bobath therapy – what is it?

8. A patient requires an orthotic assessment – what is it?

9. What is the purpose of an orthosis and give one example.

Facilitating good oral health

1. When providing oral health information for a person with Special Care Needs to carry out at home, give three examples of appropriate information.

2. When providing oral health information for a person with Special Care Needs about preventive dental care in the clinic, give an example of appropriate information.

3. Discuss how a carer may be supported to provide safe and effective oral care.

4. How can 'dry' tooth brushing support delivery of effective oral care in patients with diverse health needs?

5. How can oral hygiene items be adapted for a person who has limited manual dexterity?

6. State four factors to be taken into account when discussing a new toothbrush for a person with Special Care Needs.

7. Thinking about types of toothpaste for patients with Special Care Needs, state three factors that may help encourage use.

8. When advising a carer on delivery of oral care, state four considerations that need to be made in relation to both patient/carer.

9. When working with carers, what other points should be advised prior to carrying out oral care for another person?

10. What sort of 'visual aid' may assist a carer to carry out effective oral care for patients on a more personalised basis?

11. Discuss additional advice that could be included in relation to wearing of dentures.

12. Family members may request new dentures to be provided for their loved one. State two aspects that need to be considered in such discussions.

13. When supplementary nutrition (high-calorie drinks) is required, what advice can be given to reduce the risk of dental caries?

14. In relation to dietary choices, state two other 'external' factors that may influence intake.

15. What 'anticipatory' guidance could be given in relation to the risk of trauma to teeth?

SECTION I Answers: Disability awareness

Impairment and disability

1. 'Impairment' – a loss or abnormality of structure or function including psychological function.

2. 'Disability' – a physical or mental impairment that has a 'substantial' and 'long-term' negative effect on a person's ability to do normal daily activities.

3. Four main classifications of disability – Mental, Sensory, Physical, Cognitive.

4. **Mental** disability – mood swings/depression; unable to socialise/interact with people; emotional distress. **Sensory** disability – decreased hearing, poor vision, speech impairment. **Physical** disability – poor/no mobility, poor co-ordination, respiratory stress. **Cognitive** disability – reduced learning ability, unable to pay attention or concentrate, poor memory/recall ability.

5. Social Model of disability is caused by the way society 'operates' rather than by a person's actual impairment or difference. This model explores how restrictions and barriers can be removed to enable the person to have an independent life through more control and choice (more inclusive ways of living).

6. Medical Model of disability – the person is disabled due to their impairment or difference. Emphasis is more on what is 'wrong' with a person and that it is their impairment or additional need that should be 'treated' rather than identifying changes which could be put in place to support the person more effectively. Reinforces low expectation and aspiration leading to people losing independence and restriction of choice.

Related legislation and guidelines – consent

1. Mental Health Act (1983), Disability Discrimination Act (1995), Disability Equality Duty (2006), Human Rights Act (1998), Mental Capacity Act (2005), Principles of Mental Capacity Act (2007), Deprivation of Liberty Safeguards (DOLS), Equality Act (2010), Health and Social Care Act (2012), Care Act (2014).

2. Eliminate discrimination of people who are disabled. Be proactive in equality of opportunity. Foster good relations between people who are disabled and those who have no disability.

3. NICE Guideline 19 Dental Recall (2004).
Choosing better oral health: An oral health plan for England (Department of Health 2005). Meeting the challenges of oral Health for Older People: A Strategic Review (commissioned and funded by Department of Health 2005). Guidelines for the Development of Local Standards of Oral Health Care for People with Dementia (funded by Department of Health 2006). Valuing people's oral health: A good practice guide for improving oral health of children and adults with disabilities (British Association for the Study of Community Dentistry, British Society of Disability and Oral Health, British Society of Paediatric Dentistry 2007). Guidelines for the Oral Healthcare of Stroke Survivors (British Society Gerodontology 2010). Clinical Guidelines and Integrated Care Pathways for the Oral Health Care of People with Learning Disabilities (Princess Diana Memorial Fund, British Society of Disability and Oral Health, Royal College Surgeons 2012).
Delivering Better Oral Health: An evidence-based toolkit for prevention, 3rd edition (Public Health England June 2014).

4. Health and Social Care Act 2012

5. Equality Impact Assessment – one tool for examining main functions and policies of an organisation (whether potential exists for people to be affected differently). Purpose is to identify and address any existing or potential inequalities.

6. Equality Act 2010

7. Mental Capacity Act

8. MCA – statutory requirement in 2007. This law applies to everyone involved in care, treatment and support of people older than the age of 16 years in England and Wales who lack capacity to make all or some decisions for themselves.

9. Adult with Incapacity (Scotland) Act

10. 2000

11. Independent Mental Capacity Advocate

12. Independent Mental Capacity Advocacy may be called upon when serious medical treatment is being provided, withdrawn or stopped (unless in an emergency situation and referral may still be required afterwards);for a hospital stay of more than 28 days; during care reviews or adult protection proceedings and if the NHS or local authority propose changes to accommodation arrangements leading to a stay of more than eight weeks in a care home.

13. Independent Mental Health Advocate – introduced in 2009 – legal duty to provide Independent Mental Health Advocacy to patients who qualify under the Mental Health Act 1983.

14. Deprivation of Liberty Safeguards

15. Always work within legal, societal and ethical frameworks. Use of Mental Capacity Act. Work with other agencies/family members towards patient 'best interests'. Share information as necessary (especially regarding safeguarding concerns). Work confidentially and be aware of situations when confidentiality may be broken. Use of a translator if English is not the first language or other alternative communication tool. Record all interventions.

Barriers to access

1. Patient anxiety may be increased via unfriendly attitude of reception team. Patient can hear items of equipment being used (especially the dental handpiece) or due to the 'clinical' smell from some of the dental materials. Dental team is running late so appointment is delayed (this could also lead to additional stress for the patient particularly if they have another appointment to get to after their dental visit).

2. 'Environmental' barriers include clinic is too difficult for patients to get to – could be due to lack of transport, that is, the practice is not on a bus route or patient is non-driver. Also due to health needs, patient may not be able to travel for too long or for too far (risk of pressure sores or anxiety level will be increased too much). Clinic building may have steps up to the front door or, once in the building, there is no ground floor clinic. Actual dental surgery is too small to accommodate people who are wheelchair users (may be carer/s too).

3. 'Organisational barriers' – Clinic opening times is too restrictive, for example, not open at weekends (this could be particularly difficult if the patient and/or carer works during the week).
Certain type of 'patient image' portrayed via practice literature, range of services offered (mainly implants rather than 'family' access), type of posters and magazines in the waiting room. Treatment needs of patients are outside the role of GDP – factors include lack of confidence and experience, not enough appropriate training (or access to training). Skill mix in dental team is restricted or not enough staff. Lack of treatment facilities such as being unable to offer sedation. No funding to cover costs for Special Care facilities. Treatment delivery can be time-consuming and too costly to provide in General Dental Practice.

4. 'Social' barriers include poverty – poor lifestyle choices leading to higher dental disease risk (use of tobacco products, convenience foods). Financial – patients are unable to afford cost of treatment. Cost of taking time off from work resulting in loss of income (This can apply

to carer also). Lack of knowledge regarding health cost exemption criteria – unable to access forms (as many online) or if have the form, unable to complete (poor vision, low literacy).

5. 'Cultural barriers' – Dental team attitude – lack of understanding, lack of empathy towards patient/caregiver needs. Patients may have low health literacy and lack knowledge on how to access services and their eligibility for care. Dental care has a low priority due to own cultural background and influence of primary socialisation. Parent/carer has a lack of knowledge about dental disease and this can be more difficult if 'shared care' is in place as this is likely to be inter-generational so will be an even wider difference in attitude. Dental team may not understand requirements for certain religious practices (for example dental treatment during Ramadan may be too risky for some patients because if any water is swallowed then their period of 'fasting' will be broken).

6. Medical barriers – actual consideration in relation to complexity of medical history, for example, bleeding disorders, poly-pharmacy and timing of medications. Risks can be higher if a patient newly diagnosed (so condition may be 'unstable') also if the patient has challenging behaviour as can be very unpredictable. Difficulties can result from involuntary movements (tremors) and level of frailty (can patient cope both during and after dental treatment?). Mobility impairment may require patients to be treated in their wheelchair – can lead to difficulty in being able to adopt best practice 'posture' for both patient and clinical operator/s. Patient coping skills/mechanism – may have reduced tolerance on the day of treatment. Health needs necessitate dependency on Care givers – applicable to both young and old patients.

7. Communication barriers – Dental phobia – time and skills needed to support anxiety management. Difficulty between patients and clinicians leading to inability to understand treatment options or requirements; patients unable to consent because English not first language or because of medical challenge (dementia). Visual and/or hearing impairment.

SECTION II Answers: Facilitating access

Providing special care dentistry

1. Special Care Dentistry provides preventive and treatment oral care services for people who are unable to accept routine dental care because of physical, intellectual, medical, emotional, sensory, mental or social impairment or a combination of these factors.

2. **General Dental Practice** – depending on the patient treatment needs and Practitioner skills/equipment, care may be shared between GDP and Community Dental Service (CDS)/Special Care Service. This could include patients having treatment with Special Care Service and return to their GDP for their dental examinations. **Community Dental Service (Special Care Dental Care Services)** – usually have fully accessible facilities. Several services now have 'wheelchair platforms' so that patients do not need to transfer from their wheelchair to the dental chair. Some may also have specialist dental chairs in situ so that care and treatment for bariatric patients (up to 70 stone) can be provided safely. Much treatment is also carried out under Conscious Sedation (RA/IHS IV) as well. **Domiciliary Dental Team** – very important dental care. Mainly routine, minimally invasive dental care carried out in the 'non-clinical' setting subject to the patient's medical/social history. Care may be

delivered in the patient own home, sheltered accommodation, support living arrangements, a residential or nursing care home. There is also the **Prison Dental Service** where the dental clinic will be within the prison environment. The dental team undergoes further training in accordance with the prison induction procedures and related operational policies. Various other dental care services are offered to our very vulnerable groups in society such as people who are homeless. An example of this would be 'Crisis at Christmas'.

3. Hospital – various dental specialities providing care for more complex cases. Relates to Oral Surgery – Maxillofacial – Orthodontics – Restorative (treatment of complex periodontal disease and provision of implants/special prostheses). Head and Neck Cancer treatment (including provision of prostheses such as obturators). Orthognathic Clinics – assessment and surgery. Cleft Lip and Palate Care. Dental treatment under General Anaesthesia is carried out in the hospital setting (for example patients who require multiple tooth extraction or complex surgical extractions, also dental restorative work).

4. These are well-equipped dental surgeries 'on wheels', that is, lorries. They have their own power generators but need to be 'plugged in' somewhere. Can deliver a range of dental care directly 'on site' within a variety of care settings and some 'special schools'. Also used for oral health promotion work, for example, Mouth Cancer Action Month – could offer mouth cancer screening opportunities within a local shopping area. Can create dependency on dental team as treatment is being delivered on doorstep so patients will not be used to attending the clinical environment. If more complex treatment is needed, then they may need several visits to get used to 'true' clinical environment prior to actual treatment delivery.

5. Common to have paper record keeping in place due to lack of access to computerised system. Legible handwriting is very important. Dental notes will then need to be typed up onto IT systems on return to clinic. Limited storage facilities so need good stock control and rotation procedure in place (including carriage of water). Will need to be able to park near enough to a power supply. May have restricted X-ray facilities. Staff 'rest area' can also be limited. Need to factor in travelling time to get to venue and set up and closing down time to clinical working day. Mobile units may have a lift for wheelchair access but access is usually via steps. Clinic floor can become very slippery and dirty very quickly due to the nature of coming in 'straight off the street'. Can be very difficult to keep warm during winter months or to keep cool in the summer.

Reasonable adjustments

1. Environmental reasonable adjustments to gain access to venue include parking bays for people who use wheelchairs or require assistance for getting out of their vehicle (includes patient transport vehicles, which could be in minibus size). Also provision of appropriate space and access for actual emergency vehicles (ambulance and fire service) – due to complexity of patient base, risk for medical emergencies may be increased. There should be a clear pedestrian area within car parks. Doors to building should open automatically – especially important for wheelchair users. A 'meet and greet' service would be even more invaluable.

2. On entering dental clinical setting – Flooring – non-slip, non-shiny and suitable for wheelchair users (no thick pile carpet). Handrails should be provided throughout the building and doors/doorframe.

Colour should contrast with the surrounding area. Ensure that corridors are as clear as possible of any obstacles, for example, avoid having plants in pots. If at low level, a wheelchair user may catch their eyes. All signage to be clear – use of Braille to reinforce signage also. Black on yellow is good or the highlighting of an important button (for example emergency call bell) with a different colour. Visual alarm system, that is, ensure flashing lights for fire – use of screen for 'calling next patient' (could be via a number system to take turns so need to confirm with each patient that they can use a system like this). If required, ensure the patient is approached directly to advise of their turn, that is, not stand and just call out their name.

3. Waiting room seating arrangements – allow room for wheelchairs to fit into the actual seating area (this will facilitate easy access for manoeuvring the wheelchair and help the person to feel included). Chairs need to be varying in height and size (including height of the back of chairs). Some chairs should be able to be moved if necessary. Ensure that some have arm rests – this will provide assistance for a person to be able to get up from the seated position and assist in guiding people who may have visual impairment to be able to orientate themselves and to sit down safely. Also helpful for people who may have co-ordination difficulties or poor balance/postural control. Think about being able to accommodate Guide/Hearing dogs also. All coverings should be able to be cleaned in accordance with infection control measures.

4. 'Reasonable adjustment' and information provision – consider large print, easy to read, audio (taped), various coloured overlays, texting information to patient, use patient phone to photograph/record Oral Hygiene Instruction being carried out with them. Hearing loop facility is available.

5. Completion of medical history support – copy of form available in a different font size/colour paper (if needed). Member of staff to assist as a 'reader' while patients write their responses. Assist recording patient responses (write/type up) exactly as patient reports. Provide variety of pens with different thickness handles and writing nibs (felt tips alongside biros). Dental teams are trained in how to check hearing aids are switched on.

6. 'Toilet for people with disability' or an 'accessible toilet'.

7. 'Disability etiquette' and wheelchair users. When interacting with people with disabilities, etiquette is the same as for any person. It is primarily based on respect and courtesy. Assess the patient's ability to communicate by addressing the patient first rather than their carer. Confirm the patient's 'preferred' communication method – do not assume. Ask persons if they would like some assistance – do not assume that they do require help. Always ask permission to touch or move a person's wheelchair – the wheelchair is included within the area commonly defined as 'personal space'.

8. If a person can walk and requires assistance, always ask how she or he would like assisting, that is, would she or he like to be guided. Do not attempt to lead the individual or take her or his arm; offer to act as a guide by offering your arm at the elbow, keeping your upper arm straight at the top. Allow the person to hold to control her or his own movements and pace of walking. Talk to the person while walking, explain where you are going and of any variations in floor level (slopes or steps) or doors. Think about how you advise the person about things, for example, instead of saying 'Here is the Dentist', it would be better to say 'Mr Smith is in front of you – he is the dentist who will be caring for you today'.

Oral health screening

1. Oral Health screening is known as Epidemiology – Epi – around, Demos – related to people. Specific dental health data collected by 'calibrated' dental teams is used to help inform future funding requirements regarding resources and workforce skill mix. Information helps identify trends in dental disease and where dental services need to be set up.

2. Advantages – ensures that people who cannot express health needs or routinely able to access health care are provided with an opportunity for health screening. Will provide data to support re-direction of services as/if necessary and to secure both amount and type of resources necessary for the target group in the future. Can help focus resources on any target (high-risk) groups. May provide opportunities for much wider inter-agency collaborative working using the common risk factor approach. This could include links with local NHS Stop Smoking teams.

3. Disadvantages – expensive to provide (both in staff costs and time). Unable to see/inspect oral cavity as clearly as would be able to be done in the dental clinic and can increase health inequalities as only people already be known to be at risk are screened. People who do not need dental care (or help with accessing care) will be screened so reduced opportunity for change to be implemented. People may not attend on the day of the screening so true reflection of dental needs of target group may not be achieved. Requirement to have appropriate resources available to provide the treatment after dental need has been identified.

4. Planning considerations – ethics – why/how screening will be carried out. Items required for actual screening activity. Find suitable venue/setting – arrange dates/timings/rotas. Ensure that whole dental team is aware of screening activity – calibration needed? Consent – gain valid consent – offer opportunity for 'opt out' – who will send consent letters out? Who will collate responses? Onward referrals if necessary – to whom and how will this be done/by whom? Collating and presentation of data – who will do this and who needs the data and by when? Storage of data throughout – managing patient confidentiality (anonymised as required).

5. Confirm own details and identity. Follow any venue induction requirements. Check if any fire alarms or similar planned. Go through details of activity (purpose, timings). Assess suitability of delivery area for procedure regarding privacy and confidentiality as far as possible. Collect up-to-date participant name list and check all absentees have already been noted. Consider how to access participants, for example, if school children in various classes, is there a member of school team who can assist with keeping an efficient flow of children. This may also assist with pupil management (and support for any who may have behavioural needs). Consider how to manage any untoward incidents, for example, a participant refuses to open the mouth.

6. Ensure plenty of disposable, latex-free gloves, mouth mirrors, pen torches (additional batteries) or mobile light (upright 'portable' type plus spare bulb – ensure PAT tested), alcohol hand rub. Related paperwork and pens/boards to lean on. Infection control items – consider cleaning of pen torches, disposal of waste, clean and dirty boxes.

7. Time required for collating data. Who needs the data, by when and in what format? How will 'non-participants' be managed – how to facilitate recall opportunities and/or organise alternative screening date? Onward referrals if necessary – how will clinical need be triaged?

SECTION III Answers: Communication

Pre-visit information – supporting patient and carer

1. What is the best time/day of week for patient and carer. Whether there will be a requirement for any 'patient-specific' support before, during and end of visit. Timing of when the patient takes , if any, medications (Diabetes, Warfarin, Parkinson's), so that the regime will not be disrupted too much and the patient is likely to cope with dental intervention more positively. Location of clinic to patient home – are any transport needs. All information and care provided is on a non-judgemental basis in the best interests of patients. All people (with and without disabilities) will have good and not so good days, so it is important to maintain a flexible and adaptable approach.

2. May need transport so provide a list of taxi companies that accommodate wheelchair users. Offer details of bus routes too. Details on how to access the building with the offer of support on arrival should this be required. Advise on procedure for cancellation and/or rescheduling of appointment (may be necessary especially if the patient health needs change). Provide information about who the patient will be seeing and format of the appointment (what will happen, any tests to be done, how long the appointment will be).

3. Confirm how the patient will be accessing the clinic and check whether it will be appropriate. Confirm that the patient's medical and social health needs are unchanged. Provide information about who the patient will be seeing and format of the appointment (what will happen, actual treatment planned, any tests to be done, how long the appointment will be). Whether a chaperone is needed post-operatively and for any period of time thereafter.

4. **Background noise** – keep to a minimum, no radio, interruptions to be kept to a minimum, that is, put appropriate notice on surgery door. **Clutter** – dental work surfaces to be cleared as far as possible so less distractions. **Safety glasses** – is there a preference for wearing darkened glasses rather than clear ones? **Coping mechanisms** – patients may have certain ritual to go through before treatment commences. Use of music/own headphones. **Comforters** – patients may wish to bring own blanket or pillow. **Dental chair** – patients may not like dental chair moving when sitting in it so put chair into best position prior to the patient taking a seat so only need minimal adjustment. **Timekeeping** – Unable to be kept waiting – important not to run late over their 'appointment time'. **Disposable gloves** – preference for non-coloured or a specific coloured clinical gloves. **Meeting people** – people may not wish to see male members of dental team. Keep the number of people in the surgery to a minimum.

5. Listen carefully to what a person has to say – treat with dignity and respect at all times. Be patient, do not try to finish off sentences for the person. If unsure of what to do or say – ask/confirm with the person first and/or carer. Use positive 'non-verbal' body language and behaviour. Be aware and respectful for what may constitute 'personal space'. Negotiate when providing support and joint agreement and setting of SMART objectives. Offer assistance as appropriate and do not be offended if the offer is refused. For greeting a person who wears an artificial upper limb/has limited manual dexterity, it is acceptable to shake hands with the left hand. Use appropriate language taking into consideration both

biological/chronological age and cognitive ability. Networking and ability to work within an inter-disciplinary care team approach towards holistic/ patient centred care (useful to find out what other health-care colleagues do).

6. Communication may be impaired due to cognitive or expressive impairment (Stroke) or learning disability. Anxiety (impact of stress levels as a result of patient trying to accept dental treatment). Hearing loss – congenital or acquired. Visual – will not be able to view pictures/literature – paper/computerised or watch toothbrushing demonstrations on mouth models. Unable to read 'non-verbal' body language.

7. Four modalities of language – Reading, Writing, Comprehension and Expression

8. Dysarthria – imperfect production of sounds used in speech due to lack of muscle control from damage to peripheral nervous system.

9. Aphasia – impaired ability to process information. Primarily with 'expressive' language (how a person speaks). Also can affect 'receptive' language (how person understands). Several types – Global (most severe, minimal recognisable words/unable to read or write). Broca's (better understanding but with limited vocabulary – words such as 'and' or 'the' get missed out). Wernicke's (long sentences with no meaning – can include 'newly created' words). Anomic (understanding is good but short supply of words in relation to topic being talked about – sometimes only occurs when a person is under stress).

10. 'Environmental' barriers – too noisy (radio on in background). Interruptions – other people coming into surgery to get stores and so on. Too much clutter. Poor lighting or light too bright – also difficult when light is placed behind the person. Uncomfortable temperature – room too hot/cold. Strong smells (filling materials). Use of gloves (smells/texture – keep to minimum). Not facing patient when talking – NB eye level is also important – try to maintain at an equal level. Wearing a face mask when speaking may hinder someone who lip-reads or be difficult for those with hearing impairment.

Sensory impairment

1. Broad definition – defined as partial sight or blindness in the better-seeing eye.

2. Broad definition – partial sight is defined as best-corrected visual acuity of <6/12 to 6/60 in the better-seeing eye. It is categorised as Mild – best-corrected visual acuity of <6/12 but better than or equal to 6/18 – or Moderate – best-corrected visual acuity of <6/18 but better than or equal to 6/60.

3. Broad definition – blindness, also called severe sight loss, is defined as best-corrected visual acuity of <6/60 in the better-seeing eye.

4. Sight loss can be due to nerve damage, disease or accidents. Also include uncorrected refractive error, age-related macular degeneration, cataract, glaucoma and diabetic retinopathy.

5. Include age-related macular degeneration, glaucoma, cataract, diabetic retinopathy and uncorrected refractive error.

6. Visual disability that cannot be corrected by the wearing of glasses.

7. Clarity of vision.

8. Myopia is the term used for short sightedness (long sightedness is Hypermetropia).

9. Also known as an optician – a specialist trained to examine the eyes to detect eye problems.

10. Medically qualified doctor who specialises in eye disease, treatment and surgery.

11. Specialises in children's vision and binocular vision problems.

12. Can be congenital, inherited or acquired – as a result of damage to the auditory nerve or cochlea. Could be as a result of Meningitis.

13. Commonly described as 'ringing' in the ears or other noises that can be heard. Can vary in pitch from low to high.

14. Hearing impairment – gain the person's attention by touching gently on their arm. Face the person directly. Think about any light behind you. Remove dental face masks. Confirm whether the person lip-reads too. Speak clearly in short sentences. Do not raise voice unnecessarily. Ensure that any hearing aid worn is switched on. Keep your hands away from your face. If necessary, repeat what you say. Consider using pen and paper. Talk to the person, not sign language interpreter (sign language – there are hundreds of sign languages in use. In linguistic terms, they are as complex as oral language). Find out how to use Text Telephone service (relays calls between you and the individual). Make use of appropriate visual aids.

15. Helps a person to hear the 'source' sound (a person speaking) more clearly by removing or reducing background noise. Hearing aid microphone is turned off while the sound from the loop is received by the hearing aid. It can be used on a portable basis (desktop version).

16. Uses a microphone to pick up sounds that are processed and delivered to surgically implanted electrodes in the inner ear.

17. Visual impairment – confirm the level of visual impairment and preferred communication method. Know correct etiquette when offering 'guiding support'. Be aware that the patient may need reassurance re: clinical noises/smells. Adopt 'hands-on' approach, for example, tactile – gentle positioning of toothbrush in the mouth so that the patient can 'feel' where to place the brush. Reassure the patient if notice 'different' taste in the mouth (bleeding on brushing), this is short-term/will reduce with good oral hygiene. Always let the patient know who is in the room and if anyone leaves. Speak to the patient when you approach them and talk clearly in normal voice. Never touch a 'service/assistance' dog without the owner's permission. Provide 'descriptive' information, that is, when bringing dental light towards the patient's face, advise what you are doing and that they may feel the heat on their face from the light.

18. Information to be available in a different format such as hard copy in large print. Use of a computer screen, which can be adapted re: font size and shape, background colour. Have the document transcribed into Braille. Information can be recorded onto audio tape/CD.

19. Cognitive disability – confirm the level of cognition. Find a quiet place to talk with minimum distraction (no phones ringing, other people talking). Repeat what is being said either orally or by writing. Use simple words and short sentences. Allow time for further discussion especially if decisions are to be made. Provide support notes/photographs for home use. When making appointments, avoid using 24 hours clock – also provide a photograph of the building.

20. 'Sequencing' – enables a procedure to be broken down into small stages. Each stage in the procedure is identified by the use of directional arrows or letters in alphabetical order or numbers.

21. Speech impairment – be sure to listen fully and carefully. Do not be tempted to speak on behalf of the patient – allow the patient to finish her or his sentence. Ensure that you do fully understand what the person is saying – if you don't, do not pretend you do. If acceptable, try using a pen and paper to help clarify. Ask questions that require short or 'closed' answers (such as Yes or No) or that can be easily understood through the shake or nod of the head.

22. Mobility impairment – find appropriate seating so both can be at eye level. Allow time for the patient to get seated (may include a transfer from their wheelchair as/if appropriate) If the patient is wheelchair user, do not lean on wheelchair or move it without permission. Do not pat a person on head or shoulder – neither of these would be actioned if the patient was standing upright. If you need to phone a patient at home, remember to allow time for the phone to be answered.

23. **Sound** (noises can be too loud or 'hurt'). **Spatial awareness** (may have difficulty understanding personal space). **Sight** (difficulty in processing and responding to information being received). **Social situations** (learning the 'unsocial rules' when in new or different social settings). **Depth perception** (judging distance between self and objects). **Body awareness** (difficulty with touch sensitivity and orientation). **Balance and sound** (difficulty in focusing on a task when there are multiple distractions – can create anxiety and confusion).

Alternative communication

1. British Sign Language (BSL) – visual form of communication by using hand signs and facial expression. It has its own 'word order' and grammar.

2. A speech-based communication – often used by people with vision and acquired hearing loss. This is based on lip shapes, gestures and facial movements.

3. Use of symbols, facial expression, body language, photographs, drawings, intonation, technology, objects of reference.

4. Communication method that uses signs, symbols and speech. Its aim is to develop communication, language and literacy.

5. Widgit and Mayer Johnson. Picture symbols used to support language – may be used on own or with text.

6. Raised dots that represent letters and numbers identified by touch used to communicate with people who have visual impairment. Used as digital aid to conversation via some

smartphones, which offer Braille displays and software links when communicating by Skype.

7. Similar to Braille as is dependent on touch. Less commonly used. Letters are represented by 14 raised letters at different angles – easier to learn.

8. This refers to a method of spelling out words onto deaf-blind person's hand. Each letter has a particular sign or place on hand. More straightforward to use than receive.

9. Block alphabet is a simpler and slower method of spelling words on palm of deaf-blind person's hand. Each letter is traced as block capital letter using whole of palm of hand for each letter. Letters are placed on top of each other with a pause at the end of each word.

10. Blinking of the eyes or pointing by eye, changes in breathing pattern, squeezing the hand, more direct and meaningful use of pointing and gesturing. It also includes leading people to objects.

11. Mobile phone, voice recognition computers and voice output device.

12. A picture board is variable in design and serves as a communication tool. Images are selected to support emotional, personal, health and social care needs. Person can point to an image or use letters to spell out key words.

13. AAC system may be used for people who may not be able to communicate using their voice. People will need to have some cognitive awareness.

14. May be operated through the use of 'input systems' such as sip and puff, eye gaze, large buttons or wheelchair-mounted touchscreens.

15. Screen magnification (including change in font style/size and colour), change in colour of the screen background, increased amplification, compatible with hearing aids.

16. British Sign Language – can be via visual frame signing, hands on signing, Sign Supported English (order of words being signed follows spoken English). Deaf-blind manual interpreters. Speech-to-text reporters – listen to what is said and type words on keyboard for relay.

17. (1) Tell, (2) Show and (3) Do

18. Palatal lift (training) device – dental prosthesis designed to improve articulation and pronunciation.

SECTION IV Answers: Diversity of need

Medically compromising conditions

1. Sign is what the dental professional notices. Symptom is what patient is experiencing or 'complaining of', that is, reports to dental professional.

2. Ventricular Septal Defect – defect in ventricular septum, which is the wall dividing the left and right ventricles of the heart. Commonly known as a hole in the heart – present at birth (congenital).

3. General term describing a disease of the heart or blood vessels.

4. Coronary Heart Disease, Peripheral Arterial Disease, Aortic Disease, Stroke.

5. Reduced blood flow may occur due to a blood clot (thrombosis) and build up of fatty deposits inside an artery, which causes the artery to become narrow and hard (atherosclerosis).

6. Chronic Obstructive Pulmonary Disease.

7. Ask the patient how many pillows they use for sleeping.

8. Asthma is a common long-term condition in which the small tubes that carry air in and out of the lungs (bronchi) become inflamed. A patient who has asthma may cough a lot and sound wheezy and also may have chest tightness and breathlessness.

9. People who have been hospitalised for their Asthma.

10. Creation of an opening in the trachea (windpipe) in the front of the neck to assist a patient to breathe. This is carried out as a surgical procedure.

11. Reduction in the oxygen-carrying capacity of blood, resulting in fatigue and decreased resistance to infection.

12. Conditions – such as glossitis – red tongue with loss of papillae (may be the first sign of folate or vitamin B12 deficiency), recurrent bouts of mouth ulcers, candidal infections and angular cheilitis.

13. Condition arises if there is a problem with any part of haemostatic and clotting mechanism. Can be acquired as a result of liver disease, platelet disorders or anticoagulant therapy or congenital.

14. Group of inherited bleeding disorders in which blood does not clot properly. Person may bleed severely from slight injury, surgery or trauma due to reduced clotting ability. Caused by mutation on X chromosome (sex chromosome).

15. Haemophilia A (caused by missing or defective factor VIII, a clotting protein). Normal bleeding time and INR (prothrombin time) but prolonged activated partial thromboplastin time (APTT) and low levels factor VIII. Severity of Haemophilia A is dependent on plasma levels of active Factor VIII.

16. Haemophilia B, a genetic disorder caused by missing or defective factor IX.

17. Purpura of mucous membranes and gingival bleeding (more common than in haemophilia). The disease is caused by poor platelet function and low levels of von Willebrand factor (vWF), ristocetin co-factor (which promotes collagen binding) plus low levels of factor VIII.

18. International Normalisation Ratio. If INR is too high, then blood is too thin – versus the risk of clotting or thrombosis if the INR is too low or blood too thick.

19. INR checks are carried out regularly to monitor Warfarin (Coumarin therapy).

20. Type 1 Insulin Dependent Diabetes (or Juvenile Diabetes/Early Onset) – usually under 40-year age group. The patient will need insulin for life.
    Type 2 Non-insulin Dependent Diabetes (NIDD) – may be able to control symptoms by diet only. Type 2 is a progressive condition so the patient may need to take medication.

21. Metformin.

22. Irreversible loss of normal liver tissue due to necrosis and fibrosis.

23. Liver cirrhosis may be caused by excess alcohol consumption and infection by viral hepatitis B/C.

24. Dental Erosion, Dental Caries.

25. Parotid salivary gland enlargement, Ulceration, Angular Cheilitis, Glossitis – in common with poor nutrition.

26. Hepatitis is inflammation of the liver and may progress to cirrhosis or liver cancer. It is commonly caused by hepatitis viruses but also due to other infections, toxic substances (certain drugs/alcohol) and autoimmune disease.

27. Main hepatitis viruses are types A (HAV), B (HBV), C (HCV), D (HDV) and E (HEV).

28. Hepatitis B, C and D via contact with infected body fluids. Hepatitis A and E typically via ingestion of contaminated food or water.

29. Can be protected against Hepatitis B. There is no vaccination for Hepatitis C.

30. Human Immunodeficiency Virus.

31. Candidosis (erythematous, hyperplastic, thrush), Hairy Leukoplakia, HIV–gingivitis, HIV–periodontitis, NUG (necrotising ulcerative gingivitis), Kaposi's Sarcoma. Due to improved drug therapy and drug adherence, some oral signs have now reduced.

32. Acquired Immunodeficiency Syndrome (also known as Late Stage HIV).

33. CD4 count below 200.

34. General term for any damage that reduces kidney function (primarily failure to adequately filter waste products from blood). It is also known as Renal Disease.

35. ERSD occurs due to permanent damage of the kidneys, resulting in the need for dialysis or a kidney transplant in order to live. Chronic Kidney Disease also involves some permanent

damage, but the kidneys will have enough function for the person to stay alive. Further damage may lead to ERSD.

36. Peritoneal dialysis uses lining in abdomen (peritoneum) and special solution to remove waste and extra fluid from blood. Haemodialysis (the most common type of treatment) also cleans waste and extra fluid from blood, but this time it is via a filter on a dialysis machine.

37. Any disease involving the gastrointestinal tract – digestive process begins in mouth and continues through oesophagus, stomach, small and large intestines to rectum. This also includes accessory organs of digestion (liver, gallbladder, pancreas).

38. Chronic inflammatory disease of lining of gastrointestinal tract – also called Inflammatory Bowel Disease. This can affect any part of digestive system, commonly occurs in the last section of the small intestine (Ileum) or large intestine (Colon).

39. Buccal mucosa having cobble stone effect; swelling of labial, gingival and mucosa; angular cheilitis; mouth ulcers and mucosal tags.

40. Gastroesophageal Reflux Disease – reflux of gastric contents due to incompetent lower oesophageal sphincter.

41. A common inflammatory condition affecting the main joints of the body.

42. Patients with Rheumatoid Arthritis may have difficulty and discomfort with chewing (especially if Temporomandibular joint involved) and may have poor oral hygiene due to limited manual dexterity.

43. An autoimmune disease of salivary and tear glands, leading to dryness of mouth and eyes (characterised by sicca syndrome, keratoconjunctivitis sicca).

44. Due to dry mouth, patients can have thick, mucinous saliva, stickier plaque and increased caries risk. Patient can also have difficulty in wearing dentures, swallowing and eating plus increased risk of yeast/fungal infections. Tongue may have cobblestone effect due to loss of papillae.

45. An autoimmune, rheumatic and chronic disease – cells produce additional collagen and continue to make more.

46. Patients have difficulty in opening mouth for daily oral care (toothbrushing and flossing) and for dental care. Patients have dry eye and mouth membranes. Also, hands are likely to be stiff.

47. Neurodisability is a group of long-term conditions (congenital or acquired) leading to limitation of function. It is attributed to impairment of brain and/or neuromuscular system. Conditions may vary, occur alone or in combination. Level of severity and complexity is wide ranging.

48. Difficulties with emotion, behaviour, movement, cognition, hearing/vision, communication.

49. Parkinson's Disease, Multiple Sclerosis, Motor Neurone Disease, Dementia.

50. Trauma, Stroke and Hypoxia.

51. The correct term for lack of oxygen is Hypoxia.

52. Traumatic brain injury (ABI) and Dementia.

53. The correct term for Stroke is Cerebrovascular Accident (CVA). Two main reasons: a blockage in a blood vessel (Ischemic) and a break or bleed in a blood vessel (Haemorrhagic). Both result in the brain being deprived of blood and oxygen leading to death of cells in brain.

54. Transient Ischemic Attack (mini stroke) caused by temporary disruption in the supply of blood to part of the brain. Symptoms can appear and last for about 24 hours before disappearing.

55. Set of symptoms may include deterioration in memory, thinking, behaviour, problem solving or language and social abilities severely enough to interfere with daily activities.

56. Alzheimer's, Vascular, Frontotemporal and Lewy Body.

57. This disorder of brain and spinal cord affects muscle control, vision, balance. This may also cause fatigue. It is an autoimmune disease in which the body's immune system turns on itself and attacks the myelin sheath (which covers nerves), so signals to and from the brain are disrupted.

58. Relapsing remitting – patient has flare ups of symptoms and can then go into remission until next flare up. Secondary progressive – relapsing remitting MS, which progressively worsens. Relapse periods do not allow full recovery from symptoms. Primary progressive – least common, symptoms worsen and no periods of remission.

59. Neurones in brain send one another electrical impulses. During a seizure, impulses become disrupted, affecting how the brain and body reacts.

60. Convulsion, hallucination, mood or behaviour change (for example blinking or slurred speech).

61. Absence means brief period of unresponsiveness (can appear as 'day dreaming' or 'trance like').

62. Tonic – body spasm, head and spine extension. Clonic – repetitive jerking movements and possible bruxism. May also be partial seizures. Simple – motor, sensory or psychic features. Complex – impaired consciousness/automatic repetitive acts. Also Myoclonic and Atonic seizures.

63. Spina Bifida – failure of the neural tube to form fully. For reducing the risk, it is recommended to take 400 micrograms (mcg) Folic Acid every day at least one month before trying for a baby. Babies may also get hydrocephalus (water on the brain); this extra fluid in and around the

brain needs to be monitored carefully to prevent injury to the brain. A shunt may be inserted to help the additional fluid drain away.

64. A condition in which certain brain cells become increasingly damaged over time. This disease is inherited via an autosomal dominant pattern where only one parent needs to carry the mutation. If one parent has mutation, there is 50% chance that it will be passed on to each child the couple has.

65. A genetic condition in which lungs and digestive system become clogged with thick, sticky mucus. This is inherited via autosomal recessive pattern – both parents must have a copy of faulty gene (they are 'carriers' of the condition).

Cancer and palliative care

1. Purpose of chemotherapy is to kill cancer cells. Used to treat disease with chemicals that have a specific toxic effect upon disease-producing microorganisms or that selectively destroy cancerous tissue. Usually used to treat patients with cancer that has spread from the primary site.

2. Treatment of disease with ionising radiation. Used to damage cancer cells and stop them from growing and dividing. Destroys cancer cells in the area that is being treated.

3. Inflammation of mucosal membrane, which increases patient risk of infection. If infected, patients may require antibiotics or anti-fungal treatment.

4. Pain (often described as burning sensation), inflammation and ulceration (sometimes bleeding also present). Lack of saliva can result in both taste disturbance and dysphagia. It can also be severe enough to prevent eating and drinking totally. Speech can also be impaired.

5. Restricted ability to open the mouth. May be due to inflammatory changes or fibrosis of the muscles of mastication.

6. Benign – mild, non-threatening character of an illness or, in the case of a neoplasm, non-malignant. Malignant – having the characteristics of dysplasia, invasion and metastasis.

7. An injury or wound of diseased tissue.

8. Study of disease at cellular level.

9. A temporary restoration intended to relieve pain.

10. Of benefit – goal is the elimination or control of a disease or other abnormal state. Could be therapy or treatment.

11. Aim of palliative care is to make a person as comfortable as possible during the end stage of life. It includes pain relief and management of any other symptoms (dry mouth for example) while also providing psychological, social and spiritual support. Action is not curative.

12. Mattresses may be filled with fluid or air (pressure active mattress). Foam overlays for the mattress (eggbox style) can also be used. Pillows can help prevent deformity and are available in various shapes (V-shaped), sizes and contain variable fillings.

13. Doctors, nurses, social workers, chaplains.

Learning and physical disabilities

1. Significant impairment of intelligence (reduced ability to understand new or complex information and to learn new skills) and social functioning (ability to cope independently), which started before adulthood, with a lasting effect on development. In 2012, estimated 1.14 million people in England had learning disabilities (908,000 adults aged 18 or over).

2. Within education services, 'learning difficulty' includes people with 'specific learning difficulties' for example, dyslexia (but who do not have significant general impairment of intelligence).

3. Special Educational Needs – different codes correspond to the different levels of 'learning difficulty'. People with 'specific' learning difficulties such as dyslexia do not have 'learning disabilities'.

4. PMLD – patients may have more than one disability in relation to sensory/physical/complex health and/or mental health needs along with Profound Learning Disability.

5. Intelligence Quotient – this is a score derived from tests, which assess human intelligence.

6. A specific learning difficulty, not related to intelligence. Classed as a 'hidden' disability and is common. Difficulties with processing and short-term memory. Patients may have poor organisational and planning skills. Conditions associated with learning difficulties or disabilities do not automatically mean that the person will have a learning difficulty or disability (for example Cerebral Palsy).

7. A genetic condition caused by mutation on X chromosome (sex chromosome). People with Fragile X Syndrome may have long face, large ears and flexible joints. They may also have intellectual disability, behavioural and learning challenges.

8. Neuromuscular condition caused by mutation on X chromosome (sex chromosome). Condition that causes increasing and severe disability through the progressive weakening of muscles.

9. Usually 46 chromosomes in each cell (23 from mother and 23 from father). In Down's Syndrome, there is an extra copy of chromosome 21 in all or some of the cells. Extra copy changes how baby's body and brain develop, resulting in mental and physical challenges. Medical term for an additional chromosome is 'trisomy' (hence Down's Syndrome is also known as Trisomy 21).

10. Short neck and small ears. Large tongue often protruding from the mouth. Flat face and bridge of nose, eyes that slant upwards. Poor muscle tone (floppiness very apparent at birth), short in height, small feet. Chubby fingers and single line across palm (palmar crease).

11. May have 'atlantoaxial instability' in cervical region of spine (first cervical vertebra slips forward over the odontoid peg of second vertebra, the axis).

12. Fetal Alcohol Syndrome – linked to developmental delay, learning disability, hyperactivity, poor memory and attention.

13. Infancy – typically within first three years of life.

14. Autistic Spectrum Disorder (ASD) – Group of developmental disabilities associated with varying degrees of social, behavioural and communication challenges.

15. **Impaired communication** – both verbal and non-verbal. People have a very literal understanding of language – need to provide direct clear instruction. Not helpful to say 'You can't stand on the chair' as person with Autism will stand on chair to show they can do it! Better to say 'Do not stand on chair'. **Impaired interaction** – people do not understand 'unwritten rules' around social functioning – not know when to speak or listen. Unable to interpret or 'read' non-verbal body language. **Have restricted interests** so routines and rituals are key 'coping' mechanisms. Prefer set procedures – may need to see same dental team. Self-centred rather than selfish.

16. Neurodevelopmental disorder within ASD. By definition, people may be defined as 'high functioning' due to above average intelligence.

17. Attention Deficit Hyperactivity Disorder – a common neurodevelopmental disorder of childhood (often lasts into adulthood). Have trouble paying attention (fidgety) or taking turns, controlling impulsive actions (make careless mistakes or take unnecessary risks) or be overly active.

18. Osteoporosis.

19. A bone disorder in which the normal repair cycle (osteoclast and osteoblast activity) is disrupted and results in increased bone size with irregular and weakened structure. Common sites are skull, spine, pelvis and femur.

20. An abnormal curvature of the spine usually in an S shape.

21. Monoplegia – impairment of one limb; Paraplegia – impairment of legs only. Quadriplegia – impairment of all four limbs.

22. Hemiplegia – one side of the body affected by paralysis. In addition to motor function, sensations of touch and pain may also be affected.

23. The way an individual walks.

24. Fine – small muscle movements such as those used in writing. Gross (large) – muscle movements such as those used in walking.

25. Cerebellum.

26. Impairment of the power of voluntary muscle, resulting in incomplete movements.

27. Difficulty in carrying out purposeful movements on demand, not related to weakness in muscles. Associated with problems of perception, language and thought and manifests as a motor disorder so may impact on ability to carry out effective oral hygiene regime.

28. Hypertonia is too much muscle tone resulting in stiffness. Hypotonia is too little muscle tone leading to floppiness.

29. Slow, twisting, writhing repetitive movements in arms, legs or body as a result of changes in muscle tone (from stiffness to floppiness).

30. Name of the toxin for patients with Dystonia (excessive muscle activity) is Botulism. There are two types available: A and B. Botulism is rendered safe for use after purification and when administered in small, controlled doses. It is effective in reducing excessive muscle contraction.

31. Cerebral – to do with brain. Palsy – muscle problems or weakness so a disorder of movement and posture due to non-progressive damage or lesion to the immature brain. Most common motor disability in childhood.

32. Abnormal brain development or damage to brain (lack of oxygen). Infection in early part of pregnancy.

33. Difficult or premature birth (less than 37 weeks), twins or multiple birth. Low birth weight (less than 2.5 lb).

34. Type of Cerebral Palsy determined by whether there is Spasticity (stiff muscles), Dyskinesia (uncontrollable movements) or Ataxia (poor balance and coordination). **Spastic** – most common, some muscles become very stiff and weak **Ataxic** – characterised by Ataxia, problems with balance, co-ordination, shaky hands and jerky speech. **Athetoid** – characterised by athetosis, involuntary movements resulting from rapid change in muscle tone from floppy to intense.

35. Malocclusion – impact on feeding. 'Drooling' from poor posture/control of oral musculature.

SECTION V Answers: Preparing for patient visit

Patient assessment

1. Children, young people and older people.

2. People who could be on a low income, economically inactive, unemployed, workless or unable to work due to ill health.

3. People with physical or learning disabilities or difficulties. Refugee groups. People seeking asylum. Travellers. Gypsies. Single parent families. Lesbian and gay and transgender people. Black and Minority Ethnic groups. Religious groups.

4. People living in areas that may be **isolated** (**rural** areas) or areas that are **over populated**. People living in areas of **poor economic** opportunity and/or **poor health** and **limited/no access** to health and social care services or facilities.

5. Referral letter received and patient is appropriate for service. There is system in place for follow-up on future referrals (both in house and externally). Patient information is as comprehensive as possible – need to liaise with GMP, Social Worker and so forth around patient psychological and socio-economic circumstances. Prepare main dental records and any related documents, plus main medical (hospital) notes. Are there any test results available, for example, previous radiographs, INR levels? What is the preferred communication method for patients?

   Any coping strategies used by patients – could be that patient may prefer to wait in their car until actual appointment time.

6. Access to building, clinic and fully accessible toilets. Patient ability to transfer into dental chair – can they do this and if so, how? Actual type of treatment being carried out – how long (is patient able to sit in the wheelchair for period of time or need to bring a different seating cushion?). Care of patient if medical emergency arises – what to do and is there space to manage needs? Also if need to evacuate building quickly, confirm route suitable for all wheelchair users. If building has lifts, be aware of where refuge areas are in case of fire.

7. Confirm that an appropriate dental clinic is indeed available – suitability for wheelchair access (if patient can transfer to dental chair) or a wheelchair platform is required (if patient cannot or does not wish to transfer). If the patient is obese, then he or she may need to access a bariatric dental chair. Check clinical rota so that an appropriate skill mix within dental team is available, that is, sedation trained dental nurse to work with Dentist. Post-operative recovery arrangements will also be in place. Do not book any complex treatments too late in the day.

8. Ability to communicate – need for a translator, dementia, learning disability. Ability to co-operate – additional time, requirement for sedation or GA. Medical status – degree of impact of medical or psychiatric condition. Oral risk factors – ability to self-care, dietary needs, Xerostomia. Access to oral care – support needed – transport required, ability to transfer of use of hoist, appropriateness for domiciliary visit. Legal and ethical barriers – consideration in relation to degree of capacity – is the best interest meeting or case conference necessary?

9. Ensure up-to-date and accurate medical history at all times – take a photocopy or scan most recent repeat prescription documents or drug charts. Ensure that the patient has all drugs currently necessary with them for example, inhalers, GTN spray. Timing of appointments to fit in with any other medical care being delivered for example, Dialysis, IV antibiotics cycle for person with Cystic Fibrosis. Adopt a realistic approach (according to the patient's medical health and social needs) to both treatment planning and delivery. Confirm coping strategies used by patient/carer, for example, if tend to be anxious. Strategies may include being able to use numbers to countdown to a break/rest in intervention, for example, use of handpiece and could also communicate by slowly raising a hand on dental nurse side (so as not to knock dentist). Patient/carer need to be kept informed if dental team running late; agree how best to manage any additional waiting for patient (patient/carer can go for short walk or best to cancel and reappoint for another day).

10. American Society of Anaesthesiology Classification of Physical Status (ASA).

11. Modified Dental Anxiety Scale (MDAS). Levels of anxiety are determined by responses given by patients to a short questionnaire: MDAS 5–9, mild; 10–12, moderate; 13–17, high; and 18–25, very high.

12. A swallowing disorder usually resulting from a neurological or physical impairment of the oral, pharyngeal or oesophageal mechanisms.

13. Neurological compromise due to disease or injury or abnormality of central nervous system. Physical impairment, due to Head and Neck Cancer therapy (including surgery, e.g. glossectomy). Also respiratory illness (COPD) and psychological factors.

14. Poor oral hygiene, drooling, coughing/choking, nasal regurgitation, poor chewing ability, taking a long time to eat, food spilling from mouth. Patient reports dry mouth, feeling of food sticking in throat, need to have drinks to hand when eating.

15. It enables inspection of both anatomy and physiology of swallowing.

16. IV bisphosphonate therapy is associated with osteonecrosis of the jaw.

Organising patient transport

1. How far and for how long is the patient able to travel for? Is there a risk of pressure sores or an increase in anxiety level if transport runs late? (Book as early as possible in the morning so less risk of being held up.) Timing of appointment: agree a convenient time for the patient and then book a pick-up time, which will allow appropriate time for patient collection. Does the patient require help in and out of their home – if so, what sort of assistance is needed? Who will meet the transport team? Ask whether patient goes out at all – do they visit the hairdresser, are they able to go shopping, for example? Can the patient use a private car or taxi – are they ambulant? If need to use a taxi, do they have a preferred choice of company? Confirm any travel costs for patients and whether they will be able to claim any costs back.

2. What is the type of appointment being offered – is it for a check up, routine treatment or emergency (unknown) needs? Will a carer be required to accompany the patient especially in relation to post-operative care? If so, who would this need to be (for example someone with parental responsibilities) and how long will the patient need to be supported for post-operatively?

3. Amount of physical mobility the patient has – are they ambulant or require use of a wheelchair? What type of wheelchair – consider size and how powered (manual or battery)? How many people will be attending for appointment and will a carer be travelling with patient?

4. Book well in advance to allow adequate timeframe for interagency collaborative working. If a patient needs an ambulance – confirm the patient's needs. Check the best time for travelling to fit in with any drug regime or behavioural needs. Is the patient able to walk, using a wheelchair or requires a stretcher? Remember that patient mobility and fitness may deteriorate post-treatment (for example ME patients) so allow for this with return journeys.

5. What will actually be involved in the treatment, that is, will sedation be used, if so, what type? Is there a possibility that the patient is likely to become more tired or unwell post-treatment? Consider that there could be a requirement to change the transport type at short notice for example from car to wheelchair access. Remember to allow time for patients to be collected and to arrive home at an acceptable time (ideally not travelling home in the dark). Ensure the patient is kept somewhere warm and safe whilst waiting for their transport to arrive.

6. Carry out 'patient experience' questionnaires on completion of appointments. Feedback can be collected over the phone, by email or by letter. Monitor patient 'delivery' and 'collection' times – are patients arriving on time? If not, why? Lack of information, that is, postcodes missing. Are there traffic problems? Arrange appointments to miss rush hour periods. Is appropriate transport being booked? Be sure to collaborate with transport services also. Share patients' feedbacks but also ask for feedback in relation to service organisational procedures overall.

Domiciliary care

1. People who would find it difficult or impossible to attend the dental clinical setting. Physical and learning disabilities, Mental health needs such as dementia, depression or agoraphobia. Medical conditions including terminal health needs. Those with severe difficulty in walking any distance – Emphysema, chronic obstructive pulmonary disease. Patients in hospital or in other settings such as nursing or residential care.

2. Pros – Supports people who are anxious or unable to attend a dental clinical setting. Provides a service for people who may be very frail or unable to travel. Can be very rewarding as get to know more about patient social circumstances (family, day-to-day activity level and abilities). Working as part of the wider health care team to contribute towards an holistic approach to general health and well-being. Opportunity to liaise with district nurses, carers.

3. Cons – Time-consuming (particularly in relation to time taken out for travelling between visits) hence an expensive service to provide. Lots of planning and organisation is required. Only limited range of treatment can be offered for example no access to take X-rays. No back up support available should a medical emergency arise or if patient becomes agitated, distressed or angry. May be pets to contend with in the home. Can be difficult to collect payment for treatment at time of appointment.

4. Lone working, Chaperoning, Environmental (fire, electrical, external access), Manual handling (both for people and equipment), Vehicle insurance, Emergency equipment including oxygen (carriage and use)

5. Emphasis on team approach – ensure workplace knows about all visits (all addresses). Leave full details of vehicles being used (registration number, model and colour) along with mobile phone number. Have an agreed time for returning to workplace before the end of the working day; if running late, advise workplace as appropriate. Have an agreed 'alert' system if have a problem during visit. Have as much detail as possible about patients (both social and medical history) – liaise with a wider health care team – CPN (Community Psychiatric Nurse), GMP, social worker, district nurse. Check whether a third party will be present; if so, find out who this will be (relationship to patients). Who will answer the door to dental team? What parking facilities are available and how best to access the property? Confirm any animals at the address

will be put into another room during visit. Request that there will be 'No Smoking' for the duration of the dental visit.

6. Confirm visit is still necessary and patient fit enough to cope. Get as much information as possible regarding Medical and Social History; have there been any changes since appointment arranged? Confirm address and check access to building. Agree to phone ahead and explain to the patient that the dental team will have their official ID cards. Provide the name of the dentist to the patient. Check whether third party is present – if so, who this will be (relationship to patient). Be mindful of being able to carry out adequate infection control for both the patient and dental team; is there access to hand washing for example? Confirm patient is able to give valid consent – if not, how will this be managed?

7. Ensure the correct patient is being seen and confirm level of overall health and well-being. Ask to see any patient held records – check for any recent visits or change in drug therapy. Ongoing risk assessment in relation to environment and manual handling. What access is there to see the patient (are they seated or lying in bed). Are there any animals wandering around? Carry out comprehensive dental assessment as far as possible, plan or review the dental treatment plan. Work in the patient's best interests at all times; weigh up benefits of treatment versus risk of delivery within the context of the patient's overall health and well-being on the day. If need to move any furniture, ensure all items are replaced in exactly the same place afterwards; this is very important for people with visual impairment.

8. Dental examinations, supply of prescriptions, provision of dentures and related care (denture ease) temporary dressings, scale and polish, oral hygiene instruction.

9. Minimal Intervention approach to treatment – use of Carisolv, denture reline/copy denture technique. Choice of dental materials used will be those that require minimal preparation or management that is use of topical fluoride varnish rather than fissure sealants, use of dental materials that do not require light curing. Use of temporary dressings as necessary with follow-up arrangements made to bring patients into clinic. Timing of treatment: try to offer majority of appointments in the morning or early afternoon, avoid extracting teeth at end of the day (to reduce the risk of having to seek emergency care). Continually reassess the need and coping ability and may need to review treatment plan and re-schedule delivery format. Appointment times may be shortened and more frequent rather than one long appointment.

10. Infection control risk (unclean/unhealthy environment around patient). Patient health on the day is not good or begins to deteriorate during treatment. Maintaining a safe working position when delivering care for the patient is very important. If the patient is in bed then this can make treatment more difficult for both patient and the clinical operator. Good suction indicated during treatment or an X-ray may be required. Poor lighting and visual working field – due to patient posture or ability to open mouth (both in terms of how wide the mouth can be opened and for how long the patient is able to keep the mouth open).

11. Along with emergency care kit, will require PPE items (latex free gloves, safety glasses, mask/visor, disposable apron), clinical waste bags, sharps container, gauze swabs/cotton wool rolls, selection of dental materials and instruments according to dental intervention (for example Examination, Prosthetic, Periodontal) Suitable and labelled container/box for safe carriage of contaminated instruments, disposable paper covers/bibs, headlamp and pen torches (spare batteries), vomit bowl, tissues, alcohol hand rub, hand mirror, dental model/spare toothbrushes.

12. Dental team identity cards, mobile phones, pens/pencils/plain papers, BNF, patient record cards, medical history forms, consent forms, FP17DC forms, laboratory forms, prescription sheets and stamps (serial numbers logged with workplace), appointment cards, change for car parking, oral health education information, contact numbers for dental team.

SECTION VI Answers: Patient care during treatment

Role of the dental nurse

1. The dental nurse can welcome the patient and their carer, making particular use of any personal preference information that may have been supplied in advance. Following on from acclimatisation visit prior to the treatment appointment, it is useful to confirm whether there are any questions from the patient (and carer). A support book containing photographs of the activities covered to date can be used to initiate and support discussion. The main role of the dental nurse is to ensure patient comfort, care and safety.

2. Support can be provided in different ways, which include the following four main headings: Emotional, Physical, Communication and Monitoring.

3. Collect as much pre-visit information as possible especially around the preferred communication method and language level. Ensure use of lay terms throughout treatment as appropriate to both age and cognitive ability. Facilitate casual chat as necessary but keep to the minimum so as not to distract the patient too much. Ask closed questions that require Yes or No answers (the patient can indicate by a thumbs up or down action).

4. Desensitisation (this could be acclimatisation and/or exposure to the key 'trigger'), Hypnotherapy, Use of Imagery, Cognitive Behavioural Therapy (CBT) or Neuro-Linguistic Programming (NLP). Meditation or Mindfulness training may help to change how patients may think and feel about their dental experiences.

5. Provide a checklist for what is going to happen; patients can 'tick off' each part. Allow use of headphones to reduce background noise down to one source. Offer use of tinted/dark safety glasses. Encourage patients to wear their most 'comfortable' clothing. Ensure items to be used on the day are the same as any samples that have been provided in advance of the appointment for use in the home (disposable glove or piece of dental chair fabric). This will help support the patient, during the appointment, in relation to being able to cope with smell, colour and texture.

6. Direct physical contact with patients – dental team member holds the patient's hand. Use of treatment, materials or equipment to restrict movement for example sedation, papoose board, splints. In care settings, this may include use of doors with bolts placed out of reach of service users or requirement for use of double handles (one at top and one at bottom of door).

7. Relaxation techniques such as deep breathing (including Mindfulness) and self hypnosis. Distraction techniques such as squeezing a ball or counting back from number ten down to one. A TENS machine (transcutaneous electrical nerve stimulation) may also help.

8. Oral function and/or structure preventing access to the mouth may include restricted opening of the mouth for example trismus due to post Head and Neck cancer therapy (including surgery to soft/hard facial tissue). TMJ difficulties due to arthritis (unable to open the mouth fully or for long periods of time) so dental treatment may need to be delivered in shorter sessions. Oral musculature: There may be difficulty in controlling movement so there is a risk that the mouth may clamp shut suddenly without warning. Muscle tone reduced (hypotonia) or may be variable level of spasticity. Also, the actual size of the mouth and related oral structures, if small, can be a barrier.

9. Very small lower jaw – micrognathia

10. Macroglossia

11. Patients may have a strong tongue thrust that can make use of dental instruments difficult. The tongue may well 'drape' over the lower teeth so will need to be retracted out of operator working field of vision. It can also impact on swallowing, breathing and saliva control.

12. Minor strands of muscle tissue, which can be found in different parts of the mouth attaching cheek, lips and/or tongue to the related dental mucosa.

13. Access to the mouth can be difficult (particularly low anterior region) due to very strong and tight oral musculature, which will include any related frenum or frena. These oral structures may also complicate oral feeding in infancy. Sometimes, a frenum may be attached 'high' or very near to the actual gingival margin; this can mean effective disruption of the dental bacterial biofilm with a tooth brush could be more difficult.

14. Attachment of lingual frenum, which may result in 'tongue tie'.

15. Use of the Bedi™ wedge – plastic wedge to prop mouth open. The patient head's may be supported by using a neck cushion or the dental nurse may gently support. Two toothbrushes can be used – place brush heads together (bristles to bristles) and place between teeth. Photographic cheek retractors are useful for holding soft tissues away from teeth.

16. Dental Nurse can provide ongoing reassurance, explanation and guidance to patients throughout the appointment. Monitor the patient at all times (especially non-verbal body language): taking note of any change in breathing, increase in restlessness or if becoming more agitated, any tightening of the oral musculature (may notice during aspiration). Ensure effective suction as far as possible. Participate in an approved clinical holding technique as may be required according to the agreed best practice protocol for example hand over hand.

Ongoing risk assessment

1. Special Care Dentistry, Conscious Sedation, Consent (especially MCA), Infection Control, Medical Emergencies, Moving and Handling, Conflict Resolution, Personal Safety, Storage and Handling of Medicines.

2. Need to minimise or totally remove any actual need for the 'lifting of patients' whenever possible to protect both the patient and the dental team. Be sure to check or confirm weight

of the patient. Ask patients what assistance they need to transfer in and out of the dental chair. Find out what they are able to do for themselves and whether there may be a better time of day for them to carry this out. Clarify whether the patient able to lie flat for long periods – how far can they lay back? Encourage patients to use their own equipment whenever possible – this will help provide confidence. Continually risk assess patient situation throughout the delivery of care.

3. Enables patients who are wheelchair users to remain in their own wheelchair for dental care. Wheelchair is positioned on the platform (an area of floor that can move) up against the support framework. When the platform (floor) is activated, both the wheelchair and the patient are slowly tipped upwards and backwards. Once this has been done, the wheelchair is in a reclined position, which provides a much safer working position for both the patient and clinician. Some wheelchairs have their own facility to recline the wheelchair back.

4. If there is loss of sensation in lower limbs, the dental team needs to be aware of the risk of trauma or knocks (to legs) as the patient will be unable to advise if this happens. Also be aware of changes in body temperature – again, the patient may not notice that he or she is getting cold.

5. Transfer board (banana board): This is used as a 'bridge' for the patient to slide across from the wheelchair to the dental chair. Hoists (large slings) can be fixed, which run on a track from a ceiling or portable (frame on wheels). A portable rotating 'turntable' can be used for patients who can weight bear/stand upright. Use of a 'swivel' cushion can assist as whole body is able to be rotated around in one move.

6. Face – any sign of change: does one side droop? Arm – can both arms be lifted? Speech – can the person repeat something you ask them? Tongue – can this be moved from side to side?

7. Monitor the patient on arrival and throughout appointment. If necessary, check if a carer is present.
   Confirm drug list up to date – ask the patient to bring repeat prescriptions (photocopy/scan into notes). Check health condition/s are well controlled/stable. Ask if the patient has brought any self-administered drugs with them (inhalers, GTN spray). Do not run late for appointments.

8. Epilepsy, Asthma, Heart conditions.

9. Physical disabilities, Parkinson's disease, Gag reflex (patient can become more anxious).

10. Vascular problems (Stroke/Thrombosis risk) as medication taken may require monitoring (INR levels). Look at overall stability – check the patient's record book and check INR on the day of treatment. Epilepsy: ask about date of last seizure, frequency, type, how managed. Ask if any triggers and whether any are associated with dental care. Check whether the patient is able to recognise any aura. Diabetes: Check whether the patient's oral health has deteriorated and gingival inflammation increased (be difficult to place restorations at gingival margin).

11. Complexity of medical history – any bleeding disorders or polypharmacy. Patient has challenging behaviour, so actions may be unpredictable. Dental phobia – prevent further anxiety and anxiety management. Limited coping skills and ability due to both involuntary actions and reduced tolerance. Profound multiple communication needs – unable to understand the

need for treatment and/or the treatment delivery requirements. Not able to sit still for any period of time, poor attention span or unable to keep mouth open for long enough.

Treatment modification

1. Due to the complex and diverse needs of Special Care patients, any changes in patient health and social care needs (since the previous appointment) can have a huge impact on patient care and management. It is not uncommon for planned treatment interventions to require full re-evaluation. Reasons for this include unable to gain appropriate consent on the day. There may be physiological deterioration in general and/or oral health – patients may have a very sore mouth so unable to even open the mouth. Patients may have become unwell – more frail or tired with reduced coping skills. Changes in physical health can make a patient more anxious about letting anyone touch the area of pain. Patient behaviour can then become even more unpredictable, which can make the whole treatment session quite stressful for everyone involved. If there are any changes in the patient medication regime such as a new medication being taken, an increase in dosage or change in timing, then all of this will be 'unknown territory', which again can be unsettling.

2. Carry out a full review of the planned interventions according to clinical need along with how the interventions will be delivered. Modifications around delivery timeframe can include the following: changing the day of the week or time of day, reducing the actual number of appointments, increasing the length of each appointment, reducing the length of each appointment or facilitating longer periods of time between each appointment.

3. Consider whether to carry out less treatment than was planned for the visit, that is, just carrying out scaling of lower anterior teeth only rather than whole mouth. Working on anterior teeth will be easier for the patient to cope with and, in turn, will help support the patient to be able to experience dental treatment. It is better to attempt a little and praise the patient especially if they have always only had dental treatment previously under sedation for example. Alternatively, using the appointment to offer a 'show, tell, do' opportunity (in preparation for carrying out the procedure at next visit) can be very beneficial as this will enable a patient to experience a positive dental intervention. Take time to be able to explain everything and be sure to allow patients to assimilate information. Include sensory experiences where possible such as patients hearing the handpiece far away from their face initially and then bring it closer. Finish appointments on a positive activity such as the provision of oral hygiene instruction or helping the patient to carry out some toothbrushing – this is an activity that the patient will be able to continue with and to link back to the dental clinic (and become part of daily thought processes).

SECTION VII Answers: Pain and anxiety management

Different types of pain

1. May be moaning, crying or shouting out. Could be mood swings along with a change in behaviour – person may become agitated, pacing up and down or sitting rocking to and fro. Could also become withdrawn and not participate in daily activity. May also include self-injurious behaviours such as 'pulling' at or 'hitting own face' or self-harming (biting own

hand or banging forehead). If the person starts to refuse food and drinks or ceases to wear their denture/s, dental pain should be considered. Another sign could be disturbed sleep.

2. Acute periodontal infection (ulcerative gingivitis/periodontitis). Abscess. Carious lesions. Cracked tooth (transient acute pain, mainly during chewing). Dentine hypersensitivity. Dry socket (infection or loss of clot leading to osteitis). Delayed shedding and eruption of teeth.

3. Clenching – clamping the teeth (and jaws) together in occlusion due to stress or physical effort. Bruxism – parafunctional grinding of the teeth.

4. Outside of the oral cavity.

5. Lining of the oral cavity as well as other canals and cavities of the body, also called mucosa.

6. Referred – caused in one area of the body but felt in another. Psychosomatic – due to mental or emotional problems rather than physical disease. Neuropathic – pain (neuralgia) from problems with signals from nerves. Neurovascular – headaches (group of pain disorders felt in head). Musculoskeletal – affects bone, muscles, tendons, nerves; can be mild to severe, acute or chronic.

7. A therapy, originated from China, involves insertion of very fine, thin needles into specific points of the body to reduce pain, induce anaesthesia or reduce nausea (acts mainly by stimulating nervous system).

8. Therapy involving the application of pressure (using thumbs or fingertips) to relieve tension or pain. Uses same points on the body as for Acupuncture.

9. Hyperalgesia – the pain sensation can be either localised or widespread.

10. Allodynia is pain caused by a stimulus that would not normally cause pain. Believed to be a hypersensitive reaction, particularly in people who have fibromyalgia. Types of allodynia include tactile (from being touched), mechanical (from clothing on skin) and thermal (temperature related).

Non-pharmacological pain and behavioural management

1. Psychological and physical interventions. Not intended as an analgesic but can be beneficial in the own right.

2. Full assessment of patient needs and treatment being planned. How the patient will respond to the suggested intervention. Clinician confidence, skill and experience.

3. Includes the use of a technique or therapy to alter or control the action of person receiving treatment.

4. Use of a papoose board, provision of education or use of an anxiety relief technique.

5. It can support behaviour management as it provides patient support during dental treatment through immobilisation.

6. Diverting the patient attention to stimuli other than pain sensation. Does not remove the pain but may enable it to become more bearable (less pain intensity). Includes the use of imagery or listening to music.

7. Allow the patient to guide the level, type and number of questions. Show an active listening approach to provide reassurance. Encourage an opportunity for the patient to raise any concerns whether on a personal and/or treatment-related basis.

8. Wearing of a splint. Giving an indication when feel it is necessary to change position such as rubbing an area that is starting to stiffen. Limping when walking can also alleviate pain.

9. Heat – increase in blood flow due to vasodilation. May help reduce muscle spasms.
   Cold – reduces bleeding and oedema due to vasoconstriction. Can decrease inflammation.

10. Ensure patients can indicate when they need to change position. Factor in additional time to facilitate this. Use of support items in the dental chair (cushions/wedges) will help maintain body alignment and positioning of limbs. Agree a method of communication with patients to indicate when a rest may also be needed during treatment; this will help alleviate anxiety and reduce risk of any further stress. Allowing a patient to bring a pillow or comforter from home also offers psychological support.

11. This approach is used for carrying out dental examination or simple treatment (fluoride varnish application) in young children. Parent/carer sits facing the clinician knee to knee with child head on clinician lap and lower part of body on carer lap.

12. A short-term talking therapy used to help persons manage their problems by changing the way they think and behave.

13. Neuro-linguistic programming – an alternative therapy used to educate people in self-awareness. Exploration of three influential components in producing human experience, neurology, language and how we are programmed.

14. Allow time as necessary, not on a busy clinic day. Patient to watch dental chair being operated up and down, back and forth. Facilitate hands-on experience – touch and smell gloves, noise of suction (allow the patient to suction water out of a glass), see how dental light works (shine on hand first), warn the patient that they will feel some heat from the light on their face, use of powered toothbrushes can familiarise patients with the sensation of mechanical procedures and sensations in the mouth. Using a rubber cup to polish a fingernail will assist introduction of the dental handpiece.

Mental health

1. Mental health impairment is the term used to describe people who have experienced psychiatric problems or mental ill health or illness.

2. Disorders of mood or feeling states – can be either acute or chronic.

3. Likely to have low self-esteem, poor sleep pattern and diet resulting in poor general health all round. Unlikely to be interested in 'self-care' with oral health a low priority. Clinical

depression is a severe form of depression and can be life threatening (with feelings of suicide). Another form of depression is post-natal depression (occurs after childbirth).

4. Bipolar disorder (extreme mood swings – from being highly excited or 'manic' versus a deep depression. There may also be periods of 'stability' on occasion.

5. Psychotic illness characterised by disturbances of thinking, mood and behaviour is called schizophrenia. Includes loss of contact with real world and lack of insight. Linked to structural brain abnormality and genetics. Person may hear voices telling them what to do or warn of danger (say they receive messages through amalgam fillings). May hallucinate, be delusional and have disorganised thinking (lack of logic). Negative symptoms include loss or reduction of normal functioning leading to withdrawal, apathy, lack of emotion (no facial expression).

6. Ability to self-care is diminished due to low self-esteem with an increased risk of mouth cancer due to tobacco and alcohol use along with poor diet. Poor compliance with oral health advice, irregular attendance and short notice cancellations. May have xerostomia so increased risk of dental disease or hyper-salivation. Tardive dyskinesia – disorder of central nervous system – resulting in involuntary muscle contractions so may be in pain (including facial muscles and jaw). Frequently involves tongue (thrusts and protrusion).

7. It would be difficult for the person to change their feelings or actual behaviour. May have limited emotional response. If severe, it can cause significant impairment of day-to-day activities.

8. Very deep distress. Self-harm is any act of self-poisoning (with medication) or self-injury (by cutting). It is a form of communication of feelings that are too difficult to think or talk about.

9. Anxiety disorder – an abnormal fear of being in crowds, public places or open areas, sometimes accompanied by anxiety attacks. Fear of being in situations where escape might be difficult, or help would not be available if things go wrong.

10. An exaggerated or unrealistic (irrational) fear or sense of danger about a situation or an object (including people).

11. Increased heartbeat, upset stomach, feeling tense and/or shaky. A panic attack may also accompany high anxiety.

12. Difficulty in breathing and feeling of heart beating hard. May have choking sensation, begin to tremble or feel faint. Can occur at any time so are different from a 'natural' response to danger.

13. A term used to describe someone who may be neurotic – socially acceptable term – feelings of being stressed, anxious. Non-psychotic.

14. Obsessions may be due to unpleasant thoughts or images. Obsessive thoughts cause anxiety, leading to ritual or repetitive actions. Compulsion due to thoughts or actions that person feels must be done. Not fully understood – multifactorial. Person is usually aware they are having OCD. Typically starts in adolescence.

15. Prader–Willi Syndrome – genetically based, affects both sexes, linked to disorder of chromosome 15. Associated with oesophageal reflux, moderate cognitive impairment, hypotonia (affecting motor skills), delayed speech and hypogonadism.

16. Persistent eating of non-nutritive items (chalk, soil) – must persist for more than one month and age must be that where eating such items would be developmentally inappropriate. Can be considered as form of self-harm also.

17. Eating Disorders – seen in both males and females. Due to extreme emotion and behaviour around food and weight issues, can have serious physical and emotional consequences. **Anorexia Nervosa** – 'lost' appetite for 'nervous' or psychological reasons (anxiety, body image distortions). Unable to maintain body weight through intentional restriction of food. Two types: Restrictive (food intake restriction is sole behaviour) and Binge/Purging – restrictive practice accompanied by self-induced vomiting, excessive exercising, use of laxatives. **Bulimia Nervosa** – usually undetected for a long period. May see calluses (Russell's sign) on back of hand/fingers due to induced vomiting. **Binge Eating Disorder** – recurrent binge eating without compensatory purging.

18. Having an 'unhealthy obsession' with otherwise healthy eating. Starts out as trying to eat more healthily but then becomes a 'fixation' on actual food quality and purity rather than weight loss or being 'thin'.

19. A simple five-question screening tool for use to assess possible presence of an eating disorder.

20. Lanugo.

21. Abrasion of knuckles on hand. Soft palate trauma. Loss of enamel on teeth due to dental erosion (from regurgitation of stomach acids) and abrasion (from brushing teeth immediately after vomiting).

22. Solvent abuse – red, sore areas around nose. Alcohol – dental erosion, also may drink lots of fluids (fizzies) due to needing to keep hydrated through the use of Ecstasy. Methadone (heroin substitute) – high in sugar but can get sugar free now – risk of caries increased. Localised areas of gingival inflammation or recession – rubbing cocaine topically into gingivae. Legal Highs are now a frequent factor for increased risk of poor mental health.

23. Risk of erosive gastritis, upper gastrointestinal bleeding, peripheral neuropathy, brain disorder (Korsakoff's Syndrome). Chronic alcoholic may have recurrent bouts of jaundice leading to episodes of alcoholic hepatitis. Trauma to teeth from falls and fights. Poor nutritional state (malnutrition) so impaired wound healing.

SECTION VIII Answers: Promoting good oral health

Whole life spectrum

1. Infant: Birth to 1 year; child: 1 year to puberty (12/13); adolescent: puberty to 18 years.

2. 28th week of pregnancy to 28th day after birth.

3. 'Present at birth' – a prenatal condition.

4. Can be found before birth, at birth or any time thereafter. May vary from mild to severe and affect any part of body and how that part may look, work or both.

5. Heart defects – such as Ventricular Septal Defect, Tetralogy of Fallot, Coarctation of the Aorta (aorta narrower than usual). Cleft Lip and Palate (can have cleft lip, cleft palate or both cleft lip and cleft palate).

6. It is a congenital deformity occurs due to lack of fusion of soft and/or hard palates and may present as partial or complete lack of fusion of these tissues.

7. A disability caused by an impairment that occurs after the developmental years.

8. Arthritis, Multiple Sclerosis.

9. Begins anytime during the development period to around 18 years; usually lasts through-out life.

10. It refers to slow or impaired development of a child younger than 5 years of age at the risk of having a developmental disability.

11. 1. Cognitive (learning, memory, thinking and reasoning skills).
    2. Language and Speech (ability to communicate, express and receive information, form sentences, follow instructions).
    3. Motor (fine and gross skills – hand and eye coordination, ability to walk).
    4. Social and Emotional (interaction with others, recognition of social cues).

12. It is significant delay in two or more developmental domains, late in reaching developmental milestones.

13. Most begin before baby is born, but some can occur because of injury, infection or other factors. Complex mix of factors including genetics, parental health (smoking/alcohol) or ill-ness, for example, infection in uterus during pregnancy, complications during birth (lack of oxygen), infection in early life (Meningitis) or illness (untreated newborn Jaundice). Low birthweight, premature birth and multiple birth are associated with increased risk.

14. 'Intellectual' disability is a disability characterised by limitations in ability to learn at an expected level. Children with 'intellectual' disability may take longer to learn to walk and talk, may have trouble remembering things and may be unable to understand social rules.

15. In relation to the ageing process, it is useful to ascertain whether the patient is 'functionally' dependent or independent.

16. Paediatric.

17. Gerodontology.

18. The functional relationship of maxilla and mandible.

19. Artificial replacement of any part of the body.

20. A prosthesis to close an opening in the palate; may be disc or plate to close the opening.

Interdisciplinary and multi-agency working

1. Multidisciplinary team – also known as inter-disciplinary team (the word 'inter' is suggestive of more collaborative engagement, that is delivery of patient care being 'shared' between disciplines, rather than having 'many' disciplines all providing their part of the care).

2. To encourage communication between the General Dental Practitioner and General Medical Practitioner in relation to sharing care and management of patients who have Diabetes.

3. SALT: Speech and Language Therapy; CPN: Community Psychiatric Nurse; OT: Occupational Therapy.

4. Nutritional tool – The Malnutrition Universal Screening Tool (MUST). The MUST was developed in 2003 by a multidisciplinary Malnutrition Advisory Group (MAG), a standing committee of the British Association for Parenteral and Enteral Nutrition (BAPEN).

5. Enteral Nutrition (EN) is tube feeding achieved via different types of tubes. Parenteral Nutrition is intravenous feeding to get nutritional requirements into the body through veins. Commonly referred to as Total Parenteral Nutrition (TPN) despite the fact that some patients may need to receive only certain types of nutrients intravenously.

6. Enteral Nutrition (EN), tube feeding via different types of tubes: Nasoenteric feeding – tube placed down through the nose into the stomach or bowel, which includes naso gastric (NG), naso duodenal and naso jejunal (NJ) feeding. Nutritional requirements may also be provided directly through the skin into the stomach or bowel (enterostomy feeding) known as Percutaneous Endoscopic Gastrostomy (PEG) or Percutaneous Endoscopic Jejunostomy (PEJ) feeding.

7. A physical therapy to improve movement and posture.

8. An assessment for need and provision of a surgical appliance (Orthoses) to either remedy or relieve a medical condition or disability.

9. An apparatus (appliance) used to support, align, prevent or correct deformities. Also includes support for improving the function of movable parts of the body so may prevent the development of a more disabling condition. Examples are footwear, compression stockings, knee or spinal braces.

Facilitating good oral health

1. Remember to include and involve family members as appropriate with patient consent. Ensure all key oral health messages are given according to *Delivering Better Oral Health*, 3rd edition (Patients with Special Concern). All messages have to be provided in an accessible

(for example easy read, large print, audio) format. Promote the use of sugar-free medicines whenever possible. If not sugar-free medication, protect oral health where possible for example by trying to have medicine as near to a meal time as possible/rinse mouth with water after use of inhalers. Encourage regular soft tissue checks by care giver for mouth cancer, trauma.

Consider the impact of any snacks and drinks being offered to patients by carers – are they 'safer for teeth' choices? NB check if special dietary needs. Advise never too late to quit smoking, the single most important action a person can take to help reduce ill health. Be alcohol aware – advise on recommended daily unit intake for both men (3–4) and women (2–3).

2. Topical fluoride varnish can be applied according to clinical indication. Teeth can be fissure sealed as appropriate as soon possible post eruption. Continuing care visits to dental team will be implemented in a timely manner according to the health need and dental disease risk. Dental team is available for advice and support on an ongoing basis. Also advise that any advice given may indeed change and that all advice will always be in the best interests of patients according to the current evidence base (an example for this would be when guidelines for Antibiotic Cover were changed by NICE).

3. Involve carer in actual delivery of oral health care according to the patient's clinical need; this should be via a 'hands-on' demonstration in the clinic. Encourage the carer to ask any questions they may wish to. Ensure all appropriate items are available as necessary (gloves, oral hygiene aids, towel) and the patient has given consent. Involve the patient as much as possible and be guided by both the patient and carer as to how much may be achieved in each visit. Demonstrate suggested brushing technique for the carer to observe and then ask the carer to demonstrate back whilst under observation of a dental professional. Feedback to the carer as appropriate, taking into account all/any feedback from the patient (NB take note of both verbal and non-verbal feedbacks of both the patient and the carer).

4. Operator visual field will be clearer due to lack of froth from toothpaste so it will be easier to see where to brush. Will be able to monitor pressure of brushing (watch for gentle blanching of gingival tissue) and also enable more effective positioning of actual toothbrush bristles at gingival margin. There will be less risk of gagging as will be able to see where the head of the toothbrush is actually in the mouth of the recipient at all times. Sometimes it is useful to start brushing in the posterior region of the mouth so the patient knows that the 'fiddly bit' has been done (and can relax) and likely be more receptive to the rest of the care continuing. If any bleeding on brushing does occur, it will not appear so evident, which will be less stressful for the patient. Remember, a small amount of blood mixed with toothpaste can look much more than it really is – mention this to both the patient and carer.

5. Toothbrush handles – brush handle may be pushed through the middle a soft ball (like tennis ball) or the handle can be made longer by tying the brush to another item for example a ruler covered in tape. A stretchy strap can be wrapped around the hand to assist with keeping toothbrush in place (and lower risk of brush being dropped). Use of specialist toothbrushes such as those with heads that have three sides of bristles for example. Check if the patient is using any other adapted items such as eating utensils so that a consistent approach can be implemented (to ensure the same diameter for the width of handles). For inter-dental cleaning, *one-handed* oral hygiene aids such as bottle brushes, wood sticks, pre-loaded floss picks may be useful.

6. Why is a new brush required? Problem with technique (brushing too vigorously so risk of trauma and/or abrasion) or health needs (unable to move brush around the mouth). Does the person prefer a manual or powered brush? Ascertain whether any limited manual dexterity, if so, is it due to reduced strength and/or grip ability or poor co-ordination? Be aware of the actual length, width and texture (i.e. covering) of the brush handle. Total weight of item (if battery powered, remember to include the weight of batteries and the brush head attached). How is the brush operated – it is easy with one button for 'on/off' or is there a need to press a button several times for different brushing modes? Can the buttons be seen easily or operated by purely by touch? What is the speed of the brushing action – how fast does it rotate/will it be too vigorous for the person to control at gingival margin? What sort of noise level and what are the types of noises associated with different models?

7. Explain why fluoride toothpaste is important (and that fluoride does not have any taste or smell). Choose toothpastes that do not contain any flavours or colours nor have any texture. These will be more acceptable for people who have high sensory needs (Autistic Spectrum Disorder). A non-foaming toothpaste will remove the risk of frothing so less risk of aspiration if swallow impairment or no ability for spitting out. Dental bacterial biofilm will be mechanically disrupted and mouth can be wiped out as necessary afterwards. No need for rinsing. Remember to show how to apply the correct amount of paste onto the toothbrush.

8. Provide support to both the patient and carer – the aim is to be able to achieve good oral health using an effective, safe and non-traumatic brushing technique. Check medical history for changes – consult with Dentist as necessary. Confirm the patient's medical needs – is there any swallow impairment? Check position of patient especially if in bed (NB risk of choking). Use a non-foaming toothpaste so that it is easier to see where to place the brush during toothbrushing – this will help ensure brushing can be more focussed at gingival margins. If the patient is taking many medications (poly-pharmacy), is there a better time to carry out oral health care so that the patient may cope more easily? Could half of the mouth be brushed in the morning with the other side being brushing at night for example? Explain about safe and effective plaque control ensuring infection control risk for both the patient and carer is addressed as appropriate (whether talking to a family carer versus professionally employed carer). If the toothpaste has a high content of fluoride (such as those which are POM), remind the patient/carer about safe handling and storage.

9. Persons must be treated with dignity and respect at all times. Has consent for the intervention been given? Allowing someone else to clean your teeth is a very trustful thing to do. Carer to confirm how much the person can do on 'self-care' basis versus what care the carer will or need to provide. Ensure maximum independence is facilitated as far as possible through discussion with the patient. Evaluate whether an adapted brush or specialist brush may be needed due to any limited manual dexterity needs. Also consider the ability to open the mouth – how wide and for how long (could be restricted due to arthritis). Perhaps brush half of the mouth in the morning (for example one side) with other half (side) completed at the night-time brushing. Look at the timing of medications, depending on when medication is taken may mean person will have more ability to cope with the oral care intervention (such as reduced tremors).

10. Provision of a 'mouth map' for each patient accurately indicates exactly which teeth are actually present in the mouth. This will assist carers greatly when looking in the mouth as they will see what they are expecting to see (as indicated via the mouth map). Many carers

do not know where all retained teeth will be for example if a single upper posterior molar tooth is present, it may well be missed as will be tucked far away in the back of mouth. Also include notes (and names) of any recommended oral hygiene products and aids for the patient to use.

11. Ensure people who wear dentures are seen by a dentist as often as clinically indicated. Check that dentures are named. If dentures do not fit very well, it may be due to dry mouth (as a result of Xerostomia) or loss of muscle tone (facial paralysis due to a Stroke). Explain how some certain foods, such as tomato pips, can get underneath dentures. A dental opinion should be sought so that a full oral health assessment can be carried out; this is especially important if the patient has an unexpected weight loss or has started to remove their dentures or the patient is now refusing food and drink. Oral tissues need to be checked for any sores or discomfort (denture may need 'easing'). It has also been known for previously unerupted teeth to have grown in the mouth thus interfering with denture fit. Advise on denture hygiene and care of any remaining natural teeth too.

12. Treatment to be carried out must be in the best interests of the patient at all times. However, family members may also need to be reassured and supported throughout the care of their loved one. It can be very distressing for a family member to see their parent with no teeth especially when, prior to progression of the illness (such as Dementia), the parent would never have been seen without their denture/s in place. Need to advise that sometimes when new dentures are provided, it can be very difficult for the person to 'learn to wear' them. Many factors need considering when determining whether or not to supply new dentures (or would a reline be more appropriate). Also it is not uncommon for dentures to be misplaced – they may be removed and then the patient may forget to put them back in or the patient actually forgets where they have left them.

13. Ensure a suitable toothbrush and appropriate fluoride toothpaste is used at night and at least on one other occasion. Higher fluoride level content toothpaste may need to be prescribed. Use a straw as much as possible. Rinse mouth with water after high-calorie drink. Keep other sugary foods and drinks to mealtimes as far as possible.

14. A person may be living in a care setting (could be residential care, nursing care or supported living). Depending on the care setting and health needs, a person may not be able to choose 'when' they eat or drink (especially if fully dependent on care team) nor will they have much influence on 'what' they eat and drink. It is not uncommon to see glasses of squash on hand for people to sip all day; whilst it is important that fluid is being maintained, there will be no nutritional value (provides empty calories only). Continually sipping on such drinks can impact on appetite, resulting in the person not feeling hungry at mealtimes. Meals may be being provided by 'Meal on Wheels' and ability to self-feed is crucial; if not able to eat (unable to cut meat up for example), then person could start to supplement with 'easier to handle' foods especially those that do not require any preparation (biscuits). Loneliness can also lead to loss of interest in preparing meals.

15. Risk of trauma may be increased due to seizures or motor skills/co-ordination deficits/self-hitting. Suggest a mouth guard to be worn if possible particularly when out and about of usual accommodation setting. Provide advice on what to do in the event of a tooth being fractured or knocked out.

CHAPTER 2
Oral health education

Post Registration Qualifications for Dental Care Professionals: Questions and Answers, First Edition.
Nicola Rogers, Rebecca Davies, Wendy Lee, Dominic O'Sullivan and Frances Marriott.
© 2016 John Wiley & Sons, Ltd. Published 2016 by John Wiley & Sons, Ltd.
Companion Website: www.wiley.com/go/rogers/post-registration-dental-care-questions

SECTION I Questions: Society and oral health

LEARNING OUTCOMES

At the end of this section, you should be able to identify any gaps in your personal knowledge associated with:

- General and oral health needs
- Collating data
- Socialisation and interdisciplinary team working

General and oral health needs

1. Different aspects of health contribute towards 'holistic' health and well-being. Describe two 'types' of health.

2. Define what is meant by the term 'oral health'?

3. Define Epidemiology in one sentence.

4. What is the purpose of Epidemiology?

5. What is an Index?

6. Why are Indices used when carrying out surveys?

7. In relation to Epidemiology, define the terms Screening, Prevalence, Incidence and Distribution.

8. Which dental professional group is responsible for oral health epidemiological surveys?

9. What do the letters ADHS stand for?

10. What do 'DMFT' and 'dmft' stand for?

11. In relation to Public Health, what do the letters HWB and JSNA stand for?

12. What is meant by the term 'Evidence-Based Prevention'?

13. In relation to dental and oral health, state what is meant by Primary, Secondary and Tertiary Prevention and provide one example of each.

14. Define what is meant by Normative, Felt and Expressed need.

15. What is the Common Risk Factor approach?

16. Thinking about members of the dental team, what does the abbreviation CDPH stand for?

17. What are the five strategic points of the Ottawa Charter?

18. State two determinants of health.

19. State four 'social' factors that may impact on oral health.

20. State four 'health' factors that may impact on oral health.

Collecting data

1. Questionnaires are a common way to collect data – name two types of questionnaires.

2. In relation to patient feedback, what are PROM and PREM?

3. Name a main dental health survey of particular interest to an OHE.

4. What name is given to data that is collected in a numerical or easy to 'count' form?

5. What name is given to data collected in a format allowing respondents to express their feelings, experiences and/or opinions?

6. Questions requiring either a 'Yes or No' response are known as what type?

7. In relation to health data, how does the role of an epidemiologist and clinician differ from each other?

8. How can IT assist in collating and presentation of oral health information?

9. Which UK public department collates information and statistics about socio-economic grouping?

10. In relation to socio-economic grouping, what is the NS-SEC?

11. What is the Cochrane Collaboration?

Socialisation and interdisciplinary team working

1. Define Sociology.

2. Define Socialisation.

3. When thinking about how society lives, what are 'values' and 'norms'?

4. Primary Socialisation is carried out by whom?

5. Name two types of Secondary Socialisation.

6. What is meant by the term 'reconstituted' family?

7. List at least six health professionals who may be involved in delivering oral health advice to the public.

8. State two important points for all health professionals to remember when giving advice.

9. Mention two factors to be considered when giving oral health messages to non-dental health professionals.

10. State two sources of Oral Health Promotion resources that can be recommended to health professional colleagues.

11. How could an Oral Health Educator achieve effective 'interdisciplinary' working?

SECTION II Questions: Implementing oral health education and promotion

> **LEARNING OUTCOMES**
>
> At the end of this section, you should be able to identify any gaps in your personal knowledge associated with:
>
> - Standards informing the practice of an oral health educator (and GDC registrant)
> - Educational principles and evaluation
> - Social theories and models of health promotion
> - Role of the media in oral health messaging

Standards informing the practice of an oral health educator (and GDC registrant)

1. Name three of the nine GDC Standards for the Dental Team.

2. What is the GDC 'Scope of Practice' document?

3. Who developed the concept of Clinical Governance?

4. Service quality can be checked by three main aspects of 'care delivery' – what are they?

5. Service and care standards are checked by the Care Quality Commission (CQC) – what is it?

6. What is the NHS Constitution?

7. What is the Health and Social Care Act 2012?

8. What is the name of the key evidence-based toolkit for prevention for use in dental practice?

9. State six topic areas in the current key evidence-based prevention toolkit.

10. What does SIGN stand for and what is it?

11. What do the letters NICE stand for and state one purpose of NICE.

12. Name two Oral Health related 'strategy' or 'guidance' documents.

Educational principles and evaluation

1. How do Oral Health Education (OHE) and Oral Health Promotion (OHP) differ?

2. State the three key domains of learning.

3. What is the difference between an Aim and Objective (learning outcome).

4. Objectives should be SMART – what do the letters stand for?

5. State two considerations that need to be taken into account when setting objectives?

6. Give an example of a 'doing' word in relation to setting an objective.

7. Which words are not recommended for objectives?

8. When working one to one with a patient – state two ways that can help enhance and facilitate patient 'interaction'.

9. Define Evaluation in one sentence.

10. Evaluation of OHE and OHP activity is important – discuss two **types** of evaluation.

11. Evaluation of OHE and OHP activity is important – discuss two **methods** of evaluation.

12. Suggest two ways an OHE could 'process evaluate' during a one to one OH session.

Social theories and models for health promotion

1. Give the names of two well-known health educational theorists.

2. State two other 'models' of Health Promotion.

3. Name the two Clinical Psychologists who developed the 'Process of Change'.

4. What is 'Process of Change'?

5. Describe what is meant by the 'Iceberg Effect'.

6. In relation to the Iceberg Effect – describe what is meant by the term 'Performance Gap'.

7. Describe what is meant by 'Victim Blaming'.

8. State two reasons for lack of uptake in dental services on a 'continuing care' basis.

Role of media in oral health messaging

1. State three examples of different forms of 'Media'.

2. Explain what is meant by 'viral' marketing.

3. State one limitation of 'viral' marketing.

4. Thinking of 'positive' impact, state one way how the media can aid Oral Health messaging.

5. State one example of how the media may create 'negative' Oral Health messaging.

SECTION III Questions: Communication

LEARNING OUTCOMES

At the end of this section, you should be able to identify any gaps in knowledge associated with:

- Effective communication
- Communicating with individuals
- Providing oral health–related information
- Design considerations for a preventive dental unit (PDU)

Effective communication

1. Define Communication

2. Communication is said to consist of words, voice and facial cues – what are the percentages for each of the three aspects listed?

3. State three different types of 'relationships' for which communication is used.

4. State two Social/Cultural factors that could negatively impact on 'communication'.

5. Communication is influenced by differing levels of 'understanding' and 'feeling' – what other words may be used to describe these two aspects?

6. In relation to communication, what do the letters SOLER stand for?

7. State two aspects of 'non-verbal' communication.

8. In relation to talking, what does the term 'paralinguistics' refer to?

9. What three qualities in a person may help facilitate communication?

10. What are the three main rules of communication?

Communicating with individuals

1. State three reasons why a patient may have a negative attitude towards the OHE.

2. Give two reasons why a patient may have 'limited receptiveness' when oral health advice is given.

3. After an OHE, a person may still have 'limited understanding'. Give two reasons why.

4. State three reasons why 'Information Fade' may occur.

5. State three alternative methods of communication.

6. When caring for patients whose first language is not English, state one resource or technique that could be used to assist effective communication.

7. Describe how an OHE can support people with hearing impairment receive oral health advice.

Providing oral health–related information

1. State four points to consider when planning a one to one oral health session in the dental surgery.

2. Name one type of oral health 'clinical data' that may motivate a patient towards improving gingival health.

3. State four considerations needed prior to delivering an OHP session for a small 'external' audience.

4. State three factors that may enhance effectiveness of an OHP session for a small 'external' audience.

5. State four considerations when planning and delivering an Exhibition in the dental setting.

6. What do the abbreviations FOG and SMOG stand for and what are they?

7. Before using commercially produced OH leaflets, state two factors an OHE would need to consider.

8. Describe six ways in which information can be made more 'accessible'.

9. Give three ways Information Technology (IT) can be used to support Oral Health Education in the dental surgery.

10. Information Technology can be used in preparing actual OHE resources – give an example of this.

11. Discuss the pros and cons of using Posters and Leaflets.

12. Apart from the dental team, name four other groups of people who may be providing oral health messages.

Design considerations for a preventive dental unit (PDU)

1. When planning a PDU, state four 'organisational' factors that will need to be considered.

2. State three 'environmental' factors that could negatively influence how a PDU operates.

SECTION IV Questions: The oral cavity

LEARNING OUTCOMES

At the end of this section, you should be able to identify any gaps in knowledge associated with:

- Dental and oral structures
- Saliva and Xerostomia
- Dental bacterial biofilm

Dental and oral structures

1. At what age has the deciduous dentition normally fully erupted by?

2. At what age has the permanent dentition normally fully erupted by?

3. Describe Enamel and state the percentage of inorganic and organic materials it contains.

4. Describe Dentine and state the percentage of inorganic and organic materials it contains.

5. Describe Cementum and state the percentage of inorganic and organic materials it contains.

6. Describe the tooth pulp.

7. What is a Cingulum and why is this of interest in relation to oral health?

8. What is the name of the additional cusp commonly found on upper first permanent molar teeth?

9. What is a Frenum and why is this of interest in relation to toothbrushing instruction?

10. The periodontium is made up of which four oro-dental tissues?

11. In health, what is the depth of the gingival crevice?

12. What is the Periodontal Ligament primarily made up of?

13. Describe the main parts of gingival tissue that surround the teeth and cover the alveolar bone.

14. What is the upper surface of the tongue is called?

15. What is the under surface of the tongue is called?

16. State the role of the intrinsic and extrinsic muscles of the tongue.

17. List at least four of the main functions of the tongue.

18. State two common oral conditions that can affect the tongue.

19. Which structure makes up the floor of the mouth?

20. Why is it important to take care of lips?

Saliva and xerostomia

1. What are the main components of saliva?

2. What role does saliva play in the role of dental bacterial biofilm development?

3. Name the three main salivary glands and state how saliva enters the oral cavity from each.

4. State the approximate amount and type of saliva secreted by the three main salivary glands.

5. What component of saliva gives it it's 'viscous' property?

6. What are the two main enzymes found in saliva?

7. Name the two main inorganic salts found in saliva.

8. List at least five functions of saliva.

9. What is the normal resting pH of the mouth?

10. Salivary pH levels may be used in patients' caries risk assessments – how can pH levels be measured?

11. What component of saliva is involved with its buffering action?

12. What is the daily average amount of saliva produced by an adult?

13. Name the famous experiment involving dogs who produced saliva on the ring of a bell?

14. What does the term 'hypo salivation' mean?

15. What term is used for 'hyper salivation'?

16. Briefly describe Sjogren's Syndrome.

17. A commonly reported symptom of Sjogren's Syndrome is Xerostomia – define Xerostomia.

18. Discuss some factors that may contribute to Xerostomia.

19. Briefly state some effects of Xerostomia on the oral cavity.

20. Suggest some ways in which Xerostomia may be managed.

21. What is the Challacombe Scale?

22. In relation to salivary flow, what is the difference between 'lubrication and stimulation'?

23. Describe how salivary flow may be 'stimulated'

24. State two ways in which the oral cavity may be moistened.

25. Artificial saliva preparations contain different ingredients. State two reasons why it is important to keep updated on these products.

26. What is the term Dysphagia used to describe?

27. Describe what is meant by a 'texture-modified' diet.

Dental bacterial biofilm

1. Define dental bacterial biofilm (plaque).

2. What is the Salivary Pellicle?

3. What percentage 'microorganisms' and 'matrix' are found in mature plaque biofilm?

4. Name three components found in the plaque biofilm matrix.

5. What is the key distinguishing factor between Aerobic and Anaerobic bacteria?

6. Give an example of both Aerobic and Anaerobic bacteria.

7. State three plaque retentive factors found in the mouth.

8. Explain what is meant by 'chemical' control of plaque biofilm.

9. Explain what is meant by 'mechanical' control of plaque biofilm.

10. State two potential side effects from the use of products containing chlorhexidine digluconate.

11. To aid effective disruption of plaque biofilm, how could it be made more visible?

12. State two Plaque Indices.

13. Define Calculus.

14. In which areas of the mouth is Calculus commonly found?

15. What percentage 'inorganic salts' and 'microorganisms/organic materials' are found in Calculus?

16. How does supragingival calculus form and where is it commonly found?

17. Where is subgingival calculus found and why is it dark in colour?

18. What is the role of Calculus in Periodontal Disease?

SECTION V Questions: Oral diseases and conditions

LEARNING OUTCOMES

At the end of this section, you should be able to identify any gaps in knowledge associated with:

- Dental caries
- Periodontal disease
- Non-carious tooth surface (Tissue) loss
- Sensitivity, staining and oral piercing
- Oral malignancy
- Other common oral conditions

Dental caries

1. Define dental caries in one sentence.

2. List the four factors required for the development of caries.

3. What is the role of bacterial plaque in the development of dental caries?

4. State two common sites for dental caries to occur.

5. What is the least common site for dental caries to occur?

6. Describe the key stages in the dental caries process.

7. Explain what is meant by the term 'demineralisation'.

8. Explain what is meant by the term 'remineralisation'.

9. What is the 'ionic seesaw'?

10. What pH level is deemed to be the 'critical pH'?

11. What is the role of fluoride in relation to the 'critical pH level'?

12. Explain the Stephan Curve.

Periodontal disease

1. What is the difference between a sign and a symptom?

2. Name the four main signs of inflammation.

3. What do the letters BPE stand for and what is its purpose?

4. What is the range of BPE codes that may be used for young people aged 7–11 years?

5. Certain teeth (index teeth) are used for the BPE in young people aged 7–11 years – what are the index teeth?

6. What is the range of BPE codes that may be used for young people aged 12–17 years?

7. In relation to BPE scoring, what is the * now used to denote only?

8. What does BPE code 0 indicate and what is the suggested initial patient care?

9. What does BPE code 1 indicate and what is the suggested initial patient care?

10. What does BPE code 2 indicate and what is the suggested initial patient care?

11. What does BPE code 3 indicate and what is the suggested initial patient care?

12. What does BPE code 4 indicate and what is the suggested initial patient care?

13. What does BPE code * indicate and what is the suggested initial patient care?

14. Define Gingivitis in one sentence.

15. In relation to Gingivitis, state three signs that may be seen.

16. In relation to Gingivitis, state one symptom a patient may report.

17. What is the primary cause of chronic gingivitis?

18. A secondary factor in chronic gingivitis may be 'plaque retentive factors' – state two.

19. Name one systemic disorder that can result in an increased risk of gingival inflammation.

20. A secondary factor in chronic gingivitis includes 'hormonal change' – state one.

21. A secondary factor in chronic gingivitis includes dry mouth – state one cause.

22. A secondary factor in chronic gingivitis includes the use of 'long-term medication' – state one.

23. Define Gingival Hyperplasia.

24. During pregnancy, a 'localised' area of gingival swelling may be seen – what is it?

25. What is the primary cause of Chronic Periodontitis?

26. What secondary factors can influence development and progression of Chronic Periodontitis?

27. State three signs that dental professionals may notice in patients with Chronic Periodontitis.

28. State two signs or symptoms a patient with Periodontitis may complain of.

29. What do the letters NUG stand for?

30. State two signs or symptoms of NUG.

31. What advice could an OHE offer in relation to reducing the risk of Periodontal Disease?

32. State the two types of Aggressive Periodontitis.

33. What is the main distinguishing feature between Gingivitis and Periodontitis?

Non-carious tooth surface (tissue) loss (not involving microbial activity)

1. In relation to non-carious tooth surface loss, what is Erosion and how may it happen?

2. State two signs of dental erosion.

3. Name the main acid in the following items – a fizzy drink, vinegar, apple and orange.

4. Which type of patients may present with Erosion?

5. In relation to non-carious tooth surface loss, what is Attrition and how may it happen?

6. Which type of patients may present with Attrition?

7. In relation to non-carious tooth surface loss, what is Abfraction and how may it happen?

8. Which type of patients may present with Abfraction?

9. In relation to non-carious tooth surface loss, what is Abrasion and how may it happen?

10. Which type of patients may present with Abrasion?

11. Name two indices used to measure non-carious tooth surface (tissue) loss.

12. How can monitoring of non-carious tooth surface (tissue) loss be carried out? State two methods.

Sensitivity, staining and oral piercing

1. Tooth sensitivity is a common symptom of non-carious tooth surface (tissue) loss – what is the correct clinical term for this symptom?

2. Which type of patients may complain of sensitive teeth most frequently?

3. What symptoms do patients with 'sensitive teeth' usually mention?

4. What seems to trigger 'tooth sensitivity' (pain)?

5. Which teeth are most commonly affected?

6. Which part of the tooth is usually involved?

7. List three actions an OHE might advise a patient to carry out to help reduce tooth sensitivity.

8. Name two desensitising agents that can be found in a toothpaste for sensitive teeth.

9. What is meant by intrinsic staining of the tooth and when may it occur?

10. List three factors or substances that can cause intrinsic tooth staining pre- or post-eruption.

11. Where does extrinsic staining occur and why does it happen?

12. List three substances that can cause extrinsic staining.

13. What colour stain is commonly seen on the labial aspect of upper anterior teeth in children?

14. In relation to 'oral' piercing, state three sites it may involve.

15. State one possible risk to oral health *immediately after* tongue piercing carried out.

16. State three longer term risks to oral health from oral piercing.

Oral malignancy

1. Where may oral malignancy (cancer) be found?

2. State three main risk factors for oral malignancy.

3. Describe two signs or symptoms of possible oral malignancy.

4. What advice could an OHE provide to help a patient reduce their risk of oral malignancy?

Other common oral conditions

1. Herpes Viral infections are common in the oral cavity – state two common types found.

2. What do the letters HPV stand for?

3. What is the clinical term for the common oral condition known as a 'cold sore'?

4. Oral Thrush is a common oral condition – what organism causes it and how can it be treated?

5. What is the clinical name for sore, cracked areas found at the corners of the mouth?

6. Name the red, symptomless area commonly seen under an upper denture that is not removed or cleaned regularly?

7. Koplik spots found inside the mouth are a sign of which childhood disease?

8. Describe Aphthous Ulcers.

9. Describe Lichen Planus.

10. Describe Nicotinic Stomatitis.

SECTION VI Questions: Patient groups

LEARNING OUTCOMES

At the end of this section, you should be able to identify any gaps in knowledge associated with:

- 'Seeing' a patient
- Patient target groups – some considerations
- Some additional considerations for 'at-risk' patients
- Safeguarding and Mental Capacity Act (MCA)

'Seeing' a patient

1. People may not visit the dentist due to three A's – 'attitude, access, ability' – give two examples of possible 'difficulties' under each heading.

2. When planning Oral Health Education for a patient, many factors need to be considered in relation to Medical History – state three.

3. When planning Oral Health Education for a patient, many factors need to be considered in relation to Dental History – state three.

4. When planning Oral Health Education for a patient, many factors need to be considered in relation to Social Circumstances – state three.

5. In conjunction with 'person-centred care', state some key considerations to be made for all patients?

6. What key Dental Public Health messages need to be included for all patients?

Patient target groups – some considerations

1. State three key points when delivering OHE to Pregnant/Nursing Mothers.

2. State three key points when delivering OHE to Parents of pre-school children.

3. State three key points when delivering OHE to Parents of school children.

4. State three key points when delivering OHE to an Adolescent (13–17 years).

5. State three key considerations when delivering OHE to an Adult.

6. State three key considerations when delivering OHE to an Older Person.

7. State four oro-dental conditions which Older People may be prone to.

8. What type of patients may be classed as being Medically Compromised?

9. Give four examples of risks to oral health for people who are Medically Compromised.

10. State three key considerations when delivering OHE a person with Special Needs.

11. State three key considerations when delivering OHE to Health Education Professionals.

12. State three key considerations when delivering OHE to a person from an Ethnic Minority Group.

Some additional considerations for 'at-risk' patients
NB Key information and advice according to DBOH 3rd edition should be given for all.

1. A person with additional (special) needs may have one or multiple health needs – state three types of impairment and give two examples for each.

2. When is a SCOFF questionnaire used?

3. What hard and soft oral tissue changes may be seen as a result of an Eating Disorder?

4. How can an OHE support patients on continual (long-term) medication?

5. What advice can an OHE provide to patients worried about dental treatment costs?

6. How can an OHE support patients living with Diabetes?

7. How can an OHE support patients living with Epilepsy?

8. How can an OHE support patients living with Dementia and their carer?

9. How can an OHE support patients who are homeless/living in temporary accommodation.

10. How can an OHE support patients from Gypsy and Traveller communities?

11. How can an OHE support patients with dental phobia?

12. How can an OHE support patients who are involved in substance misuse?

13. State two ways 'poor lifestyle and dietary choices' may impact on oral health.

Safeguarding and Mental Capacity Act (MCA)

1. Describe current definition of 'dental neglect' according to British Society of Paediatric Dentistry.

2. What is the general role of an OHE in relation to Safeguarding?

3. State two different types of abuse.

4. State the five key principles of the Mental Capacity Act (MCA).

5. In relation to Mental Capacity, what is an IMCA?

6. In relation to Mental Capacity, what do the letters IMHA stand for?

7. In relation to Mental Capacity, what does DoLS stand for?

8. The Enduring Power of Attorney has been replaced by the Lasting Power of Attorney (LPA) – what are the two types of LPA?

SECTION VII Questions: Self care skills for effective oral hygiene

---

LEARNING OUTCOMES

At the end of this section, you should be able to identify any gaps in knowledge associated with:

- Toothbrushes, Toothpaste and Interdental Aids
- Care of Dental Prostheses and Appliances

Toothbrushes, toothpaste and Interdental Aids

1. What two purposes are served when teeth are brushed with fluoride toothpaste?

2. According to Delivering Better Oral Health, 3rd Ed, when should teeth be brushed?

3. State two different toothbrushing techniques.

4. Which toothbrushing technique is generally considered suitable for a young child?

5. Up to what age should young children received supervision and support for their tooth-brushing?

6. From young adulthood, toothbrushing techniques advise bristles are aimed towards gingival crevice – what degree of 'angle' is commonly recommended?

7. What generic advice can an OHE offer a patient in relation to buying a new toothbrush?

8. How could a toothbrush be adapted for someone with limited manual dexterity?

9. State three functions of toothpaste.

10. Fluoride is described as a 'therapeutic ingredient' – name two common types of fluoride that may be found in toothpaste.

11. What is meant by PPM?

12. What is the maximum level of fluoride concentration allowed in 'over-the-counter' tooth-pastes?

13. According to Delivering Better Oral Health, 3rd Ed, what amount and level of fluoride tooth-paste should be used for 0–3 year olds?

14. According to Delivering Better Oral Health, 3rd Ed, what amount and level of fluoride tooth-paste should be used for 3–6 year olds?

15. According to Delivering Better Oral Health, 3rd Ed, what amount and level of fluoride tooth-paste should be used for 7+ years?

16. Duraphat® 2800 ppm and 5000 ppm toothpaste may be used from which ages respectively?

17. Duraphat® 2800 ppm and 5000 ppm toothpastes are POMs – what does this mean?

18. State one other type of 'therapeutic' ingredient that may be found in toothpastes or gel.

19. In toothpaste, what do the letters SLS stand for and what purpose does it serve?

20. 'Humectant' is an ingredient found in many toothpastes – what is it?

21. According to Delivering Better Oral Health, 3rd Ed – when should interdental cleaning be carried out?

22. Interdental cleaning can be carried out in a variety of ways. State four types of interdental cleaning aid.

23. In relation to providing OHI, what is the purpose of a 'disclosing agent'?

24. State the name of an index that can be used to gain a 'Plaque Score'.

Care of dental prostheses and appliances

1. How should full or partial acrylic dentures be cleaned?

2. Before recommending how dentures with metal parts are cleaned, what should be checked?

3. During cleaning of dentures, how can the risk of damage be minimised?

4. When not being worn, how should dentures be stored?

5. How can 'disinfection' of dentures be carried out?

6. An obturator is type of dental prosthesis – what is it?

7. Thinking about orthodontic treatment – what is a 'retainer'?

8. Apart from a 'fixed' appliance, what other types of orthodontic appliances are used?

9. State four pieces of advice an OHE can provide in relation to care of a 'fixed' orthodontic appliance.

10. What type of dental treatment would be classed as an 'advanced restoration'?

SECTION VIII Questions: Improving public 'response ability'

LEARNING OUTCOMES

At the end of this section, you should be able to identify any gaps in knowledge associated with:

- Fluoride Products and Fissure sealants
- Sugars and Sweeteners – COMA – Vipeholm Study – Hopewood House
- Tobacco – Alcohol
- Balanced Diet – NACNE – SACN
- Dental Recalls – NICE

Fluoride products and fissure sealants

1. Define fluoride and state where it may be found.

2. Which type of fluoride occurs naturally in water supplies?

3. Which type of fluoride is added to artificially raise the level in water supplies?

4. Fluoride can be administered systemically or topically – what is the difference?

5. State two ways in which topical fluoride may be administered.

6. How can fluoride be administered systemically?

7. What is the most cost–effective method of delivering fluoride to population groups?

8. State two ways how fluoride may reduce the risk of dental caries.

9. What is the 'critical age' for potential enamel fluorosis?

10. Fluoride mouthwash can be used daily or weekly – state % fluoride concentration for each.

11. What % fluoride concentration does Duraphat varnish contain?

12. What is deemed the 'optimum' level of fluoride in water?

13. Other than by water fluoridation, give two other ways fluoride may be administered.

14. Who noticed 'mottled enamel' in dental patients in early 1900s in Colorado Springs, America?

15. Who carried out extensive research on 'mottled teeth' in the United States in the 1930s?

16. What is the correct term for 'mottled teeth' due to fluoride?

17. Describe how 'mottled enamel' can occur.

18. Who was the first dentist to remark on possible connection between fluoride and incidence of caries?

19. In what year was fluoride first added to toothpaste in the United Kingdom?

20. An important court case about water fluoridation was held in Scotland – give the name of both the place and the Judge.

21. The Judge deemed the outcome of this court case was *'Ultra Vires'* – what does this mean?

22. What was the 'Knox Report' about and when was it published?

23. When was the York Report published?

24. Define the purpose of Fissure Sealants and state where they may be placed.

25. State two types of patient group for which fissure sealing' would be advisable.

26. In relation to the stages for placing a fissure sealant, what stage comes immediately after 'etching' of the tooth surface?

27. A tooth surface that has been 'etched and dried' takes on what sort of appearance?

28. Clinical trials have been carried out to show effectiveness of Fissure Sealants in prevention of caries development – name one.

Sugars and sweeteners – COMA – Vipeholm study and Hopewood House

1. In relation to advising on policies for nutrition – what does COMA stand for?

2. Explain the COMA Classification of Sugars.

3. In a sentence, explain the difference between intrinsic and extrinsic sugars.

4. Which sugars are regarded as less cariogenic and why?

5. When was the COMA committee set up and when did the COMA Panel provide their report on 'Sugars in the Diet'?

6. List three recommendations from the COMA Panel report.

7. Which sugar is most widely used in the Western diet?

8. How might an OHE advise people to find possible 'hidden' sugars in food/drinks?

9. Give the names of two 'hidden' sugars.

10. Why is Lactose regarded as least cariogenic?

11. Products used to prevent caries may contain CPP-ACP. What do the letters stand for?

12. What is a Sugar Substitute?

13. What is a Bulk Sweetener and when is it used?

14. State three Bulk Sweeteners.

15. What is an Intense Sweetener and when is it used?

16. State two Intense Sweeteners.

17. In relation to reduced caries risk, why is Xylitol of interest?

18. What advice could an OHE give when advising patients about reducing sugar consumption?

19. What was the purpose of the Vipeholm Study and in which year did the study commence?

20. What was the main conclusion of the Vipeholm Study?

21. What was the purpose of the Hopewood House Study and in which year did the study commence?

22. What was the main conclusion of the Hopewood House Study?

23. Name two other sources (studies) that show a relationship between sugar and caries.

Tobacco and alcohol

1. State two reasons why people smoke.

2. In relation to providing smoking cessation information, what does 'VBA' mean?

3. State the three steps for carrying out 'VBA'.

4. What two ways can a smoker be supported during a quit attempt?

5. State four ways in which Nicotine Replacement Therapy can be administered.

6. State two forms Pharmacological support that do NOT contain Nicotine.

7. What are E-Cigarettes?

8. State four effects from smoking on general health in relation to Pregnancy.

9. State four ways 'passive smoking' may impact on general health in relation to Children.

10. State four ways smoking may impact on general health in relation to Adults and Older People.

11. State four effects of smoking on oral health.

12. How can an OHE support a patient who may be making a 'quit' attempt?

13. What is the recommended daily intake of alcohol units for men?

14. What is the recommended daily intake of alcohol units for women?

Balanced diet – NACNE – SACN

1. What does NACNE stand for?

2. What key suggestion was made in the NACNE report of 1983?

3. According to NACNE, what should people be eating MORE of?

4. According to NACNE, what should people be eating LESS of?

5. In relation to nutritional policy and advice, what does SACN stand for?

6. Give two examples of the type of advice SACN provides in relation to nutritional policy.

7. What commonly used health 'resource' helps show what a balanced diet should include?

8. State the five main food groups that support a balanced diet.

9. What does the health initiative 'GRAB 5' relate to?

10. What is Non-Starch Polysaccharide commonly known as and why is this important in the diet?

11. Give four 'dietary constituents' required for the body to function effectively.

12. Vitamins are required for health. State four and give an example of where each may be found.

13. Minerals are required by the body for good health and well-being – name four.

14. What is Phenylketonuria?

15. In relation to food labelling, in what order would the ingredients be listed?

16. Give three examples of other information that may be found on a food label.

17. What is the difference between Best Before Dates and Use By Dates?

18. What foods are not required by law to be labelled?

19. What does this letter 'E' signify on a food label?

Dental recalls – NICE

1. What do the letters NICE stand for?

2. What is the purpose of NICE?

3. State NICE recommendations for recall interval periods between routine dental examinations for both adults and children.

4. What sort of data could an Oral Health Assessment typically include?

5. Name two key documents that may help inform management of oral disease.

SECTION I Answers: Society and oral health

General and oral health needs

1. Physical – concerned with full body functioning. Mental – ability to think clearly and coherently – separate from emotional/social health. Social – complete well-being. Emotional – recognition of fear, joy, grief, anger and able to express the range of emotions appropriately. Spiritual – religious beliefs, personal qualities and behaviour – able to achieve peace of mind. Societal – healthy society providing basic physical and emotional needs.

2. 'The standard of health of the oral and related tissues enabling an individual to eat, speak and socialise without active disease, pain or embarrassment all of which contributes to general health and wellbeing.' Department of Health. An Oral Health Strategy for England. London: Department of Health; 1994. World Health Organization (WHO) definition is more detailed 'Oral health is a state of being free from chronic mouth and facial pain, oral and throat cancer, oral sores, birth defects such as cleft lip and palate, periodontal (gum) disease, tooth decay and tooth loss, and other diseases and disorders that affect the oral cavity. Risk factors for oral diseases include unhealthy diet, tobacco use, harmful alcohol use, and poor oral hygiene'.

3. *Study of prevalence and distribution of disease within population groups NEBDN 2001*
   Comes from Greek words *Epi* (upon) *Demos* (people) *Ology* (to study)
   Who is getting disease, when and where disease is occurring, identify patterns of disease to be able to consider both causes and measures needed for prevention.

4. Data received helps teams (e.g. NHS England Area Teams) to plan dental services and health improvement teams to tailor programmes for groups where oral health is poor. This also includes consideration of optimising wider dental team skill mix such as 'Use of fluoride varnish by dental nurses to control caries' – Primary Care Commissioning document, July 2009.

5. A 'numerical' scale by which variables, such as the levels of plaque, can be measured and compared with each other or with some base level. The scoring can act as evidence for individual oral health assessment, along with the monitoring of change (which can help motivate patients). The plural of Index is Indices.

6. The use of indices enables collection of data via 'reliable and reproducible' methods of measuring and grading. Calibration of team members prior to data collection facilitates accuracy in areas such as decision making regarding disease presentation (type, amount, location) and the consequent recording of that same data.

7. Screening – an activity carried out to identify disease in members of a defined population, irrespective of individual risk. All members of the defined population would be invited to participate. Prevalence – indicates how widespread a condition is within a defined population group usually at a *single point* in time. Number of people or proportion of cases can be identified. Incidence – measures how often a condition occurs in a defined population over a period of time. Actual incidence 'proportion' or incidence 'density' can also be measured. Distribution – indicates range (dispersal) and pattern (classification) of disease in a defined population.

8. British Association for the Study of Community Dentistry (BASCD). Local fieldwork teams from the Community Dental Service teams usually carry out these surveys. National and regional training is provided to ensure all are calibrated to support robust, high standards and reproducibility through all stages of each survey. Overall aim is to improve oral health and dental care provision and ultimately reduce inequalities in health. Statistics are collected/collated/recorded and eventually published on North West Observatory website http: //www.nwph.net/dentalhealth/.

9. ADHS stands for Adult Dental Health Survey.

10. DMFT stands for Decayed, Missing, Filled, Teeth. Use of capital letters indicate permanent dentition with the lower case letters (dmft) relating to deciduous teeth. For more accurate data in relation to levels of treated and untreated caries, actual tooth 'surfaces' may be counted, for example, DMF-S. Here the 'S' stands for Surfaces with a score of 1–5 allocated depending on the number of surfaces involved. If there is one surface decayed = score 1. A score of 2 would be allocated for a DO filling (as covers two surfaces). Thinking about deciduous dentition, the def(t) or def(s) Index may be used where the letter 'e' relates to loss of a tooth due to extraction rather being shed naturally, that is, exfoliated.

11. In relation to Public Health, HWB and JSNA stand for Health and Wellbeing Board and Joint Strategic Needs Assessment, respectively. Local authorities now, for example, have responsibility for the provision of Oral Health for Children and Young People along with the requirement to plan preventative measures for future generations. Health outcomes to be achieved are set for both the NHS and Public Health, for example, there is a Public Health outcome specifically to address tooth decay in 5 year olds.

12. Evidence-Based Prevention – tangible proof that a particular health strategy is effective.
    'Effectiveness' however can be measured in many ways depending on context. Examples can include actual reduction in disease and related savings to both the individual (saving their life) and NHS (saving treatment costs). Other factors can be 'social impact' (unintended outcomes such as gaining employment due to increased self-esteem and confidence) or value of 'legacy' (sustainable due to an individual being better able to carry out 'self-care' skills). Cost–benefit analysis is also important – the cost of intervening now versus treatment costs in the future (consideration of value of overall savings).

13. **Primary Prevention** – action taken to prevent the development of a disease in an individual who is well and before they get the disease. Main aim is to prevent disease and thus reducing both incidence and prevalence of disease. Includes delivery of key dental public health messages at all opportunities (to 'make every contact count') such as the following:
    - Brush teeth at night and at least one other time with a suitable sized toothbrush and fluoride toothpaste.
    - Keep sugary food and drinks to mealtimes.
    - Visit a dentist for an oral health assessment as often as advised.
    May also include more 'direct' working with different target population groups such as the following groups:
    - New parents – to encourage establishment of an effective oral hygiene regime for their children.
    - Young people – to facilitate informed decision making regarding oral health risks from oral piercings, tobacco and alcohol use.

    Secondary Prevention – identifies people with existing disease or conditions (people with 'higher risk') at an early stage in disease progression. The aim is to facilitate early intervention so that the treatment given can be more effective to prevent further deterioration.
    Examples of focussed, more individualised interventions include:
    - early caries lesions via effective use of fluoride toothpaste and dietary advice;
    - preventing gingivitis from progressing to periodontitis through effective plaque control (particularly relevant to Diabetes management).

    Tertiary Prevention aimed at people who have already developed a disease, condition or disability. Aims at preventing further damage and pain to slow down disease progression and prevent complications, help people to regain as much of a healthy life as they can.
    May require help such as:
    - special care items to achieve an effective oral hygiene regime;
    - more information on managing complex dental restorations (for example implants).
    Important to note that 'recommended or best practice action' is different from 'evidence-based' activity.

14. Normative – from perspective of the professional – what they think is desirable in accordance with their professional definition of health. Felt – what the lay person feels they need or what they want. Often linked to previous experiences and can be very different

from the professional definition. Expressed – these are the demands people may make via words/actions. If perception is that no solution or service is available, then 'expressed need/s' may not be raised.

15. The Common Risk Factor approach can be implemented in different ways, usually within a wider health policy context. Rather than focus purely on one specific disease, it is more effective to deal with common risk factors such as smoking, alcohol, poor dietary choices (for example high sugar/fat/salt, low fibre) along with stress and lack of exercise. These are common to chronic conditions such as obesity, type 2 diabetes, cardiovascular disease, cancers, respiratory disease and mental illness. Impact of environmental and social factors also need consideration along with ensuring collaborative interdisciplinary and multi-agency working. A Smoking Cessation policy could cover Cardiac and Respiratory diseases for example.

16. The abbreviation CPDH stands for Consultant in Dental Public Health.

17. The Ottawa Charter is a framework for the promotion of health based on the:
   1. Building of healthy public policy – organisations to take account of health effects in policies.
   2. Creation of supportive environments – make a healthy choice an easy choice.
   3. Strengthening of community action – identifying own needs to plan strategies.
   4. Development of personal skills – providing individuals with skills to cope with everyday life.
   5. Reorientation of health services – more prevention than treatment towards goal of health gain.

18. Determinants of health can be environmental (social, economic or physical) and influenced by characteristics unique to each of us as an individual. In detail, these can be broken down into:
   - Income – rich versus poor.
   - Social status – higher level linked to higher level of health – social networks important too.
   - Physical – clean air and water, housing, workplaces, employment.
   - Education levels – low level linked to lower life choices and self-esteem.
   - Genetics and gender – determines lifespan, disease risk.
   - Personal choices and attitude – lifestyle, diet, exercise.
   - Health care – ability to access, self-care skills.

19. Social factors that may impact on oral health include:
   - Poverty – unable to afford dental care and oral hygiene products for home use/self-care.
   - Poor dietary choices – use of processed/convenience foods – healthier food items perceived expensive.
   - Access to NHS dental services (no service available/long waiting lists).
   - Fear of cost of dental treatment.
   - Embarrassed about the state of teeth/mouth (low self-esteem).
   - Cultural influence and socialisation – diet, oral hygiene not priority, poor dental experiences.
   - Education – low health literacy.

20. Health factors that may impact on oral health include:
- Systemic conditions – Diabetes, Hepatitis, HIV, Post-cancer therapy.
- Medication – drug induced gingivitis – commonly due to drugs such as high blood pressure (Nifedipine), beta blockers (Atenolol), anti-convulsants (Phenytoin, Epilim), anti-organ rejection (Cyclosporin). Dry mouth – very common side effect of many medications.
- Genetic.
- Pregnancy – hormonal imbalance, exaggerated response to plaque, cravings.
- Eating disorders – soft tissue trauma, non-carious tooth surface loss – erosion.
- Physical and mobility impairment, for example, Arthritis – possible limited manual dexterity.
- Sensory impairment – hearing and sight (includes 'tactile' – loss of touch/sensation).
- Mental health – may be depressed so oral health is not a priority, effects of medication.
- Learning disability – due to poor short-term memory, alternative communication needs, anatomical challenges, in mouth (such as mal-occlusion, high palate, large tongue).
- Dementia (may be unable to recognise what a toothbrush is or what used for).

Collecting data

1. Two types of questionnaire include:
> **Pilot** questionnaires can be used to explore the local community needs (could be in relation to dental treatment needs or development of service provision). Using data collected, further questions can be designed to gain more detailed and specific information.

> **Pre** and **Post** session questionnaires can be used with patients either on a 1–1 clinical treatment basis or during delivery of an exhibition. Also suitable for OHP visits in the community setting.

2. A PROM (Patient Reported Outcome Measure) is a validated questionnaire that patients may be asked to complete pre and post session from a health-care organisation. More detailed data can be captured via a PREM (Patient Reported Experience Outcome) as it may include topics such as how well the health professional is able to deal with the patient needs, how well they communicate with the patient and so forth. The Patient Reported Outcome Measures (PROMs) programme reports on results at provider, Clinical Commissioning Group (CCG) and national level. Data collected and published via the Health and Social Care Information Centre (HSCIC).

3. Adult Dental Health Survey (usually carried out every 10 years). Surveys need to be easy to carry out due to the amount of data collected. For results and data to be easily collated and compared, surveys also need to be reproducible – protocols for implementation are determined for use on a national basis.

4. Numerical or easy to count data is called Quantitative data.

5. Data that captures information about feelings, experiences and opinion is called Qualitative data.

6. Yes or No responses are given in response to 'closed' questions.

7. An Epidemiologist is concerned with collating data in relation to screening, prevalence, incidence and distribution of disease in population groups. A clinician uses health data along with disease presentation to determine treatment need in individuals.

8. IT can be used as a resource (show patients oral health topics on computer) as well as to produce resources (use of software packages such as publisher and alternative communication signs and symbols). There are also many software applications which support alternative communication methods. It can assist in clinical research and literature reviews. Data can be collated to show trends of disease mapped to geographical areas or postcodes.

9. Office of National Statistics is responsible for collating information about socio-economic groups within the population.

10. NS-SEC stands for National Statistics Socio-economic Classification – an 'occupationally' based classification. By showing the employment relations and conditions of different occupations, the structure of socio-economic groups in modern society is seen that helps explain various social behaviours. Categories distinguish positions (not people) as defined by social relationships in the workplace. Socio-economic classifications are grouped into 1–8 categories as shown in the following list:
1. Higher managerial, administrative and professional occupations.
     Large employers and higher managerial and administrative occupations.
     Higher professional occupations.
2. Lower managerial, administrative and professional occupations.
3. Intermediate occupations.
4. Small employers and own account workers.
5. Lower supervisory and technical occupations.
6. Semi-routine occupations.
7. Routine occupations.
8. Never worked and long-term unemployed.

11. Cochrane Collaboration – an international independent network of groups (health practitioners, researchers, patient advocates and others) with the aim of bringing evidence together to support clinical decision making. Systematic reviews of scientific evidence from a range of health topics (including dentistry). Investigations into effects of interventions for prevention, treatment and rehabilitation are carried out to the highest standard. Reviews are then published via the online Cochrane Library. Originally set up in the 1970s by British epidemiologist Archie Cochrane (1909–1988).

Socialisation and interdisciplinary team working

1. The science or study of the origin, development, structure and functioning of human society.

2. A continuing process whereby personal identity is acquired through learning of norms, values and social skills necessary for participation in relationships and society as a whole.

3. Values are the 'ideal' standards a community would like to embrace and live up to based on what is good and just in society. Being deeply embedded, they are critical to the establishment of 'collected beliefs'. Norms are the behaviours and cues within a society or group of people. They are a way of behaving (can be positive or negative), which has become accepted by the group as an unwritten rule.

4. Primary socialisation is carried out by parents and carer givers including close family members such as grandparents and starts as soon as a child is born. It is important that 'values' and 'norms' of family life are embedded as early possible.

5. This learning happens outside of the close family unit and usually starts at school (nursery onwards). The two types of secondary socialisation are **Formal** secondary socialisation – this is carried out by people such as teachers and health-care professionals. **Informal** secondary socialisation – it occurs by interacting with peers and work friends. Outside of the family, a child learns the 'values' and 'norms' of society.

6. Reconstituted family is the sociological term for the joining of two adults via marriage, cohabitation or civil partnership including the children from previous relationships. Also known as a blended family.

7. Health professionals who may be involved in delivering oral health advice include:
   • Community and District Nursing Teams
   • GPs and Practice Nurses
   • Hospital Teams (Nursing, Speech and Language, Occupational Therapy, Physiotherapy)
   • Carers (Family, Residential, Nursing and Supported Living settings)
   • Dieticians
   • Health Visitors
   • Community and Hospital Midwives
   • Social Workers
   • Pharmacists
   • Teachers and School Nursing Services
   • Childminders, Playgroup, Crèche leaders
   • Health-trained representatives from commercial companies selling oral health aids, etc.
   • Health-trained reporters for magazines and newspapers.

8. All providers need to give consistent messages to avoid confusion among recipients. Keep information updated.

9. Reduce/limit the use of dental jargon – do not assume they will know dental terminology. May be embarrassed about not knowing much and/or standard of own oral health.

10. Sources of Oral Health Promotion resources for health professional colleagues include:
    • Delivering Better Oral Health, 3rd edition – many aspects of advice on lifestyle, fluoride, sugar-free medicines and importance of checking product information when actually providing advice on use of the product.
    • Scientific Basis of Oral Health Education, 7th edition – the British Dental Association.
    • British Dental Health Foundation – independent information, advice and helpline service.
    • NHS Choices website.

- Local Oral Health Promotion unit (may be linked to or based with health improvement teams).

Also it is important for the dental team to keep up to date with other health professional literature too.

11. Effective interdisciplinary working involves links with other health professionals. They will be knowledgeable on health-related matters such as an actual disease process so OHE will need to share and inform of the impact of poor oral health on general health and well-being. Ensure dental information is evidence based and up to date. Important to offer information on all core dental disease topics and to introduce both 'lay' and technical terminology, for example gums and gingivae. Identify useful visual aids to support recognition of dental conditions – think about how they show links with common concepts such as 'inflammation and infection'. Offer to participate in wider, general health promotion work, for example, No Smoking Day. Carry out regular self-reflection – what did you learn from taking part? What do you need to learn more of and why? What could/will you do differently and why? Share with other members of your dental team as well so that everyone can be kept updated. It may even result in changes in how the practice manages patient care.

SECTION II Answers: Implementing oral health education and promotion

Standards informing the practice of an oral health educator (and GDC registrant)

1. Every dental professional has a responsibility to behave in an appropriate manner, and the General Dental Council (GDC) has very clear guidelines for this. Standards for the Dental Team is the ethical guidance for registrants. The **nine** standards (2013) are as follows:
   1. Put patients' interests first.
   2. Communicate effectively with patients.
   3. Obtain valid consent.
   4. Maintain and protect patients' information.
   5. Have a clear and effective complaints procedure.
   6. Work with colleagues in a way that is in the best interests of patients.
   7. Maintain, develop and work within your professional knowledge and skills.
   8. Raise concerns if patients are at risk.
   9. Make sure your personal behaviour maintains patients' confidence in you and the dental profession.

2. The GDC Scope of Practice document sets out the skills and abilities each different registrant group should have and also describes additional skills that may be acquired after registration to increase the Scope of Practice. Registrants should only carry out a task or type of treatment or make decisions about patient care if they are sure that they have the necessary skills and are appropriately trained, competent and indemnified.

3. Dr Avedis Donabedian (born in 1919 – Lebanon, Beruit). Recognised that social response to health was a complex process involving general principles and themes rather than a series of unrelated events. His work still informs the **evaluation** of the quality of health care. Clinical

Governance is the framework by which the NHS can evaluate and continuously improve the quality of services. High standards of care are safeguarded by the creation of a 'clinical excellence' environment.

4. Three aspects of care delivery used to ascertain service quality include the following:
   - **Structure** (facilities to provide care) organisation – access – team skills/knowledge – equipment used
   - **Process** (how the care is delivered) – ensure appropriate to patient needs – safety in delivery paramount
   - **Outcome** (evidencing service quality) – encourage/act on patient feedback (both positive and negative)
   The following areas are also commonly used:
   - **Risk Management** (look at what can and does go wrong – what is the learning from this?)
   - **Clinical Audit** (measuring standard of care delivered to check performance against agreed standards). **Education, Training and Continuing Professional Development** (updating knowledge and skills). **Evidence-based care and Effectiveness** (care for patients should be based on good quality evidence). **Patient and Carer Involvement** (gain a better understanding of those using services)
   - **Teamwork and Team Management** (skilled team working efficiently in well-supported environment)

5. The Care Quality Commission (CQC) is an independent health and social care regulator for England. Regulates health and adult social care services provided by NHS, local authorities, private companies and voluntary organisations. Also protects rights of people detained under Mental Health Act. All providers of health and social care are required by law to be CQC registered.

6. NHS Constitution was first published in 2009 (Lord Darzi review). It establishes principles and values of the NHS in England, setting out rights to which patients, public and NHS staff are entitled along with the responsibilities each of these groups owe to each other to ensure that a fair and effective NHS is achievable for all.

7. The Health and Social Care Bill gained Royal Assent on 27 March 2012 and became Health and Social Care Act (2012). This created an entirely new NHS commissioning body (framework) for provision of health care in England including provision of and proposals for both social care services and public health. Clinical Commissioning Groups (CCGs) operate within guidelines authorised by NHS commissioning body, and each CCG has a board (panel of members) with various skills and necessary experience (for example clinical/financial/policy development) to commission services for own locality areas. CCGs are supported by Local Area Teams (LATs). Partnership working is also created via Health and Wellbeing Boards (HWBs) with membership from the NHS, public health, adult social care, children and young people services, local Healthwatch and other elected representatives.

8. Delivering Better Oral Health: An Evidence-Based Toolkit for Prevention, 3rd edition (June 2014). Evidence-based messages are to be given to patients regardless of perceived risk so that social 'norms' for better home care can be established. Also useful for informing commissioners so that contracts with 'preventive activity' can be encouraged and developed. Also creates an opportunity for supporting other health, education and social work partners

to bring effective daily oral health care into diverse settings. A 'public facing' version of the document is expected.

9. Delivering Better Oral Health, 3rd edition (2014), contains the following topic areas:
    - Summary guidance for primary dental care teams
    - Principles of tooth brushing for oral health
    - Increasing fluoride availability
    - Healthy eating advice
    - Sugar-free medicines
    - Improving periodontal health
    - Smoking and tobacco use
    - Alcohol misuse and oral health
    - Prevention of erosion
    - Helping patients change their behaviour
    - Supporting references

10. SIGN stands for Scottish Intercollegiate Guidelines Network – provides evidence related to clinical practice. May come up in final examination. Information can be found at www.sign.ac.uk.

11. National Institute for Health and Care Excellence. Provides national guidance and advice to improve NHS health and social care by producing evidence-based guidance, development of quality standards and performance tools plus supplies a range of health and social care information.

12. 'Strategy' or 'guidance' documents for Oral Health include:
    - NICE Guideline 19 Dental Recall (2004)
    - Choosing Better Oral Health: An Oral Health Plan for England (DH 2005)
    - Meeting the Challenges of Oral Health for Older People: A Strategic Review commissioned and funded by the Department of Health (2005)
    - Guidelines for the Development of Local Standards of Oral Health Care for People with Dementia – funded by the Department of Health (2006)
    - Valuing People's Oral Health: A Good Practice Guide for Improving Oral Health of Children and Adults with Disabilities (2007)
    - Guidelines for the Oral Healthcare of Stroke Survivors (2010)
    - Clinical Guidelines and Integrated Care Pathways for the Oral Health Care of People with Learning Disabilities (2012)
    - Smokefree and Smiling: Helping Dental Patients Quit Tobacco, 2nd edition (12 March 2014)
    - Delivering Better Oral Health: An Evidence-Based Clinical Toolkit for Prevention, 3rd edition (June 2014)

Educational principles and evaluation

1. Oral Health Education is concerned predominately with providing new oral health–related information and skills to people on an individual or very small group basis. Oral Health Promotion may include some OHE but on a much larger, wider ranging scale. OHP potentially involves oral health policies, strategies and even legislative actions.

2. The three key domains of learning are Knowledge, Attitude and Behaviour (KAB). Knowledge-related (cognitive) – Receiving new information/explanations, increasing knowledge, for example, able to explain what causes caries to occur. Attitude-related – Forming and changing attitudes, beliefs, values and opinions, for example, person with full dentures continues to visit the dentist. Behaviour-related – Acquiring and improving skills, for example, more effective biofilm disruption via use of interdental aid.

3. Aim is a general statement of purpose or overall intention of the intervention that is to be achieved. Objectives are smaller steps or stages that are needed to be taken in order to achieve the aim, for example, what the person will be able to do at the end of the session. Not advisable to have more than two or three SMART objectives. An example would be as follows:
Aim – To raise awareness of importance of interdental cleaning.

   Objectives – At the end of session, the patient will be able to:
   - recognise the role of plaque in gingivitis;
   - state two types of interdental cleaning aids;
   - demonstrate effective plaque removal from interdental areas.

4. - Specific – clarity about what the patient is aiming to achieve.
   - Measurable – there will be a way to evidence the desired outcome.
   - Attainable – the patient has capacity and capability to achieve the desired outcome.
   - Relevant – relates to what the patient is seeking to achieve.
   - Time related – time frame is achievable.

5. Objectives need to be appropriate to the target audience (whether working with one person or many people) and suitable for use in the setting where the activity is happening. Helpful background information can be sought through a class teacher, care home manager or from local public and dental health statistics/publications (Health Profiles). Typically includes gender, age, previous knowledge, any learning needs (English not first language for example) or if there are any key health issues identified in the target group. To facilitate effective engagement, appropriate resources are necessary to support intended objectives (outcomes). Consider specific topic material that takes into account acceptability for age of group, recognition of diverse cultural needs, ability for audience to use. Also need to be aware of budget implications and time for preparation, delivery and evaluation.

6. When deciding objectives, try thinking of the following statement: 'At the end of my session the patient/person will be able to list, describe, demonstrate, answer, write, explain, state, discuss … '.

7. Know and/or Understand – this would make the objective difficult to prove or measure unless the patient is actually tested in some way. Another difficult word is 'Feel' as very subjective so hard to measure.

8. Use of visual aids (includes photographs/diagrams/computer software) such as picture of healthy versus unhealthy gingivae or stages in a treatment procedure. Dental models for demonstration of brushing technique (use of a life size model is more effective as will be a realistic comparison regarding the actual size of brush to the size of the human mouth). Selection of each type of oral hygiene aid being recommended actually allows a patient to have choice (rather than just be given an item to use). Using the patient's own mouth to discuss their oral health status can be very powerful. A patient needs to be able to see where

they need to focus for maximum effectiveness and to improve their 'response ability'. Gaining patient consent is a good indication they are receptive and would like to engage. Dental literature especially use of 'personalised mouth maps' can help reinforce the session content. Are your patients given their BPE score? If not, why? Literature can be produced 'in house' or 'commercially', but always ensure it is appropriate for target audience. Do not just hand out 'product support' information and literature – check what leaflets are being given out and why they have been chosen. Items such as a timer will remind patients of the recommended brushing time through support as a visual prompt.

9. Making a judgement on the outcome and effectiveness of an OHE session or OH programme. What worked well/not so well and why?

10. Evaluation Types:
    - **Process Evaluation** – this relates to assessing how actual session **delivery** is going and awareness of being adaptable and responsive to the 'context' where possible. Is the person or group engaged? Are they asking and responding questions or remaining silent? Awareness of audience non-verbal body language is important. Are there signs of embarrassment (looking away or covering their mouth with a hand)? or, if in a group setting, are the participants yawning/scribbling on books (or texting!)?
    - **Patient Evaluation** – non-verbal feedback especially 'open and closed' body language needs to be taken into account at all opportunities. Patient experience questionnaires (**pre** and **post** session) are important – known as Patient Reported Experience Measures (PREMs) or Patient Reported Outcome Measures (PROMs) and can be written or verbal.
    - **Outcome Evaluation** – what is the intended outcome for the patient/people participating in the OH activity? Think carefully about outcomes – what **will** participants demonstrate as outcomes? What change or changes in KAB **of participants?**
    Most questions about evaluation in OHE exam concentrate on Outcome Evaluation.
    - **Peer Evaluation** – this is feedback from your colleagues. Ask for comments and suggestions for changes/improvements and consider these when planning future sessions. Use of patient notes – what did you cover with the patient? Are there any aspects of last session that you need to revisit? Are there any notes from the dentist regarding changes in patient OH? Receptionists may pass on comments they have received from patients. How are your patient attendance levels? Do referring Dentists comment to you regarding changes in patient OH?
    - **Self-Evaluation (reflection)** – exploration and identification of how well (or not so well) the outcome of the activity was achieved. Many factors are considered, including confidence, knowledge and skills, could all questions be answered for example? If a learning need for the OHE is highlighted, make a note of this for Personal Development Plan (PDP) and action. Could also include reflecting on whether a specific resource was missing, for example, information on eligibility/how to access free NHS dental care if talking to antenatal group? Reflective practice can be carried out 'in action', that is, during an activity or 'on action' for after the activity has been carried out. It is an important part of coursework, and in order to successfully complete patient Oral Health Education logsheets/Expanded Patient Case Studies, you must show evidence of reflective practice. It is useful to keep notes on activities, thinking about why and how you would change your performance or if you would leave things same, also say why.
    Remember, it is absolutely fine to recognise something did not work … in such situations, explain what you have learnt and what you would do to change this outcome for next time.

11. Evaluation methods:
    - **Questions and Answers** – skilful questioning (remember 'open and closed' questions) will help patients give full, clear, honest answers, for example, patients could tell you that they have noticed less bleeding on brushing. As this is purely a 'verbal' approach, it is difficult to show results to other people.
    - **Demonstration and Observation** (of a new skill) – unless you have photographic evidence, it is difficult to 'prove' that patients have changed their behaviour, for example, brushing technique.
    - **Questionnaire** – most popular method. Can show results on paper – disadvantage is patients often give answer they think you are expecting, rather than what they believe.
      Questionnaires are an important part of planning in relation to putting on an Exhibition/Display and will give you immediate feedback.
    - **Clinical Records** – Dentist or Hygienist can help in assessing long-term outcomes in patient oral health. Evidence of behaviour change such as reduced BPE and Plaque scores (with use of agreed indices) and clinical records may perhaps show a documented decrease in caries rate. These are all **measurable**.

12. What can an OHE 'see' and 'hear' when working with patients? Physical presentation (such as oral health becoming poor) can be an indication that the patient may have personal worries, which could impact on the ability of the patient to participate. Listening to what patients 'say' and, crucially, what they may not 'say', for example, looking at what is missing from the food and drink diary the patient has completed is key. **Questions and Answers** (the patient asks questions about where to buy a product, says will buy new brush). **Observation** (observe the patient's body language whilst OHE is talking or when patient is watching a new brushing technique being shown on model). **Demonstration** (patient is able to brush effectively at gingival margin in own mouth).

Social theories and models for health promotion

1. Education is based on theories formulated over many years by eminent academics and the OHE should be aware of Tones and Tannahill (two expert educationalists).
   The **Tones** Model for Health Promotion (1993) is that *illness is not sole responsibility of an individual*. Emphasis that illness not responsibility of individual person alone and that many factors, both social and environmental, can have an influence. Also introduced concept of *self-esteem*, encompassing ideas about appearance, intelligence and physical skills as well as our perception of how people react towards us. Assumption that someone who feels good about themselves is likely to be more receptive to health messages.
   The **Tannahill** Model for Health Promotion has three main aspects:
   - Health Prevention – detecting problems such as smoking or alcohol abuse
   - Health Education – educating children in healthy lifestyle choices
   - Health Protection – government legislation in protecting public (e.g. drink driving laws and smoking ban in public places)

2. **Medical Model** – focuses on reducing morbidity and premature mortality through use of screening tools and immunisation programmes for example. **Behaviour Change Model** – encourages adopting healthy behaviour and lifestyles. **Educational Approach Model** – health promoter provides information so an individual can make an informed choice. **Empowerment Model** – 'Bottom-up' strategy – health promoter becomes facilitator

or catalyst to help bring about 'social' change. Focuses on environment and government policy.

3. Prochaska and DiClemente 1986 – they believed that for people to change attitude or behaviour, then several stages are needed (as a continuous cycle, rather than one off event or action). People may relapse but this is actually part of learning about themselves and necessary for preparing for the next attempt to change – it is said that people should not 'quit quitting'.

4. Process of Change is a behavioural change model consisting of key stages for each 'cycle' through which people need to go when making changes:
   - Pre-contemplation – not thinking about change (may not even be aware of a problem)
   - Contemplation – thinking about change – may be receptive to advice
   - Preparation – intending to take action – actively seeking information to support change
   - Action – modify behaviour, commit to making change (may need to revisit preparation stage)
   - Maintenance – work to prevent relapse and consolidate gains made.

   Relapse (occurs when maintenance is not achieved so will enter 'cycle' again). Remember relapse is not end of cycle, but the part that precedes the beginning again. A person may need to go through several cycles to change.

5. The concept of an iceberg is used to show the 'difference' in perception of need between what the public perceives they need versus their actual need (as perceived by health professionals). This can happen due to lack of effective communication so may be outside patient control. Thinking about an iceberg, the amount below the water line is four-fifths with the remaining one-fifth (tip) above the water line. Health professionals consider whole 'iceberg', whereas patients' perspective is tip of iceberg only.

6. The Performance Gap relates to the four-fifths of the 'iceberg' that is underwater ('actual need' of patient decided by health professional) versus the small tip of iceberg (the need as 'perceived' by the patient).

   This difference in 'perception of need' can influence how a patient may or may not respond (as is more commonly the case) to any advice they are being provided with.

7. A patient may be doing his or her best; yet due to personal, social and economic circumstances, the standard performed may not be adequate. The health professional may be unaware of the true situation and blames the patient as thinks they are not bothering to carry out advice. In this situation, the patient is a victim of personal circumstance and a breakdown in the relationship of the health professional and patient may happen. An OHE can re-educate both parties.

8. Political – many dentists have moved to private sector working so many people may no longer be able to afford.
   Cultural influence – some sections of society do not attend dentists unless in dental pain.
   Lifestyle – homeless (no support structure to guide/no address), substance misuse (chaotic lifestyle).
   Low priority – oral health is not seen in the context of general health and well-being.
   Unable to access – impairment/mobility needs/dependency on other people.
   Lack of dental services – too far to travel, no NHS service, not on bus route.
   Fear – dental phobia.

Role of media in oral health messaging

1. Radio
   TV
   Newspapers and Magazines
   Commercial leaflets and literature
   Web based – Internet (professional and social media websites)
   Adverts (bill boards, signage on buses)

2. 'Viral marketing' includes junk mails (flyers, catalogues, etc), emails (particularly 'spam') and unsolicited phone calls (cold calling) and subliminal messages via radio and television. The message being communicated is usually very generic and not targeted at any one specific group. Mass media can 'talk' to the consumer directly and can be targeted as appropriate if necessary. Can be cheap and quick to circulate. Despite this, information that is produced in large quantities (as more cost-effective to print en masse) can indeed be effective simply because of the sheer volume of copies being circulated. This results in increased opportunities for the information to be seen.

3. Can result in many people 'talking' at same time, especially between the industry and professionals. May produce a lot of unnecessary, duplicated or conflicting 'noise'. No opportunity for people to ask questions or follow up on a topic once interest is raised. Due to very nature of junk mail, majority end up being thrown away without even a cursory glance.

4. The media is very useful for the promotion of self-care awareness/health campaigns, such as 'bleeding on brushing' or 'self-check' signs and symptoms for Mouth Cancer risk. Also sharing of new research and updates on advice, such as, no rinsing out any more after brushing teeth.

5. Media reporting on scare stories such as poor dental practice or claims about poor infection control. Promotion of health claims (or health gains) for products that may be unsubstantiated by evidence-based research.

SECTION III Answers: Communication

Effective communication

1. Communication is the sending of a message by one individual and the receiving of the same message by another individual.

2. Communication consists of
   7% actual words
   38% voice cues
   55% facial cues.

3. Communication occurs informally and formally to promote different 'relationships' via exchange of information. Can be written and/or verbal (use of text/email for short communication messages as opposed to a letter). Verbal communication, for example, a telephone call enables more projection of personality and emotion (voice).

Communication via Skype facilitates verbal and visual contact over a distance. Relationships include – **Greetings** – for people meet each other on a friendly basis. Factors such as non-verbal body language, familiarity, that is, 'custom and practice' will identify/determine amount of physical contact acceptable within 'personal space', for example, handshake versus kiss on cheek. Same applies if communication is not on a 'friendly basis'. **Expressing emotion** – includes both happiness and pain. **Determining Status** – as in a learner/teacher or employee/employer situation. **Contractual** – use of communication in more formal context with a requirement for detail to ensure agreement is achieved and understood by all parties.

4. **Social Class** – judgement of a person is made very quickly upon first meeting. Influencing factors include appearance, type of clothes worn, body adornments (tattoos, piercings). **Gender** – some people feel more comfortable communicating with people of same gender. May also be a requirement for cultural reasons. **Age** – may dictate how well communication exchange takes place. Personal perception is very individual – one older person may judge a younger person as inexperienced, while another may think that as they are young, they have recently trained so should be up to date, for example, patient–doctor relationship. A young person may feel reassured with advice from an older person, while another may feel the older person is 'too old to understand'. **Speech** – accents and language (range/choice of vocabulary) can play a huge part in communication. **Ethnicity** – cultural/religious beliefs (for example hygiene/nutrition). **Values and Beliefs** – whilst differences of opinion can be healthy, they are a common barrier to communication.

5. Cognitive (understanding) and Emotional (related to feelings).

6. SOLER – an acronym useful for non-verbal demonstration of effective listening. **Square** – to effectively demonstration listening, face patient squarely. **Open** – open body position – avoid crossing or arms/legs, can be interpreted defensive/closed approach. **Leaning** – a slightly forward posture suggests eagerness to engage. **Eye** Contact – when listening good (not too focussed) eye contact will encourage the speaker to continue talking. **Relaxed** – relaxed posture is important, otherwise communication will seem artificial.

7. Non-verbal communication may involve the nodding of the head and eye contact. It is especially important that eye contact is appropriate according to the situation. For some people, maintaining eye contact can be very difficult (even impossible) to achieve. Facial expression and gesturing are indicative of interest and attention being given.

8. Paralinguistics refers to **how** something is 'said' and includes the tone of the voice, speed of delivery and volume used.

9. Three qualities to help facilitate communication are **Warmth** – indicates interest in other person achieved mainly via positive 'non-verbal' body language. **Empathy** (not same as sympathy). Empathy is the ability to see the situation from the perspective of the other person. Can be very empowering for recipient and important in facilitative communication. **Respect** – recognition of other people having different feelings and opinions from our own. Many health-care professionals give advice that may not be appropriate or welcomed instead of helping a person to find their own solution.

10. Rules for effective communication are

Tell, Show, Do

Tell – explain to patient what you are going to do

Show – show patient what is involved

Do – perform the task

These key rules of communication can also be interpreted as

Tell me … I forget

Show me … I remember

Involve me … I learn

Communicating with individuals

1. Previous experience – being told off or treated like a child. Embarrassment – patient is aware of poor oral health and does not feel ready/able to make changes (could be scared of bleeding on brushing, does not have enough money for oral hygiene aids). Attitude of dental team – OHE not properly planned/discussed, information offered as an 'add-on' within a clinical treatment appointment so no emphasis on importance, low interest or emphasis from dental professional, patients told to 'brush more' rather than being provided with individual advice, seeing same (old) oral health leaflets routinely handed out. Messages in the practice not changed or updated (same posters up in waiting room for years). Information is not age or culturally appropriate so patient will not take an interest. Attitude of patient – does not feel needs to be informed (has managed to keep teeth for years already) and feels waste of time. Family history of poor oral health outcomes, so not worth bothering about.

2. Limited receptiveness may occur as a result of the following: Mental health problems or confusion due to effect of medication (check this when planning appointments). Dementia (even in early stage) may prevent short-term memory recall. Illness – person may tire quickly or if in pain, depending on the level of pain, may become so distracted that usual coping skills are challenged. Self-care – unable to carry out self-care skills so not worth listening to advice. Low self-esteem – patients feel they are not worth bothering about or worth doing anything to improve their health. Fear of dental environment is a barrier for many people. It is preferable that OHE be carried out in a 'non-clinical' area. Lack of time – people in demanding professional roles or with many responsibilities (carers) may not concentrate fully due to workload pressure (don't like being away from work/home for too long). No interest – expectation is that dental team will deliver all necessary care.

3. Limited understanding after OHE may occur due to conflicting messages in dental practice and/or from different dental team members. Lack of interdisciplinary working – dental and medical/health-care teams still not being used to working together. Updates in research – happening so quickly that continual dissemination of new information is necessary. Family and friends – influences can be confusing – may be out-of-date information or simply the sharing of a poor 'personal' dental experience. Clinical terminology – too much used when caring for patients – this is real problem for patients who have poor language skills (for example English not first language or different emphasis on aspects of health message) and thus will not be able to benefit from intervention. Even supportive literature post-session may be 'too wordy' or include too many 'difficult' words. Low literacy levels (low level of education) or learning difficulty or disability will also impact on ability to understand. Is 'word level ability' evident? Observe patients' actual performance and their ability to

follow instructions. Memory difficulties may also result from differing health needs such as Dementia or an Acquired Brain Injury. Provide information in a written format where possible especially for Carers who need to report back to the care setting. Easy-read versions should also be available. The Accessible Information Standard is due 31 July 2016.

4. It has been shown patients do not remember much information given by dental professionals. Reasons given for information fade are as follows:
   - Too nervous to pay attention
   - Memory skills not good
   - Feeling stressed from personal problems
   - Hard of hearing (don't like to tell you)
   - Diversity in relation to ethnic/cultural background
   - Information not relevant to lifestyle
   - Information not age-group relevant
   - Professional does not explain clearly
   - Generally not interested in making any changes to oral health

5. Alternative methods of communication include Makaton, Total Foundation Communication System (includes signing, photos, objects, symbols, speech), Braille, Moon, Picture Exchange Communication System (PECS), Use of Translation Services, Use of Interpreters, Text Phone (Minicom), British Sign Language, Deaf Blind Alphabet, Audio tapes/CD, Use of IT for speech boards (assistive technology), Mobile phones – provide information via 'applications' (apps) use of texts/emails to remind patients of appointments, photographs of patient mouth during TBI (showing where to position toothbrush or for after disclosing teeth, for example). NB consent regarding the use of photography.

6. When caring for patients where English is not first language:
   - Use an interpreter for translation (Language Line);
   - Use pictures/dental models to simulate stages for planned procedures;
   - Provide leaflets in preferred language;
   - Ask questions that require Yes or No answers as far as possible;
   - Implement the Show–Tell–Do approach.

7. An OHE can support a person with hearing impairment by:
   - ascertaining the level of hearing impairment;
   - confirm preferred communication method with the person;
   - use hearing loop, pen and paper, text information via a phone;
   - check whether Sign Language used/signer required;
   - check person has hearing aid switched on;
   - ask questions that require Yes or No answers as far as possible;
   - implement the Show–Tell–Do approach.

   Also confirming how to contact patient at home, check if Text Phone (Minicom) used or written format preferred, such as, send a letter or text via mobile phone.

Providing oral health–related information

1. Referral from dentist – to indicate what oral health advice is needed. Additional needs – is there any that may impact on your session? Does patient tire easily, have a learning

disability? Previous clinical notes – read these carefully and particularly your own notes if seen patient before. Action plan – what was agreed with patient? To brush at night and at least on one other occasion or purchase a specific toothbrush? Resources you need for appointment – would a visual aid convey message effectively (remember 'a picture paints a thousand words')? Consider literature being given out for 'post-session' reinforcement. Resources patient will supply – could use their mouth and their own or your oral hygiene aids. Also completed food and drink diaries are a 'patient-supplied' resource. Evaluation – how will you know whether session has been successful or not? Will patient be asked to demonstrate a new brushing technique, aim for reduced plaque score, complete a pre and post session questionnaire?

2. Oral health 'clinical data' that may support patient motivation to improve gingival health includes Plaque and Debris Score, Bleeding Index, Gingival Index and Basic Periodontal Exam (BPE) scores. Although an OHE is restricted to Plaque and Debris Scoring, they can use other data as appropriate from the patient records to reinforce positive gingival health gain, that is, reduced BPE score.

3. Availability – date free and accessing the venue. Clarify requirements – type of target audience/what information have they had previously? Need to carry out a pilot questionnaire? Delivery costs – resources (any photocopy costs), travel (petrol and time), hidden costs such as 'clinical' downtime. Aim and SMART Objectives – what is realistic for the size/type of audience? Visual aids/resources – appropriate according to culture/age and large enough to be seen by all? Seating arrangement – is session delivery via lecture style or group working? Facilities – use of projector/laptop, will you need sink and mirror? Evaluation of the session (method/type)?

4. Timing – be on time. Set up and prepare resources – Introductions – both OHE and any helpers (plus participants if not too large a group) could ask for show of hands to questions, such as do they live locally, carry out any OHE for example. If group work involved having helpers reinforces to audience that group working is achievable. Establish ground rules – respect, confidentiality, remind 'no question is silly', opportunity for anonymous questions (use 'Post It's). Aim and Objectives – state these and how evaluation will be carried out. Session plan – when breaks will occur (many people have caring responsibilities today so important to advise when they can check in). Delivery style – use varied approach (visual, listening, writing, talking, 'hands-on' element). Finish – be on time, thank for attending/attention/participation, advise your contact details for follow-up queries, provide evaluation form/session hand-outs. Tidy up – thank venue owner.

5. Target audience – who will they be and why chosen? What topic and why? Aim and Objectives – what will participants 'gain' after seeing exhibition, for example, new information or skill? Evaluation – 'evidence' how event went, for example, pre/post exhibition questionnaire to show improved knowledge? Resources – preparation and sourcing – will you use commercially produced items or self-made? NB FOG/SMOG any literature used or designed. Use bright, eye-catching resources and include 'interactive' aspects if possible. Budget – consider actual monetary cost to purchase visual aids **and** hidden costs such as time required to be released from usual work role (for preparation and delivery of exhibition). If using questionnaires, will you need help from Reception? Where and when going to be carried out – plan carefully if work rotas require adjustment. Is it a 'one off event' or to roll on for a week? Advertising – will advance notice/invitation be sent to practice patients or hold event on

a specific day, for example, No Smoking Day? Health and Safety – no fire exits blocked/no drawing pins used if young children around/display boards are secure, etc. Team work – keep everyone involved/aware of the event/carry out peer review. Photographs (NB if any people will be in photographs seek their permission first). Photographic information serves as a good reminder/prompt of the event and resources used to assist future planning. Good idea to prepare a checklist of 'action areas', which can be adapted for any event.

6. Readability indices – FOG stands for Frequency of Gobbledygook. Using printed text and counting the number of difficult words contained within a defined number of sentences, a 'reading level' can be identified. SMOG stands for Simple Measure of Gobbledygook – the process this time involves a piece of text. Another index is the Ease of Reading Index (ERI). Readability scores can be worked out on a computer also.

7. How easy is the material to read? What is the 'real' message being given? If the information is related to oral health promotion, is it accurate and factual? Is the leaflet purely based on the product? Is the product available locally?

8. Easy-to-read font such as Ariel, Tahoma, Verdana, Calibri. Take care with using shades or shadowing. Colour – black text on off-white or yellow paper is easier to read. Avoid red and green as some people find these difficult to distinguish between. Avoid writing in capital letters as will be unable to determine start of the word, which may reduce ability to anticipate what it is. Font should be at least 14 point in size (16 point is even better). Allow a little more space between lines of text such as 1.5 line spacing instead of single. Try not to have too many short lines of text as can be harder (and tiring) to read. Text should be aligned to the left rather than centralised or justified. Margins within a document for pictures (about 8 cm wide on left of text). Matte or silk finish paper rather than high, shiny glossy sheets will be easier for people with visual impairment to read. Laminated documents can also reflect light and become 'bright'. Free space on a document can make it easier to read. Binding will help if many pages involved – choose binding (plastic comb or spiral binding), which allows the document to lay/open out flat. This will also enable the use of a magnifying glass if needed or photocopies to be made. Loose sheets can be difficult as may be read out of order (which may cause confusion). Terminology – use simple words, for example, Doctor instead of General Practitioner. Consistency in words or names being used and use numbers in figure form. Symbols – such as % – write out in full as percent and take care with acronyms (words made up of first letters of other words), for example, BPE for Basic Periodontal Examination. Readability indices should be used. Alternative formats can be used such as Makaton, sub-titling, large print, audio tapes/CD rom.

9. IT in surgery can be used for patient records to confirm oral health status and referral from Dentist. Can confirm action plan previously decided/agreed. Plaque Score – can be a good patient motivational tool. Internet – can access information and visual aids for what patient needs to know to enable discussion of options and informed choice. Information and website details can be printed for patients (NB care where access information from, use evidence based, recognised professional websites only). Computer screen in waiting room so patients can view/review information key practice messages. Practice website – provide additional oral health–related information for patients. Mobile phones – text reminders about next appointment or when to brush teeth. Can upload specific phone 'apps' too.

10. Computers and Internet have revolutionised the way resources produced. Now possible to produce material of a very high standard using *Clip Art* and pictures of teeth, mouth, foods and

drinks. Desktop Publishing can be used for leaflets and brochures. Computer programmes that explain modern dental techniques such as implants can be found using a search engine such as *Google*® and even YouTube. Dental companies often provide easy-to-follow information about their products on their websites. *PowerPoint*® is useful in a teaching session and widely used in talks and lectures.

11. Posters – can be wall mounted and seen by many people. Need to consider wheelchair users if too high on wall – may not be able to read all text. Can become tatty quite quickly and look dated. May require quite large spaces on walls. Some posters are printed for key oral health and national health campaigns, for example, National Smile Month and No Smoking Day. Having current literature on view can evidence a wider 'practice message' of being up to date and proactive about good oral health. May only provide one message or be age related so will not be of interest to some groups of patients. Leaflets – these are easily portable and can be used to reinforce oral health messages and advice. Opportunities now to design own or have practice details added to commercial copies. May be expensive to produce/purchase. Need to check accuracy of content and readability level. Will require storage facilities, for example, cupboard and the need for versions in other languages.

12. Oral health messages can also be provided by:
    - Pharmacists
    - General Medical Practitioners/Practice Nurses
    - Nursing teams and the wider interdisciplinary team such as Speech and Language Therapists, Dieticians, Occupational Therapists, District Nurses, Health Visitors, Midwives
    - Educational setting – Teachers/Teaching Assistants, School Nurses, Children Centre Workers
    - Carers – both professionally employed and family carers
    - Social Workers

Design considerations for a preventive dental unit (PDU)

1. Referrals – who will be the PDU be for? What is the demand likely to be – every patient to have an OHE session or those with high caries/periodontal risk? Activities to be carried out – only information and advice or 'hands-on' toothbrushing with fluoride varnish application? Protocol – does the practice need to develop one? Budget – what sessions can be facilitated? Cost of operator to provide sessions. How will appointments and recalls be booked? Space – will the PDU operate on a shared surgery basis or dedicated room? Overheads involved – tooth brush/paste samples, disclosing tablets, leaflets, photocopy costs? Patient base – who is attending for dental treatment? Age of patients – what range and numbers in each group (for example under 5 years, adolescents, over 50 years). Ethnicity – will leaflets in other languages be required?

2. Interruptions from other members of team (accessing stock supplies for example). Noise from surrounding activities (if situated near Reception, phones could ringing or if near clinical area, could hear noise from handpieces – not helpful for nervous patients) Smell – from use of clinical materials. Type of lighting – poor or too bright? Temperature – if not natural light or ventilation (could become too warm). Limited space to accommodate more than one person, for example, parent/carer with the patient. If only a small room, unable to be accessed by wheelchair users or family with a pram. Clutter – can be a distraction if too many leaflets or items on side. Seating – could be uncomfortable or, if unable to adjust, difficult to work at

eye level (key to effective communication). Need to also consider Operator Health and Safety. Water – no sink for hand washing/no drinking water if wish to use disclosing materials. IT facilities unavailable (so unable to show OHE programmes/videos).

SECTION IV Answers: The oral cavity

Dental and oral structures

1. Total 20 in number – usually fully erupted between 24 and 36 months.

2. Total 32 in number – usually fully erupted by 18 years+.

3. Enamel is 96% inorganic and 4% organic. Hardest substance in body and unable to repair itself. Covers the crown of tooth (part seen above gingival margin). Because of large amount of inorganic (non-living) material, it is not susceptible to stimuli such as temperature change. Subject to four main types of non-carious tooth surface wear.

4. Dentine is 70% inorganic and 30% organic (softer than Enamel so decay rate may occur more readily). Large part of tooth predominately made up of 'dentinal tubules', which run from tooth pulp out to both Enamel and the Cementum on the tooth root surface. Sensitive to stimuli – different theories about why this may occur.

5. Cementum is 45% inorganic and 55% organic and covers the root surface. Forms part of the 'anchor mechanism' securing teeth into maxilla and mandible. Periodontal Ligament fibres fix onto root surface and related alveolar bone surrounding each tooth.

6. Soft tissue (containing blood supply and mainly nerves) found inside pulp chamber in centre of tooth continuing into tooth root canals.

7. Cingulum commonly found on palatal aspects of upper incisor teeth. Can be plaque retentive factor and prone to decay.

8. Additional cusp on upper first permanent molar teeth is the Cusp of Carabelli.

9. A frenum (or frena) is a soft tissue attachment joining the mucosa usually to the attached gingivae. They can be found all around the mouth (commonly seen in the region of upper and lower central incisors). A frenum can prevent the effective use of a tooth brush at the gingival margin.

10. Periodontium consists of Alveolar Bone, Cementum, Periodontal Ligament, Gingivae.

11. Gingival crevice depth in health is 0–3 mm.

12. Periodontal Ligament is mainly bundles of collagen fibres. Width of ligament is from 0.1 to 0.3 mm with the fibres forming the attachment between tooth and alveolar bone. This allows teeth to move slightly in the socket to withstand the stress from occlusal loading during mastication.

13. The gingiva at the actual neck of the tooth is not bound down to the underlying bone and called the **Free Gingivae**. This tissue borders the teeth whilst also filling the spaces between each tooth as the **Interdental Papillae**. In health, each papilla is flat, pointed and triangular in shape (as a 'pyramid' of tissue between each tooth). The 'contoured' Free Gingivae and Interdental Papillae form the **Gingival Crest,** creating a crevice (small 'ditch') between tooth surfaces and this gingival tissue. The **Junctional Epithelium** is the point at which the gingival tissue actually attaches to the tooth surface. The attachment point can be seen as an 'indentation' line known as the **Free Gingival Groove**. Below the free gingival groove is **Attached Gingivae,** which is firmly bound down to the underlying alveolar bone. It is keratinised (toughened) gingiva similar to that found on the hard palate. This resilient tissue plays a part in digestion as it can withstand the friction created by chewing of food and formation of a 'bolus' of food (in readiness for swallowing). In health, attached gingiva is pale pink in colour with, when dry, a similar appearance to 'orange peel'. This effect is known as 'stippling' and created from the ends of the collagen fibre bundles ('stippling' is lost during inflammatory change, i.e. when swollen, ends of fibres cannot be seen).

   Gingival tissue below the 'attached gingivae' level is known as the **Vestibular Mucosa**. This 'non-keratinised' tissue covers the inside of the mouth (cheeks and floor of mouth). It has a darker pink, shiny surface. These two types of gingival tissue have a demarcation line between them called the **MucoGingival Junction**.

14. Upper surface of the tongue is the dorsal surface.

15. Under surface of the tongue is the ventral surface.

16. Intrinsic muscles in the tongue alter its shape. Extrinsic muscles move the tongue and also help alter its shape.

17. **Taste** – sweet, sour, salt, bitter, umami (described as fifth 'savoury' taste to complement conventional taste categories that the human tongue is known to detect). **Mastication** – in conjunction with hard palate, enables chewing of food to form a bolus along its dorsal surface towards back of the mouth. **Deglutition** – the tongue moves bolus towards oesophagus for swallowing. **Speech** – particularly production of different sounds. **Cleansing** – the tip of the tongue helps loosen and remove food particles from teeth and buccal sulci. **Protection** – optimise antibacterial role of saliva through the distribution of the fluid all around oral cavity.

18. **Glossitis** – inflammation of the tongue. Can be due to dry mouth, injury from a burn or irritant, Vitamin B deficiency/hormonal imbalance. **Soreness** – Vitamin B deficiency, hormonal imbalance. **Black hairy tongue** – overgrowth tongue papillae stained by chromogenic bacteria/chlorhexidine. **Geographic tongue** – irregular pattern (resembles a map hence the use of term geographic), harmless. **Median Rhomboid Glossitis** – loss of papillae in the centre of dorsum.

19. Mylohyoid muscle makes up the floor of the mouth.

20. Lip cancer is included as part of Skin Cancer – this is a Public Health priority.

Saliva and Xerostomia

1. Saliva consists of 99.5% water and 0.5% dissolved substances (made up of different types of proteins known as mucin).

2. Glycoproteins in saliva (which are substrates for plaque bacteria) form a sticky coating on teeth known as Salivary Pellicle. Bacteria then attach to the pellicle (known as colonisation) to form the biofilm.

3. Parotid Gland – via Parotid Duct on buccal mucosa opposite the upper first and second permanent molar teeth on both sides of the mouth. Submandibular Gland – via Submandibular Duct on the floor of the mouth anterior to the tongue – may see 'fountain of saliva' expressed when patient mouth open during dental treatment. Sublingual Gland – numerous ducts on ridge of sublingual fold on the floor of the mouth beneath front of the tongue.

4. Saliva can be a serous (watery) and/or mucous (thick/viscous) fluid. Parotid – 25% (serous) via parotid duct. Submandibular – 70% (serous and mucous). Sublingual – 5% (mainly mucous).

5. Glycoproteins give saliva its viscous property.

6. Salivary Amylase, which begins digestion of cooked starch, and Lysozyme, which has an antibacterial action (controls bacterial growth).

7. Calcium and Phosphate mineral salts – important in the formation of calculus and remineralisation process.

8. **Chewing** (mastication) of food items. **Digestion** – Salivary Amylase begins digestion of fermentable carbohydrates in mouth (NB caries risk increased if low flow rate or poor quality of saliva). Swallowing (deglutition) – supports formation of a food bolus. **Oral hygiene** – washing/cleansing action to remove oral debris from oral cavity. **Antibacterial** action from the enzyme Lysozyme. **Speech** – acts as a lubricant; allows tongue to move around to facilitate the formation of sounds. **Cooling effect** – oral cavity is able to withstand hot foods and drinks. **Taste** – assists in the dissolving of substances so taste buds on the tongue can identify/recognise different flavours. **Water intake** for body – helps maintain balance. (If too low, saliva is reduced leading to thirst sensation.) **Excretion** – loss occurs in small amounts as urea/uric acid. **Buffering** action – helps maintain a neutral pH usually just below 7.0.

9. Resting pH of the mouth is 6.8/7.0. The range of pH level is 0 (highly acidic) through to 14 (highly alkaline). So the lower a pH number is, the more acidic it is.

10. Saliva testing kits – contain saliva collecting pot, litmus paper and acidity grading sheet.

11. Bicarbonate ions are concerned with the buffering action of saliva.

12. 0.5–1.5 litre.

13. The experiment was carried out by Russian physiologist Ivan Pavlov in which dogs learned an association between the bell and food (resulting in production of saliva). This was a new behaviour that had been learnt, and as the response is learned (or conditioned), it is called a conditioned response.

14. Reduced or diminished flow of saliva – the term indicates the clinical diagnosis of salivary 'hypo function'.

15. Sialorrhea (ptyalism) is excessive production of saliva (may be seen in teething, acute dental infections).

16. Sjogren's Syndrome is a chronic autoimmune condition causing a person's immune system (white cells) to attack the body's healthy tissues – in this case, it is the moisture-producing glands. Main symptoms are dry eyes and dry mouth.

17. Xerostomia is dryness of the mouth due to insufficient oral secretions. Dryness (which is subjective) can result from a reduction in either a change in composition of saliva or in amount or flow.

18. Age (saliva production and flow can diminish with age). Changes in hormone levels (females).
    Drug therapy (particularly prescription drugs to treat high blood pressure, depression, allergies). Anxiety – stress or nervousness (fight or flight reaction). Acute illness – diarrhoea/vomiting. Mouth breathing – incompetent lips/lack of lip seal. Salivary calculi – calcified stones in salivary ducts. Radiotherapy – treatment for Head and Neck Cancer (especially if in the region of salivary glands).

19. Due to dryness, lack of buffering capacity, slow clearance of debris (food) from oral cavity and stickier plaque; increased risk of the following may occur – Caries, Gingivitis, Fungal and Yeast infections, Glossitis (sore tongue), Ulceration especially post-radiotherapy, Eating difficulties, for example, dry foods such as crackers or 'sharp' items like crisps along with possible altered oral sensation and disturbance in taste. May be difficulties with speech and retention of dentures.

20. Important to determine why Xerostomia is occurring. Diet high in fruit and vegetables – increases salivary flow due to the requirement for mastication plus the water content found in fruit and vegetables. Chewing of sugar-free gum – look for Xylitol as it has anti-cariogenic properties. Frequent sips of water – use of an atomiser is helpful if need to control quantity being taken in. Suck small ice chips. Use oral moistening products such as Biotene/BioXtra/Oral Balance. Lubrication of oral tissues prior to eating, for example, flavourless salad oil to assist with bolus formation and actual swallow mechanism.

21. It is a Clinical Oral Dryness Score (CODS) suitable for all health professionals to use. It has a simple numeric system to quantify the severity of Xerostomia. Treatment need is determined by the score achieved. Designed under supervision of Professor Stephen Challacombe (Kings College, London).

22. Lubrication is necessary when the ability to produce salivary fluid 'naturally' is lost or if the fluid produced is of poor quality. Usually a supply of additional (artificial) fluid is then

required. Stimulation is used when the natural production and flow of saliva is present but needs to be increased.

23. Visualisation/anticipation of food or drink. Smell of food or drink (olfactory senses). Chewing of sugar-free gum.

24. Artificial saliva. Sucking ice chips. Drinking milk/water. Use of specialised mouth care gels.

25. Some artificial saliva items contain fluoride – others do not. This would be important for people who have natural teeth rather than those who are edentulous. Mucin is used to provide viscosity – it can be derived from pig mucin, which may not be acceptable to some groups of society due to religious (Islam) and/or dietary (Vegan) preferences. Fruit-based products could have a low pH – not suitable if natural teeth are present.

26. Dysphagia is the term for swallowing difficulties. Degree of difficulty can range from problems with certain foods or liquids to a total loss of swallowing ability. Some people with dysphagia have problems swallowing certain foods or liquids, while others cannot swallow at all. If occurs in the mouth or throat, it is known as oropharyngeal or high dysphagia; if occurs in oesophagus, known as oesophageal or low dysphagia. Usually related to health condition in other parts of the body, for example, Nervous system (stroke/dementia), Cancer (mouth or oesophagus) and GORD (gastro-oesophageal reflux disease as a result of acid from the stomach going into oesophagus).

27. Texture-modified diet is when the texture of solid foods and/or liquid consistency is altered to support swallowing ability. Types of texture-modified diet include soft, minced, pureed.

Dental bacterial biofilm

1. A soft, very sticky substance containing bacteria and debris that collects on surfaces of teeth and dental appliances as a bacterial film. Enzymes and toxins of the mature plaque bacteria are main factors in the development of dental disease.

2. A transparent film of glycoproteins (complex sugars and proteins in saliva) that forms on tooth surfaces and dental appliances. Very soon after the formation, the pellicle is colonised with microorganisms to form early plaque. Colonisation continues and attracts more harmful microorganisms.

3. Mature plaque biofilm is made up of 70% microorganisms and 30% matrix framework.

4. Food debris – proteins and carbohydrates. Dead cells – oral mucosa. Red and white blood cells. Enzymes and toxins of plaque. Lactic acid. Antigens.

5. Requirement for oxygen. Aerobic bacteria need oxygen to survive, whereas Anaerobic do not.

6. Aerobic bacteria consist mainly of streptococci (*Streptococcus mutans, S. mitis, S. salivarius* and *S. sanguis*). Anaerobes are primarily Fusiforms, Vibrios and Spirochaetes (found in periodontal pockets and more pathogenic).

7. Plaque retention factors include bridges, crowns, implants, dentures, orthodontic appliances, periodontal pockets, large/uneven restorations and calculus.

8. Chemical control involves use of oral health-care products designed to suppress the growth/development of plaque biofilm formation such as chlorhexidine gluconate based products (dental gel, mouthwash, spray).

9. Mechanical control involves physical disruption of biofilm through toothbrushing and flossing. Also thought that a low sucrose diet could control plaque.

10. **Staining** – brown, extrinsic stain found on surfaces of teeth and tongue (black hair–like appearance). **Taste disturbance** – reports of altered taste (temporary basis). **Calculus** – may be an increase in the formation of calculus (supra gingival).

11. Use of disclosing agents – either in tablet or solution form. Erythrosine provides colour – check if the patient is allergic to colours.

12. Modified Silness and Löe Plaque Index (1964) – much-simplified form of earlier index produced by these Swedish researchers. The patient is disclosed and the presence of plaque is noted as follows: Code 0 = No plaque deposits visible in the gingival area. Code 1 = Plaque deposits visible in the gingival area. Turesky Plaque Index – many people use Turesky Index – relatively simple method to measure the presence of plaque, offers a high level of sensitivity and a useful patient motivation tool. Although looks complex, simple to carry out with assistance.

13. The mineralised or calcified bacterial plaque deposit found on teeth and other solid structures in the mouth. The mineral salts (calcium and phosphate) are found in saliva and taken up into biofilm.

14. Calculus found particularly in areas of mouth where salivary gland ducts are positioned close to teeth. Parotid gland – opposite upper first permanent molar teeth. Submandibular and Sublingual glands – close to lingual aspect lower anterior teeth. These are also difficult areas of the mouth to brush.

15. Calculus is made up of 70% inorganic salts and 30% microorganisms/organic material.

16. Calculus is 'calcified' plaque and formation is dependent on effectiveness of plaque control and mineral content of saliva (calcium and phosphate ions). Appears white and chalk like. Due to roughness, it attracts more plaque. Found above gingival margins usually behind lower anterior teeth and on buccal aspects of molar teeth (6's).

17. Subgingival means being below the gingival margin. It is very hard (from minerals in crevicular fluid) and difficult to remove (tenacious). Dark colouration is from the breakdown of blood components from crevicular ulceration.

18. The role of calculus in the development of Periodontal Disease is that it attracts more plaque (plaque retention factor).

SECTION V Answers: Oral diseases and conditions

Dental caries

1. Progressive destruction of enamel, dentine and cementum, initiated by microbial activity at the susceptible tooth surface.

2. Susceptible tooth, bacterial plaque, bacterial substrate (fermentable carbohydrate, food source for plaque bacteria), and time. Susceptible tooth + bacterial plaque + substrate + time = caries.

3. Maintains concentration of acid at the tooth surface. Resists salivary buffering. Provides carbohydrate reserve (food for bacteria).

4. Common sites for dental caries – Occlusal surfaces especially newly erupted molars and pre-molars (Pit and Fissure Caries). Contact areas between adjacent teeth (Interstitial). Cervical areas – near to the gingival margin (especially in children and young people). Exposed root surfaces (Root Caries). Other risk areas include molar teeth (buccally), palatal grooves on upper anterior teeth, that is, Cingulum and upper first permanent molar teeth (Cusp of Carabelli).

5. Smooth surfaces of teeth.

6. Initially small, white 'chalk-like' spot (early demineralisation) may be seen. Reversible with effective oral hygiene (optimal exposure to fluoride). If enamel constantly exposed to acidic challenge, then decay can continue under the top surface layer. This will result in a breakdown of enamel structure to allow progression of decay into dentine. Decay process can spread more quickly as dentine softer than enamel. If the pulp of the tooth becomes involved, this can lead to pulpitis (inflammation of pulp and pain) resulting in pulp death. An abscess may form (due to the infection).

7. During 'acidic' challenge, calcium and phosphate ions leave the enamel of the tooth, resulting in 'softened' enamel. When demineralisation occurs more frequently than remineralisation, caries may occur.

8. Saliva acts to dilute and neutralise plaque acids. It contains bicarbonate ions that help return calcium and phosphate ions to the enamel surface (known as 'buffering' effect). 'Buffering' can take up to 1 hour.

9. Ionic seesaw relates to the movement of calcium and phosphate ions 'in and out' of enamel.

10. Spectrum of pH levels ranges from 0 to 14 (0 being most acidic to 14 being most alkaline). Resting pH level of mouth is normally neutral at a pH of 6.8/7.0. The 'critical pH' occurs when the pH level lowers to pH 5.5 (as more acidic).

11. By incorporating fluoride, tooth surfaces can withstand even lower pH level – down to pH 4.5. This results in slower loss of calcium and phosphate ions (less risk of demineralisation).

12. Stephan Curve relates to a graph (the curve) showing how sugar frequency can impact on resting (neutral) pH level of the mouth. Intake of sugar leads to acid production, which lowers 'resting' pH level (seen as a 'dip' on graph) from 6.8 down to 5.5 critical pH and below. Demineralisation occurs at 5.5 and lower. If no more sugar eaten, that is, no more acid produced, then pH level is able to return to 'resting' pH again. This may take up to 1 hour.

Periodontal disease

1. A sign is what can be seen by the dental professional 'on examination' (O/E). A symptom is what the patient may report or 'complains of' (C/O).

2. Redness (rubor). Swelling (tumour). Heat (calor). Pain (dolour) – rare in gingivitis. Loss of function (as a result of inflammation).

3. Basic Periodontal Examination – this is a screening tool for Periodontal Disease. The BPE does not monitor disease progression nor can it be used to formulate a treatment plan. It is an indicator of whether further detailed investigation is required (such as six-point periodontal charting). OHEs should be able to 'interpret' BPE codes (in relation to delivery of accurate OHI for the patient).

4. For 7–11 years of age, use BPE codes 0, 1 and 2.

5. Index teeth for BPE in young people aged 7–11 years are all 6's, UR1 and LL1 (to avoid false pocketing).

6. For 12–17 years of age, use the full range of BPE codes 0, 1, 2, 3, 4*.

7. The code * is used to denote furcation involvement (exposure of roots on multi-rooted teeth). Can be used in conjunction with a BPE code as appropriate, for example, code 3* = probing depth 3.5 mm up to 5.5 mm PLUS furcation in sextant.

8. BPE 0 – Black band fully visible. No bleeding on probing. Healthy – no periodontal treatment needed.

9. BPE 1 – Black band fully visible. Bleeding on probing present. Oral Hygiene Instruction (OHI).

10. BPE 2 – Black band fully visible. Bleeding on probing/plaque retention factor(s), for example, calculus, overhangs. OHI and remove retention factors (supra and/or sub gingival calculus).

11. BPE 3 – Black band partially visible. Probing depth from 3.5 mm up to 5.5 mm/bleeding on probing/plaque retention factor(s). OHI/Root Surface Debridement (RSD).

12. BPE 4 – Black band fully disappears. Probing depth will be more 5.5 mm (so over 6 mm). OHI/RSD – assess complexity level also – may need to refer.

13. BPE code * – Furcation involvement. OHI /RSD – assess complexity level also – may need to refer.

14. Inflammation of the gingivae, which is reversible with effective plaque biofilm control.

15. Loss of stippling, loss of gingival contour ('knife-edge' appearance gone), swollen gingivae, soft/spongy gingivae, marked redness in colour, bleeding on probing.

16. Bleeding on brushing or when eating hard foods, for example, apple. May also see blood on pillow in morning. May report a 'bad taste' (halitosis) and sometimes pain (not common unless acute gingival infection present).

17. Poor oral hygiene results in formation of a mature biofilm. It is the enzymes and toxins of anaerobic bacteria contained in the biofilm, which cause inflammatory change.

18. Plaque retentive factors include calculus, overhanging fillings, ill fitting crowns, bridges, dentures, implants, orthodontic appliances.

19. Systemic disorders that may increase the risk of gingival inflammation include Diabetes, Blood-Borne Viruses (HIV, Hepatitis) and those affecting Gastrointestinal tract (Crohn's Disease).

20. Hormonal changes during pregnancy, puberty or menopause.

21. Mouth breathing or lips-apart posture, common side effects of many medications, damage to salivary glands (Head and Neck Cancer treatment), smoking (thermal effect).
Common side effects of medication and illness (nausea and diarrhoea) can lead to dehydration.

22. Drug-induced gingivitis – fibrous gingival tissue often seen with long-term use of Phenytoin (Epilepsy – anti-seizure), Cyclosporin (Immunosuppressant – anti-rejection organ transplant), Nifedipine (Hypertension – calcium channel blocker). Gingival enlargement seen.

23. Enlargement of gingival tissue. Results from abnormal increase in the number of normal cells leading to increase in volume. At cellular level, it is connective tissue that is involved – impact of drugs on collagenase secretion by gingival fibroblasts (resulting in excessive gingival collagen formation). Cause may be hereditary or inflammatory (often also by gingival inflammation, which masks the underlying fibrous tissue). Other terms used include gingival overgrowth, hypertrophic gingivitis, gingival hyperplasia or gingival hypertrophy.

24. Pregnancy Epulis – usually involving interdental papillae (one or more), benign, generalised inflammatory enlargement (mass) as a result of hormonal excess and poor oral hygiene. Usually resolves after childbirth.

25. Enzymes and toxins of mature plaque bacteria. Enzymes – chemical substances produced by bacteria, for example, for metabolism of fermentable carbohydrates. Toxins – poisons (waste products) from bacteria, resulting in variable levels of periodontal destruction.

26. Dental History/Family History – genetic disposition (NB age when Periodontitis diagnosed important). Medical History – host (person) response to inflammatory challenge (NB

Immunocompromise, Diabetes, Stress). Polypharmacy (dry mouth). Lifestyle risk factors – smoking, alcohol, substance misuse, poor diet. Retention factors – inability to effectively disrupt biofilm (overhangs, malocclusion, crowns). No interdental cleaning being carried out – bleeding on probing (and/or brushing), severity of inflammation. Probing depths and Clinical Attachment Loss (CAL). Bone levels – dependent on the number of sites affected/location. May be localised or general depending on the percentage of mouth involved. Furcation involvement. Mobility or drifting of teeth. Recession – amount present may make too sensitive for effective plaque control to be carried out.

27. Variable gingivitis. BPE code 2 or higher (Junctional Epithelium integrity challenged resulting in bleeding on probing, possible subgingival calculus). Loss of attachment (pocket formation). Gingival recession from previous Periodontal Disease, loss of interdental papillae, periodontal abscess (invasion of pocket organisms into surrounding tissue), loose or mobile teeth. Halitosis (bad breath). Horizontal or vertical bone levels (determined by X-rays).

28. Recession (reports a 'long in the tooth' appearance). Teeth more sensitive to hot/cold stimuli. May complain of a 'bad taste' (accumulation of bacteria in pockets) and presence of pus on gentle pressure. Varying level of tooth mobility – may report teeth have moved (drifted) as can see difference from old photos. Bleeding on brushing or when trying to eat hard food items. Pain on occasion (abscess).

29. NUG – bacterial infection Necrotising Ulcerative Gingivitis (previously known as Trench Mouth).

30. NUG – signs and symptoms classically include necrosis of interdental gingival tissue (papillae), sloughing present (grey in colour), fetor (very unpleasant odour), halitosis, very painful, fever may be present along with a feeling of being unwell. People with compromised immune system more at risk. Microorganisms include *Treponema* and *Prevotella* species.

31. Oral hygiene advice to ensure effective daily disruption of bacterial biofilm – confirm non-traumatic brushing technique and advise on appropriate oral hygiene aids. Explain correct use of any additional oral hygiene items, for example, chlorhexidine-based products. Encourage patients to quit use of tobacco. Advice on importance of balanced diet (use Eatwell Plate).

32. Diagnosis made due to rapid rate of progress or severity of disease in people younger than 35 years – characteristic vertical bone defects on radiographs. Localised aggressive periodontitis (LAP) involves some teeth. Generalised aggressive periodontitis (GAP) involves most teeth.
Sometimes no clinical signs and oral health may be good – probing pocket depths and X-rays needed.

33. Irreversible damage is a distinguishing feature. Gingivitis – superficial inflammation of gingivae, reversible with effective oral hygiene. Periodontitis – inflammation/gradual destruction of supporting tissues around teeth – damage irreversible, can be slowed or halted (through maintenance programme).

Non-carious tooth surface (tissue) loss (not involving microbial activity)

1. Erosion – irreversible loss of tooth structure due to chemical dissolution by acids not of bacterial origin. Seen on occlusal, palatal and lingual aspects of teeth. Mainly due to dietary acids. Intrinsic – due to gastric reflux (usually hydrochloric acid). Perimolysis (decalcification of tooth) occurs due to exposure to gastric acid linked to chronic vomiting or regurgitation. Extrinsic – highly acid items in diet, for example, fruit-based foods/drinks, salad dressings, fizzy drinks. Medication can be a risk (especially recreational drugs) as can lifestyle habits (for example holding fizzy drinks in mouth). Idiopathic – acids from unknown origin.

2. Particularly seen upper anterior teeth. Enamel appears smooth and glass-like due to the loss of enamel on labial aspects and incisal edge (loss of shape). Tooth can appear thin even transparent.

3. Main acids found – Fizzy drinks: Phosphoric; Vinegar: Acetic; Apple: Malic; Orange: Citric.

4. Patients with erosion include all ages – children (sucking sour sweets), teenagers (drinking alcopops), people with an Eating Disorder (anorexia, bulimia) or Hiatus Hernia, Alcoholics, people who are medically compromised (dry mouth due to lack of saliva), people who play sports sip energy drinks, which are usually fizzy (carbonated), or sucking fruit.

5. Attrition – happens due to tooth to tooth contact – results in physical wearing away of tooth surface on occlusal surfaces or incisal edges. May see 'cupping' effect on occlusal surfaces due to enamel loss.

6. Common in older people due to wear, also in people who grind their teeth (Bruxism – night-time grinding). Also seen in people who eat a 'rough' diet (rice, nuts etc). People who are continually chewing, for example, tobacco. Occupational risks now rare (used to be dust from mining mixed with saliva).

7. Abfraction – happens due to forces created from abnormal 'occlusal loading', resulting in slivers (thin chips) of enamel fracturing at cervical margin. Wedge-shaped effect in enamel at neck of tooth – wedge has 'sharp angle', which helps in differentiation from toothbrush abrasion (where 'wedge angle' is wider).

8. Patients whose teeth may be in poor alignment. May also include teeth that have a 'high' restoration.

9. Abrasion – loss of hard tooth tissue due to mechanical factors other than tooth-to-tooth contact. Mainly affects incisal edges and 'notching' may be seen due to pipe smoking, oral and facial piercing, occupational habits (opening rolls of film, holding pen or pin). Also may see shiny brown/yellow areas at gingival margin due to a poor and often traumatic toothbrushing technique.

10. Becoming more common especially in young people due to overzealous brushing in order to achieve 'white teeth'. People who smoke tend to brush vigorously to try to avoid tobacco staining.

11. Smith and Knight Tooth Wear Index. Basic Erosive Wear Examination (BEWE) 0 = No Erosive Wear. 1 = Initial loss of surface. 2 = Distinct defect < 50% surface area has hard tissue. 3 = Tissue loss > 50% surface area. * Scores 2 or 3 with dentinal involvement.

12. Monitoring can include use of photographs, study models and number of treatments (frequency) necessary in order to deal with the 'active' episode of non-carious tooth surface (tissue) loss.

Sensitivity, staining and oral piercing

1. Dentine Hypersensitivity.

2. Young adults – females especially as more OH aware – likely to brush more frequently (especially if using a traumatic technique). Patients who have a diet high in acidic foods and drinks. Patients who have conditions involving frequent vomiting and/or regurgitation of gastric acids (Eating Disorders, Hiatus Hernia). Patients with severe occlusal trauma. Patients undergoing orthodontic therapy or tooth whitening and those with a history of previous Periodontal Disease (gingival recession).

3. Short, sharp, severe painful episode – like an electric shock.

4. Temperature – cold air/sometimes heat, sweet foods/drinks, metal items that touch tooth for example, fork.

5. Dentine hypersensitivity commonly affects canine and premolar teeth.

6. Dentine hypersensitivity commonly affects buccal and labial tooth surfaces at cervical margins.

7. Optimise exposure to fluoride – confirm correct level in toothpaste and spit, no rinse method. Use fluoride mouthwash at different time to brushing (dentist may prescribe higher fluoride content toothpaste and applications of fluoride varnish).
Reduce intake of known acidic foods and drinks – identify via food and drink diary, keep to meals. If drinking fruit-based/fizzy drinks, serve chilled, use of straws, no swishing or holding in mouth. No brushing for at least 30 minutes after eating or drinking.

8. Potassium Chloride, Potassium Citrate, Potassium Nitrate, Strontium Acetate – depolarise nerve impulses. Used in conjunction with Sodium Fluoride – thought to encourage secondary dentine and occlusion (blocking) of dentinal tubules.

9. Staining within tooth structure (endogenous – incorporated in tooth matrix during development). Usually before birth or during early childhood before tooth erupts. Can also be a result of trauma to tooth post-eruption.

10. Tetracycline – darkened (grey) enamel, no longer prescribed during pregnancy or for children younger than 12 years. Fluoride (in excess) can result in staining known as 'mottling' or 'fluorosis' (varies in severity – from fine white lines to brown stain – graded via Deans Index). Systemic upset – due to episode of acute illness during pregnancy or early childhood, can

lead to enamel hypoplasia. Developmental imperfections due to rare, inherited conditions – Amelogenesis Imperfecta (enamel) or Dentinogenesis Imperfecta (dentine). Death of tooth pulp from trauma, dental infection, dental treatment – tooth becomes darker over time.

11. Extrinsic staining occurs on the surfaces of both natural and artificial teeth. Salivary Pellicle picks up pigments from various dietary substances. Can be removed by prophylaxis.

12. Tobacco – combustion (burning) of tobacco during smoking produces black/brown/orange stain (as smoke cools down – 'tar-like' sticky substance forms). Pan or betel nut chewing – red stain from Areca nut contained in the betel 'quid' or 'pouch'. Tannin – found in tea, coffee and red wine – variable levels of dark (black, brown) staining. Chlorhexidine digluconate products – brown stain (can be removed by polishing). Iron supplements – black.

13. Green/orange stain – known as 'chromogenic' – result of waste products being produced during bacterial activity.

14. Oral piercing sites include Frena (frenum) such as fold of mucous membrane and soft tissue extending from the floor of the mouth to the midline of under surface of the tongue. Also known as 'web' piercing. Lips are a common area. Tongue – usually dorsoventral (top of the tongue through to under surface) – can also be dorsolateral, that is, left to right across the tongue (not common). Cheeks and the Uvula (not a common site) may also be chosen.

15. Swelling – risk to airway. Possible haemorrhage.

16. Chipped or fractured teeth (pain) – commonly due to wearing of metal piercings. Teeth may move position – especially if ball stud pushed frequently against/between upper central incisors. Receding gingivae – abraded by rubbing from button stud. Speech impairment and possible drooling. Loss of taste. Infection risk if handling without washing hands or failing to keep jewellery clean.

Oral malignancy

1. Oral cancer can be found in any part of the oral cavity including the lips.

2. Use of tobacco (including chewing or smokeless tobacco), Alcohol, Human Papillomavirus (HPV), poor diet. Some thought also around a probable cause being environmental tobacco smoke (second-hand tobacco smoke).

3. Possible signs or symptoms for oral malignancy include any non-healing (after 3 weeks) ulcer, lump or red or white patch in mouth or throat. Persistent, unexplained pain in the mouth or if a tooth (or teeth) has become loose for no reason (remember dentures too). Bleeding or numbness in mouth or tongue. Changes in voice (hoarseness), difficulty in talking and swallowing, swollen glands (neck region especially). Unexplained weight loss. Pain in one ear without hearing loss.

4. Have a balanced diet – rich in Vitamins A, C and E. Get to know own mouth, check for changes when brushing teeth such as ulcers. Any ulcer or any red and white patches not healing in

3 weeks must be investigated by a dentist and be aware of any unusual lumps or swellings in mouth or head and neck region. Protect skin from the sun and use appropriate lip balm. Visit Dentist as often as recommended – includes people who do not have any natural teeth and even more important for people who smoke and drink. Try to stop smoking and be alcohol aware.

Other common oral conditions

1. Herpes viral infections may be primary or recurrent infections. Herpes simplex virus – causes primary herpetic gingivostomatitis or oral herpes. May periodically recur as 'cold sores'. Varicella zoster virus – primary infection is chickenpox – reactivation as Herpes zoster (shingles). Epstein-Barr virus – primary infection Infectious Mononucleosis ('kissing disease' as often acquired by young adults – infected saliva).

2. Human Papillomavirus. Known mainly in relation to cervical cancer but now implicated in mouth cancer.

3. Cold sores are Herpes Labialis.

4. Oral Thrush is caused by species of *Candida* – *Candida albicans*. Commonly due to poor denture hygiene (especially upper dentures). Nystatin is commonly prescribed (lozenges, cream).

5. Angular Cheilitis (or cheilosis) – affects labial commissures (angles of mouth) – commonly associated with *Candida albicans* and *Staphylococcus aureus*.

6. Denture Stomatitis.

7. Koplik spots are a characteristic sign for measles. Found on buccal mucosa in premolar and/or molar area. Look like tiny grains of white sand surrounded by a red ring. May persist for several days and begin to slough with the onset of rash.

8. Aphthous Ulcers – Aphthous stomatitis or recurrent aphthous ulcers (RAUs). Unknown aetiology – typically starts in childhood. Can be one or more small, round, shallow ulcers with a yellowy/grey centre – can be painful. Typically last 7–10 days. Not associated with formation of vesicles, fever or gingivitis. Ulcers that do not resolve may be associated with systemic conditions such as inflammatory bowel disease.

9. White 'lace-like' striations seen on buccal mucosa (both sides of cheeks), also tongue and gingivae. Oral lichen planus (OLP) immune response of unknown origin due to chronic inflammatory disease. May be found with other diseases of altered immunity. Blisters may or may not be present.

10. Due to smoking and is symptomless. Lots of white, slightly raised 'papules' (with central red areas due to inflammation of minor salivary gland openings) seen in palate area (posterior of hard/soft palate).

SECTION VI Answers: Patient groups

'Seeing' a patient

1. Three A's for not visiting the dentist. **Attitude** – A non-judgemental approach is required. Health Professionals (including dental team) need to promote 'person-centred care' – think about patients as 'experts through experience'. Remember oral health may also be a low priority. Is attendance on a reactive rather than preventive approach? **Access** – what type of care offered – NHS, Mixed or Private (how would an unplanned dental need be met)? Accessibility to service – can appointments be made for weekends or late evenings (when Carers may be home from work)? Is building/dental clinic fully accessible for wheelchair users (or are there lots of stairs)? What about partially sighted people – are signs clear, forms available in large print? Can the clinic be accessed by public transport or is a car necessary? **Ability** – confirm individual physical and cognitive abilities to 'self-care' or is person dependent on others? Can the person communicate/express their needs? – indicate where they may have dental pain. What coping skills does the person have to manage the dental intervention? – would sedation be needed? Is the opportunity for personal health gain promoted? – dental public health messages provided, support to make healthier choices easier, information on availability of suitable oral hygiene aids.

2. Medical history – age. Gender. Medication taken. Systemic Disorder (Diabetes, HIV). Physical or Sensory impairment (hearing and vision). Learning Disability (Down Syndrome). Impaired Memory (Dementia, Acquired Brain Injury). Pregnancy. Diabetes (early or late onset) increases Periodontitis – slow healing. Epilepsy (drugs often cause gingival problems). Anorexia/bulimia – vomiting causes tooth erosion/trauma to oral soft tissues. Chewing/swallowing difficulties/trismus – may be due to illness/trauma/ill fitting dentures. Use of tobacco and alcohol. Substance misuse – chaotic lifestyle. Chemotherapy/Radiotherapy – radiation-induced Caries, sore mouth (mucositis). Dry mouth (Xerostomia) – drug-induced, post-operative. When checking medical history, ask for repeat prescription sheet whenever possible/update records by photocopying or scanning into patient notes.

3. Dental History – current and previous treatments – how much – how often? What Caries/Periodontal Disease risk level is noted? Ability to cope with treatment – any anxiety/phobia/behavioural needs? Referral to OHE to include as much detail as possible, for example – if being asked to provide tooth brushing instruction (TBI) – state why, is it in relation to Dental Caries or Periodontal Disease? Delivering Better Oral Health, 3rd Ed, has specific TBI advice for both diseases.

4. Social Circumstances – Socio-economic background (ability to pay for treatment or oral hygiene items). Access – appointment times, access to building (wheelchair user). Dependency on Carers (are these professional or family Carers). Communication needs – English not first language, large print format leaflets. Are there any cultural needs? Preferences regarding oral hygiene items (suitable for vegetarians). Have any key life events taken place recently, for example, loss of loved one, lost job/home, divorce, recent ill health (loss of independence). Dental team well placed to note changes in patient general health and well-being too – if patient unable to recall family member names or if oral hygiene poor (when previously good) could indicate possible mental health needs (depression) or even early Dementia.

5. Ascertain how much person can do for themselves before advising or 'helping'. Facilitate informed decision making and offer choices. Allow appropriate time for person. Treat everyone with respect and dignity – no assumptions and non-judgemental approach. Practice literature in appropriate format, such as audio/large print/culturally sensitive. When forms being completed – be aware of what is not being 'openly disclosed', for example, a person who has difficulty with reading and/or writing may say have 'forgotten' their glasses. When completing forms on behalf of patients – ensure full information is given, that is, all questions are asked (even if not thought appropriate). Provide all response options, for example, for Ethnicity – offer all 'group' choices available on form – if none appropriate, ask patients to state what they prefer. Important not to 'tick a best option'. Record full responses provided by patients 'word for word'.

6. Advise key information according to DBOH 3rd Ed, for age and need. Generally brush twice daily at night and at least on one other occasion. Use fluoride toothpaste appropriate for age and suitable toothbrush. Spit – no rinsing. NB seek advice if swallow impairment. Explain risks to oral health from smoking, alcohol, poor diet, HPV. Raise awareness of risk of Mouth Cancer (3-week message – if in doubt, check it out). Encourage balanced diet and to attend dental visits as often as recommended.

Patient target groups – some considerations

1. Pregnant/Nursing Mothers – advise key information according to DBOH 3rd Ed. Encourage importance of good General Health (balanced diet, not to use tobacco or alcohol). Oral health – advise good plaque control, if problem with morning sickness advise rinse with water after vomiting, brush at another time of day, use small head toothbrush, correct fluoride toothpaste (at least 1350 ppm – spit no rinse), care with snacking especially if sugary cravings. Reassure if bleeding on brushing – explain hormonal change exaggerates plaque response. Advise on current eligibility for free dental care (during pregnancy and 12 months after baby born).

2. Parents of pre-school children – advise key information according to DBOH, 3rd Ed. Reinforce importance of deciduous teeth and supervision of toothbrushing to age 7 years. Introduce drinking cup by 6 months of age (non-valve – free flow) and cease use of bottle for infant feeding by 12 months. As soon as teeth erupt – use of correct amount and level fluoride toothpaste for age. 'Safer for teeth' snacks and drinks (milk – water). Check for hidden sugars – words ending in OSE. Not to use sweets/treats as rewards. Adopt 1 hour before going to bed to be 'food and drink' free – then teeth to be brushed. If drink through night needed – only water. Ensure all care givers are aware and involved.

3. Parents of school children – advise key information according to DBOH 3rd Ed. Use of correct amount and level fluoride toothpaste for age. Advise to be alert for first permanent molar teeth. 'Safer for teeth' snacks and drinks (milk – water). Check for hidden sugars – words ending in OSE. Not to use sweets/treats as rewards. Adopt 1 hour before going to bed to be 'food and drink' free – then teeth to be brushed. If drink through night needed – only water. Ensure all care givers are aware and involved.

4. Adolescent (13–17 years) – advise key information according to DBOH, 3rd Ed. Discuss with patients about their preferred OH routine – ensure correct amount and level of fluoride

toothpaste and being used effectively. Check toothbrush (small, medium soft texture). Provide detailed advice if undergoing orthodontic treatment. Likely to graze so at an increased risk of Caries. Encourage fresh fruit and vegetables. Use of sugar-free gum. May be experimenting with peers (and at risk of peer pressure) so explain risks to oral health (mouth cancer) from smoking, alcohol, HPV. Be prepared to discuss topics such as oral piercing.

5. Adult – advise key information according to DBOH 3rd Ed. Provide advice according to dental need (such as Caries, Periodontal Disease, Tooth Surface Loss, Denture or Implant care). Discuss at level appropriate to each adult, their preferred OH routine – ensure correct amount and level of fluoride toothpaste. Check toothbrush (small, medium soft texture). Ask patient to demonstrate (on model or in own mouth) to confirm technique is effective as could need to brush more frequently rather than to have to change actual technique. Suggest changes for those areas that require it (as more input could resolve a situation) or where there are signs of trauma (abraded gingivae). Inform of natural/vegan oral hygiene products as necessary.

6. Older Person – advise key information according to DBOH 3rd Ed. Confirm ability to hear and see (check regarding hearing aids are on/reading glasses). Discuss preferred OH routine and ability. Ensure correct amount and level of fluoride toothpaste and being used effectively. Check toothbrush (small, medium soft texture). Check manual dexterity – adapt toothbrush as necessary to maximise self-care skills. OHE according to dental need (Caries, Periodontal Disease, Tooth Surface Loss, Denture or Implant care). Write down information if needed particularly names of any oral hygiene items being recommended.

7. Older People may be prone to Xerostomia, Periodontitis, Root Caries, Dental abscess, Attrition, Trauma to hard dental tissue (broken/lost teeth due to falls). If full denture wearers – may have soft tissue trauma (due to ill fitting dentures), Denture Stomatitis, Angular Cheilitis. Oral cancer to be considered also especially if not attended dentist for many years (ability to self-check mouth may be difficult due to possible reduced vision).

8. Medically Compromised includes such needs as cardiovascular disorders, respiratory diseases, blood and bleeding disorders, diabetes mellitus, liver, kidney and gastrointestinal disease, immunosuppressed states, receiving cancer treatment and terminal care, neurological diseases, infective diseases.

9. Oral health risks due to medical compromise – dry mouth and impaired healing common to many conditions. Periodontal risk – Diabetes (inflammatory challenge). Acute gingival infection (localised) – HIV. Erosion – Gastro-oesophageal Reflux Disease (GERD) affects lower oesophageal sphincter (LES), ring of muscle between oesophagus and stomach leading to acid indigestion. Attrition – substance misuse (Ecstasy and tooth grinding). Soft tissues – Crohn's Disease – 'cobblestone' effect buccal mucosa. Pregnancy Gingivitis – exaggerated plaque response during pregnancy due to hormonal changes. Caries and Periodontal risk – Chronic Fatigue Syndrome – extreme tiredness/lack of energy to carry out oral hygiene. Soft tissue trauma – Eating Disorder (scratches from finger nail on palate).

10. Special Needs – general considerations – impact of three 'M's' – **Medical history, Mental capacity** and **Manual dexterity**. Impact of any systemic disease or syndrome and side effects of any relevant drug therapy. Determine the level of ability to 'express' need and preferred communication method. If unable to check own mouth after cleaning or unable to act

on instruction and advice, ascertain level of dependency on Carer intervention and facilitate support as necessary. High importance on prevention – ensure 'safer for teeth' choices of food and drink.

11. Health Education Professionals – advise key information according to DBOH, 3rd Ed. Do not assume they will know everything. Take care with use of too much dental terminology. May feel embarrassed if oral health not as effective as it could be as feel should 'know better'. Consider providing information on oral health for background reading.

12. Ethnic Minority Groups – advise key information according to DBOH 3rd Ed. Be aware oral hygiene may not be part of daily lifestyle. Be sensitive to cultural needs regarding use of leaflets or when recommending products (consider whether any ingredients may be of animal origin). Have an awareness of religious events such as Ramadan and consider how oral hygiene may be managed during fasting. Increased risk of mouth cancer from chewing paan (betel quid) common in religious ceremonies.

Some additional considerations for 'at-risk' patients

NB Key information and advice according to DBOH 3rd Ed should be given for all.

1. Impairments – **Physical** – mobility difficulties – unable to walk or move limbs (may be one limb or all four). Limited manual dexterity, for example, Parkinson Disease, Multiple Sclerosis, Arthritis, Stroke. Bruxism/Posture – associated problems with excess saliva – drooling/inability to control. Cerebral Palsy – poor muscle coordination. Haemophilia – increased risk from bleeding (including when giving LA) – important to minimise require-ment for dental treatment. **Sensory – Hearing** – may be variable D/deaf. **Vision** – variable sight (level of blindness may be partial/full). Both may be present from birth (congenital) or occur later in life (acquired) **Mental** – Learning Disability – 'a significant impairment of intelligence and social functioning acquired before adulthood', for example, person with Down's Syndrome (often other health needs such as heart).

   Autistic Spectrum Disorder – Asperger's Syndrome (high functioning). Attention Deficit Hyperactivity Disorder (ADHD), short attention span. Head injury or trauma – may result in inappropriate (disinhibited) or challenging behaviour including self-injury. Other difficulties include Dyslexia. Due to both variety of and different stages of Dementia – may need more time and patience particularly if loss of short-term memory. **Emotional Disorder** – phobias/unreasonable fears/depression/neuroses/mental illness can all prove very difficult for a person to engage with health services. Advice for 'Patients Giving Special Concerns' can be found in Delivering Better Oral Health.

2. SCOFF is a screening tool for Eating Disorders. The SCOFF questions*:
   - Do you make yourself **S**ick because you feel uncomfortably full?
   - Do you worry you have lost **C**ontrol over how much you eat?
   - Have you recently lost more than **O**ne stone in a 3-month period?
   - Do you believe yourself to be **F**at when others say you are too thin?
   - Would you say that **F**ood dominates your life?
     *One point for every "yes"; a score of ≥2 indicates further investigation is needed.

3. Hard dental tissue – erosion – enamel, surface smooth and shiny (glass-like), incisal edges may show loss of contour. Also, loss from palatal aspects of teeth. Soft oral tissue – may see trauma on palate – redness/scratches from finger nails.

4. Medication – OHE can support patients by working out an OH routine that fits into the medication regime. Medication may need to be taken with or after food (risk for Caries if frequent food intakes). Confirm medication timing – if first thing in morning or last thing at night could impact when toothbrushing can be carried out. Advise at night and at least on one other occasion. Be aware of side effects from medication (tiredness and inability to concentrate, gingival overgrowth, dry mouth, nausea or diarrhoea).

5. OHE can confirm person knows about availability of NHS treatment and how to find an NHS provider. Have copies of related paperwork regarding eligibility for help with dental charges for those not on benefits. Advise on availability of good quality, reasonably priced oral health aids – write down the name of items and where they can be sourced (as could be a Carer doing the shopping).

6. Diabetes – OHE can 'keep to time' re: appointments especially if insulin dependent (may have to 'eat' regularly to avoid hypoglycaemia – possibly avoid appointments around mealtimes). Explain can be more prone to Periodontal Disease (due to inflammatory change, vascular deficiencies and lower immune response). If poorly controlled diabetes – difficult to sustain good gingival health. Snacking – explain may be more prone to Caries.

7. Epilepsy – OHE can explain risk of gingival hyperplasia (overgrowth of gingivae) associated with anticonvulsant drugs (such as Phenytoin, Epanutin). Emphasis on excellent plaque control. Keep medical history updated (how seizures managed and whether well controlled?). Encourage importance of attending appointments with dental team.

8. Person living with Dementia. Find out as much as possible from record card about how patient is living with Dementia/coping skills. Ask patient and Carer if they need any specific help. Confirm Carer own dental care arrangements in place to support their own health and well-being. Keep appointments as short as necessary – try not to run late. Keep information and tasks simple. Ask 'closed' questions – try to avoid a choice of answers. Be sensitive to short notice changes to appointments when requested. Consider Carer requirements when arranging appointments. Provide appointment details and any further information in an accessible format as far as possible (can include simple photos of 'stages of toothbrushing' to support 'sequencing'). Consider use of modified toothbrushes. Ensure emergency contact information given in case of dental trauma from falls.

9. Homeless/temporary accommodation – OHE information readily available so 'every contact counts'. Appropriate dental public health messages – spit no rinse, chew sugar-free gum, signpost help to quit tobacco (free from NHS). Provide free samples of toothpaste/brushes for immediate use but also reinforce availability of 'Every Day' brands of oral hygiene items. Show where to find fluoride content on toothpaste products so informed decision making facilitated regarding budget. Also frequent snacking/poor dietary choices risk due to lack of daily routine and low health literacy.

10. Gypsy and Travellers – be aware and recognise that access to health care is not easy. Lack of permanent address makes it difficult to register with a Doctor, resulting in presentations

at A&E. Some may find it difficult to discuss health issues with a person of the opposite sex. May have low literacy levels so uncomfortable with form filling. Use of visual aids helpful.

11. Dental phobia – OHEs are well placed to support people who have dental phobia. Reduce environmental barriers, that is, 'triggers' as far as possible. Use of pre-visit questionnaires. Taking time to 'listen' to what the person is 'saying' is crucial using a SOLER approach. Establish SMART objectives – initially, could be as simple as working towards the person being able to attend for appointments with OHE.

12. OHE should be aware of what constitutes 'substance misuse' (for example use of 'legal highs') and keep informed of any local issues in their area via Public Health/Local Authority data. Substance harm reduction programmes may be in place (such as Methadone – substitute for Heroin). A 'non-judgemental' approach is crucial and recognition that chaotic lifestyles may result in poor attendance at dental clinic. May exhibit 'challenging behaviour'. When setting objectives – must be SMART according to individual ability and circumstance.

13. Dental erosion (from alcohol). Stained teeth and mouth cancer risk from smoking. High Caries rate due to frequent snacking/poor dietary choices. Poor Periodontal health – lack of daily routine and low dental health literacy. Dry mouth (side effect of drugs and smoking). Attrition from grinding of teeth (especially recreational drug use). May have trauma to facial tissues and teeth due to falls.

Safeguarding and Mental Capacity Act (MCA)

1. Dental neglect – 'the persistent failure to meet a child's basic oral health needs, likely to result in the serious impairment of a child's oral or general health or development'.

2. Sometimes patients may disclose (inadvertently or deliberately) sensitive, very personal issues. The OHE should know how and where to seek further guidance on any matters they feel unable to deal with regarding child protection, disclosure of domestic violence, protection of vulnerable adults. No matter where the OHE may be working, there should be a policy in place to manage such scenarios – be sure to follow the local policy. Recordkeeping is vitally important – notes must be contemporaneous, accurate and factual. Consider management of DNA (did not attend) rates for vulnerable patients – is recordkeeping accurate? Is the patient a DNA or CNA (could not attend)? See GDC 'Statement on Child Protection' www.gdc-org.uk and Child Protection and the Dental Team www.cpdt.org.

   May take a number of visits before patient is comfortable enough to look at oral hygiene aids and discuss any treatment but achieving a positive result can give great confidence and 'job satisfaction'.

3. Types of abuse – Emotional, Sexual, Neglect, Physical, Financial.

4. Mental Capacity Act:
   • Every adult must be assumed to have capacity to make own decisions unless proved otherwise.
   • A person must be fully supported to make their own decisions.
   • Remember a person can make an unwise decision.

- Anything done on behalf of a person lacking capacity must be in their best interests.
- Anything done on behalf of a person lacking capacity should be least restrictive of their basic right and freedom.

5. IMCA – Independent Mental Capacity Advocate.

6. IMHA – Independent Mental Health Advocacy.

7. DoLS – Deprivation of Liberty Safeguards.

8. Property and Affairs LPA – attorney makes decision about financial and property matters (bank account/sale of house). Personal welfare LPA – attorney makes decision about health and welfare needs (day-to-day care, medical treatment).

SECTION VII Answers: Self care skills for effective oral hygiene

Toothbrushes, toothpaste and Interdental Aids

1. Disruption of dental bacterial biofilm and application of fluoride to tooth surfaces.

2. Teeth should be brushed at night and at least on one other occasion.

3. Fones, Vertical, Charters, Bass, Modified Bass. 'Vertical' technique no longer recommended.

4. Fones method – easy to learn and carry out (teeth are held in occlusion – brush using large circle action to incorporate cleaning at gingival margin). Help from care giver needed for 'intra-oral' brushing.

5. Depending on manual dexterity, toothbrushing should be supervised to 7 years of age.

6. Bristles placed at 45° angle to gingival crevice.

7. Check if preference for manual or powered brush. Manual – small headed toothbrush with medium to soft texture bristles. Consider thickness and length of handle. Change every 3 months or sooner if bristles splayed. Powered – oscillating action/rechargeable rather than battery. Consider weight/length of handle. Would any additional functions be helpful such as pressure indicator/timer/selection of brush heads (interdental). Each brush head to be easily identifiable for each individual user within a family. Shop around for prices.

8. Bicycle handle grip, piece of foam tubing (insulation tubing), soft ball with toothbrush inserted through middle, Velcro™ strap, TePe™ moulded handle for toothbrush to be inserted into.

9. Three functions of toothpaste – disruption of bacterial biofilm to minimise mature plaque formation. Removal of food debris (detergent effect and mechanical action of brushing). Freshen the mouth (various flavourings – commonly 'mint'). Desensitise tooth surface (due

to active ingredient). Improve tooth colour (via extrinsic stain removal). Strengthen tooth surface against decay (via fluoride).

10. Sodium Fluoride (chemical formula NaF), Stannous Fluoride (chemical formula SnF_2), Sodium Monofluorophosphate – also called MFP (chemical formula Na_2PO_3F).

11. Parts Per Million.

12. Toothpaste on 'general sale licence' – maximum concentration fluoride 1500 ppm.

13. 0–3 years – Smear – no less than 1000 ppm fluoride.

14. 3–6 years – Pea size – more than 1000 ppm fluoride.

15. 7+ years – Pea size – at least 1350 ppm fluoride.

16. Duraphat® toothpastes 2800 ppm for 10 years and over. 5000 ppm for 16 years and over.

17. POM – Prescription Only Medicine (in this case, it is for 'Treatment of Dental Caries').

18. Strontium Chloride, Potassium Nitrate, Potassium Citrate – desensitising agent (toothpaste). Bicarbonates – neutralise plaque acids (toothpaste). Essential Oils – reduce inflammation (toothpaste). Chlorhexidine – plaque suppressant (dental gel). Triclosan – anti-plaque agent (toothpaste).

19. Sodium Lauryl Sulphate – foaming (or detergent) effect.

20. Humectant (for example glycerine) – reduces moisture loss to maintain consistency of the paste.

21. Interdental cleaning should be carried out **before** toothbrushing.

22. Types of interdental cleaning – **Floss** – may be flat, rounded or spongy. Waxed and unwaxed available with floss threaders available to assist use. 'Superfloss' – single piece of floss with different sections such as a stiffened end for passing under a bridge. Different types of floss holders are available to enable single-hand use. Some may also be 'preloaded' with floss for single use. Dental **Tape** – thicker than conventional floss – useful for wider spaces between teeth. TePe™ small **interproximal** brushes – range of size/texture – central wire plastic coated. Many other brands of 'bottle brushes' available – some have a tapered or cylindrical shape. **Interspace** (or single tuft) brush – there are a variety of brushes available with some having longer bristles. Some brushes may also have more 'angulations' for better access around implants, for example, TePe Implant Care™. **Interdental Sticks** – still available – wooden item, triangular in shape for use in areas where papillae flattened or lost. Other items include the **Air Flosser™ Waterpik™**.

23. Highlight the presence of 'biofilm' (may also include other materials such as food debris) on both natural/artificial teeth, appliances or other prostheses. Either in a tablet or solution format. Erythrosine or vegetable 'dye' commonly used (check any colour allergies). Depending on product (for example if two tone) can indicate new (red colour) biofilm and more mature

(blue colour) biofilm. Not to be confused with Gram Staining (which is a test that is carried out in laboratory).

24. Plaque Score can be based on O'Leary Plaque Control Index (British Society Periodontology 2012). Also Turesky Plaque Index (1970) and Silness & Loe (1964).

Care of dental prostheses and appliances

1. Acrylic dentures – use 'non-perfumed' household soap and soft nailbrush. Ensure any traces of dental fixative are removed daily. Rinse thoroughly. Toothpaste should not be used on acrylic dentures. Do not use hot water or any bleaching products.

2. Always check with referring dentist for manufacturer instructions on how to care for dental appliances as different metal alloys may be used in the production of these items. Take particular care when cleaning around any metal clasps – small head toothbrush may be easier to use.

3. Dentures should be transported in denture pot. Ensure cleaning over sink/bowl with water in or over a folded towel. Denture should be placed (cupped) in the palm of one hand for gentle scrubbing with soft nailbrush.

4. Wrap in a damp cloth or if overnight, store in cold, clean (fresh) water. Remember denture pot needs to be kept clean also.

5. Disinfecting dentures – confirm with dentist – commonly used 'short soak' agents include dilute hypochlorite (Milton®) for acrylic dentures and chlorhexidine products (for example Corsodyl®) for those with metal parts.

6. Prosthetic device for covering an opening in the body, for example, palatal obturator covers (occludes) a 'hole' in the palate. It serves as a 'removable' roof of the mouth to help restore speech and eating.

7. Retainer – used to prevent teeth from moving after orthodontic treatment. May be fixed or removable. Not classed as an appliance as does not 'move' teeth.

8. Removable orthodontic appliance – may be worn for varying periods of time. Orthodontic Mini Implant (TAD – temporary anchor device).

9. Fixed orthodontic appliance – cut hard foods into small pieces. Avoid particularly sticky foods, for example, toffee, chewing gum. Avoid fizzy or fruit-based drinks (use straw) – keep 'dietary' acid to a minimum. Use wax to cover any sharp areas/wires. Seek advice from a dentist as soon as possible if a bracket becomes loose. Attend for routine dental check-ups alongside those for orthodontic care. Effective daily plaque control – use small headed soft to medium texture brush, bottle brushes/single-tuft brush. Clean tongue too. Confirm effective use of fluoride-containing products (supplements to be prescribed by dentist).

10. Advanced restorations – Dental Implant, Crown, Bridge, Veneer.

SECTION VIII Answers: Improving public 'response ability'

Fluoride products and fissure sealants

1. Naturally occurring element found in water, soil, rock, air and many plants and in diet – salt mackerel, salmon and dried tea leaves. Is normal/essential component of body fluids and tissues – deposited mainly in bones and teeth.

2. Naturally occurring – Calcium Fluoride.

3. Added fluoride – Sodium Fluoride.

4. Systemic fluoride – ingested. Topical fluoride – applied to tooth surface/s.

5. Topical fluoride – Gel (not commonly used), Varnish, Tablets (as sucked before being swallowed), Toothpaste, Mouthwash.

6. Systemic fluoride – Drinking water, dietary supplements – milk or salt, tablets and 'ingested' toothpaste.

7. Water fluoridation.

8. Pre-eruption – calcium hydroxyapatite (compound of calcium and phosphate) in enamel is replaced by calcium fluorapatite (crystals more 'uniform in shape' so stronger). Post eruption, shallower pits and fissures may be seen. Tooth tissue may withstand pH level 4.5 (which is lower than usual 'critical' pH level 5.5). Topical fluoride is important for 'ionic exchange' (acts as catalyst) to support remineralisation of early carious lesions. Enzyme activity of plaque bacteria blocked so less acid actually produced (also reduces opportunity for creation of acidic environment in which acidogenic bacteria thrive).

9. Age range 22–26 months (maxillary permanent incisors at risk).

10. Sodium Fluoride mouthwash – Daily use 0.05%. Weekly use 0.2%.

11. Duraphat Fluoride Varnish contains 2.26%. 26,000 ppm.

12. Fluoride level of 1.0 ppm.

13. Toothpaste, Mouthwash/rinses, Varnish, Drops, Tablets (0.5 and 1 mg).

14. Dr F MacKay 1901 – Colorado Springs, USA.

15. Dr H Trendley Dean researched 'mottled teeth'. Looked at severity of mottling in relation to fluoride concentration. Concluded 1.0 ppm fluoride was optimal level in water.

16. Dental Fluorosis.

17. Intrinsic staining caused by fluoride ingestion at level of 2 ppm+ during tooth formation.

18. First dentist – Sir James Crichton Browne 1892 (UK).

19. 1974.

20. Strathclyde (Scotland) – Lord Jauncy.

21. Ultra Vires – 'beyond the legal powers of authority'.

22. After Strathclyde case, committee (led by Professor Knox) set up to investigate fluoride. No evidence found that fluoride added to water causes cancer. Report published in 1985.

23. York Report published in 2000 – this was a systematic review of evidence around 'fluoride and health' by University of York.

24. This is a dental preventative procedure to reduce dental caries risk. Dental material (plastic coating) is placed primarily in occlusal pits and fissures of permanent molar teeth as soon as possible after eruption (6–7 years of age). Surface rendered more smooth and easier to clean thus reducing risk of food debris retention. Also 'seals' tooth surface against effects of plaque. May also be placed palatally on incisor teeth around a cingulum (raised area of enamel) and any palatal grooves. Also sometimes on any additional cusps found on the palatal aspect of the upper first permanent teeth (additional cusp known as Cusp of Carabelli).

25. Caries history indicates increased susceptibility – high risk includes whether caries occurring in deciduous teeth and caries history of both primary Caregiver and any siblings.
Patients with a complex medical and/or social history (need to reduce/prevent dental extractions). If requirement for long-term medication as increased dry mouth risk. People with reduced 'self-care' skills to carry out effective oral hygiene (or dependency on others for oral care). Also beneficial for those who are unable to actually cope with dental treatments or have difficulty to access.

26. After etching surface for recommended time (15–20 seconds) with phosphoric acid (commonly 35%), wash tooth surface thoroughly – avoid contamination from saliva (if gets contaminated, will need to re-etch).

27. A dried, etched tooth surface should have an opaque (frost-like) appearance.

28. Rock et al. (1983). British Society for Study of Community Dentistry. British Society for Paediatric Dentistry (2006).

Sugars and sweeteners – COMA – Vipeholm study and Hopewood House

1. Committee on Medical Aspects of Food and Nutrition Policy.

2. Total Sugars include – **Intrinsic** (as in fresh fruit/vegetables) or **Extrinsic** (free or added). Extrinsic sugars may also be either **Milk Sugars** (for example, Lactose in dairy items) or **Non-Milk Extrinsic Sugars** (for example, sugar used in drinks and confectionery) – Term 'free sugars' to replace terms NMES and 'added sugars' (SACN – 2015).

3. Intrinsic sugars are held within the plant cell structure (as a 'natural' sugar), whereas extrinsic sugars have been released from plant cell structure or added. Honey is an extrinsic sugar.

4. Intrinsic sugars are least cariogenic as found inside plant cell structure and start of breakdown process (during digestion) not started in the mouth. Natural (intrinsic) sugars can become more cariogenic, for example, fresh apples processed into fruit juice. Fructose in the 'whole' apple, that is, within plant cell wall is intrinsic, whereas fructose in apple juice is 'released' from plant cell structure during processing to become extrinsic (more readily acted upon by Salivary Amylase in mouth). Same principle for dried fruit, for example, why raisins not considered 'safe for teeth' snacks, also very sticky. As with all sugars, it is both the frequency and amount consumed that must always be considered.

5. 1986 COMA committee set up. COMA Panel reported on role of sugar and obesity in 1989.

6. Non-Milk Extrinsic Sugars (NMES) consumption to be reduced – eat more fresh fruit, vegetables, starchy foods. NMES not make up more than 10% *energy (calorie intake) within daily diet. Frequency of sugary snacks/drinks should be minimised – limit to mealtimes. People providing food/drinks for others should reduce frequency of sugar intakes. Schools should promote/provide healthy dietary choices. No sugar added to bottles used for infant feeding – weaning foods to be free of sugar or low sugar. Cease use of bottles for infant feeding by 1 year of age (especially if on soya or formula milk). Older people with natural teeth to reduce frequency and consumption NMES. Sugar-free medicines requested/prescribed when possible. *SACN report 2015 – recommends reduce to 5%.

7. Sucrose (table sugar).

8. Advise to look on label for ingredients ending in 'OSE'.

9. Maltose, Glucose, Fructose, Dextrose, Sucrose, Lactose

10. Amount of lactose actually found in milk is low, so less risk. Milk has other essential nutrients such as Calcium and Phosphorous, so potential dissolution of enamel (which is made up of Calcium and Phosphate) is reduced. Also aids in remineralisation. Casein (phosphoprotein found in milk) has protective action via ability to concentrate Calcium and Phosphate in plaque.

11. Calcium Phosphopeptide – Amorphous Calcium Phosphate (Recaldent™) derived from Casein in milk. Binds to tooth/biofilm – localizing bio-available calcium and phosphate. Recaldent™ found in products such as GC Tooth Mousse.

12. Artificial sweetener – may be synthetic (manufactured) or plant (for example, Xylitol).

13. Bulk sweetener replaces sugar weight for weight, looks like sugar and used in food production when a quantity or 'bulk' ingredient needed. Not readily used by oral bacteria.

14. Sorbitol (E420), Xylitol (E967), Mannitol (E421), Isomalt (E953), Maltitol (E965), Lactitol (E966), Hydrogenated glucose syrup.

15. Intense sweetener commonly manufactured as tiny pellets. They have no nutritional value or calories and are very sweet (intensely and deceptively) sweet, despite of small size.

16. Saccharin (E954), Aspartame (E951), Acesulfame K (E950), Thaumatin (E957).

17. Xylitol – has an antibacterial effect. Disrupts energy processes of bacteria (bacteria die thus prevents growth) so less acid produced. Reduces ability of bacteria to adhere to tooth surface.

18. Reduce snacking – NB advice always in conjunction with any other health needs or advice given. Try to make healthy choices easier choices – provide information for example Change4Life™ – Sugar Swap Campaign to show water/milk as alternative to fizzy drinks. Check food and drink labels carefully for hidden sugars. Do not add sugar to daily diet. Sugar substitutes may be used appropriate to age. Avoid using food (especially sweets) as rewards.

19. To investigate the relationship between diet and caries (especially in relation to sugar frequency) – study began 1939 – Vipeholm Hospital, Sweden.

20. Consumption of 'sticky' sugary items between meals increases caries risk the most.

21. This study in 1942 was undertaken by an Australian businessman. It looked at how health improvement can be attributed to dietary habits (especially if refined carbohydrate removed)

22. Refined carbohydrates in diet contribute to the risk of caries and rate at which both caries occurs and progresses.

23. **G Toverund** – carried out studies during war time period looking teeth of Norwegian school children. Sugar was in short supply so caries rate low.
    Tristan da Cunha Study – remote island in South Atlantic with Islanders only eating what they grew/caught themselves. Once sugar imported, caries incidence increased. **Gnotobiotic** (germ-free) rats – when fed sugar, no caries recorded – highlighted requirement and role of bacteria for caries to occur. Various studies show sugary medicines on long-term basis may increase caries.

Tobacco and alcohol

1. Addiction – will be addicted to Nicotine. Young people may start to smoke due to peer pressure – want to be seen as 'grown-up'. Many believe smoking reduces stress (NB Nicotine is a stimulant). Smoking is an 'appetite suppressant' (used by women especially who wish to keep weight down). Will be a lifestyle choice (social smokers) and may even just 'enjoy' smoking (smoking identity).

2. VBA – Very Brief Advice – usually takes 30 seconds only.

3. **Ask** – about smoking status and record. **Advise** – on the best way to quit (state 'combination of support and treatment will significantly increase chances of stopping'). **Act** – all smokers receive advice on value of attending local stop smoking services for specialised help with a referral as necessary.

4. Support may be **Pharmacological** – via Nicotine Replacement Therapy (NRT) and **Non**-NRT. **Behavioural** – to implement change to daily 'habits and routines'.

5. Adhesive patches (for use over different time periods and of variable strengths). Oral products – such as inhalator (like a cigarette), chewing gum, lozenge, micro-tab (use under tongue), nasal and oral sprays. Two NRT items may be used at the same time, that is, a 'patch' plus an oral product.

6. Non-NRT – Zyban® (Bupropion) and Champix® (Varenicline). Both items only under medical advice from a doctor.

7. E-Cigarettes – electronic cigarette (or PV – personal vaporiser or ENDS – electronic nicotine delivery system). Battery powered so heat 'vaporises' liquids containing a mixture of items (propylene glycol, nicotine and flavourings) to produce 'mist' rather than smoke. 'Mist' has less toxins than cigarette smoke does – work currently in place around setting standards in relation to providing a list of the ingredients in liquids, child-proofing liquid containers and use of the items in general.

8. Affects developing foetus – increased risk of miscarriage, premature labour, low birth weight and reduced educational attainment of child. Children of mothers who smoke during pregnancy have a higher caries rate via adverse effects on developing enamel.

9. Children (Passive Smoking – term for 'involuntary' or 'second-hand' smoking). Dangers include increased risk of Sudden Infant Death Syndrome (SIDS), respiratory problems, asthma, ear infections – so increased risk of hospital admission and subsequent absenteeism from school.

10. Adults and Older People – Emphysema, Chronic Bronchitis, Cardiovascular Disease (coronary heart disease/stroke), Peripheral Arterial Disease (includes impotence), Infertility, Cancer.

11. Stickier (harder to remove) bacterial biofilm. Increased extrinsic staining on teeth – may result in abrasion due to a forceful toothbrushing technique (to prevent staining). Halitosis (may be increased caries due to sucking mints), Dry mouth, Hairy tongue, Loss of taste (and smell), Poorer periodontal health. Increased risk of pre-cancerous changes – white, *hardened* palate (*Smoker's Keratosis*) and white patches on oral mucosa (*Leukoplakia*). If smoking and drinking alcohol (particularly spirits), risk of oral cancer is increased.

12. Be supportive. Provide key oral health information (reassurance if bleeding on brushing is seen or other oral changes appear, for example mouth ulcers). Remind benefits of stopping of smoking for both oral and general health. Suggest change of toothbrush at the same time as quit attempt started. If eating sweets or chewing gum (in place of smoking) – sugar free only.

13. Men – 3–4 units daily. Maximum 21 units per week (not to be saved up to consume in one go).

14. Women – 2–3 units daily. Maximum 14 units per week (not to be saved up to consume in one go).

Balanced diet – NACNE – SACN

1. National Advisory Committee on Nutrition Education.

2. NACNE 1983 report outlined links between diet and range of conditions and diseases – suggested **quantitative** dietary targets for prevention of diseases associated with affluence.

3. Fish (especially oily types) – mackerel, pilchards, salmon, tuna and trout. Starchy and fibrous foods – bread, cereals, potatoes, rice and pasta. Fruit and vegetables – fresh, frozen and tinned.

4. Sugar and sugary foods/drinks – biscuits, cakes, confectionery, fizzy drinks. Salt and salty foods – pies, pasties, crisps, salted nuts. Fat – biscuits, cakes, pastry, fat spreads, fried foods, fatty meats and meat products.

5. SACN – Scientific Advisory Committee on Nutrition (now instead of COMA). Advisory committee of independent experts giving scientific advice on nutrition and related health issues to Public Health England and other government agencies and departments.

6. Advice covers – nutrient content of individual foods and definition of a balanced diet. Nutritional status of people in the United Kingdom and how this may be monitored. Nutritional issues that affect wider public health policy issues – common risk factor approach (for example cardiovascular disease, cancer, osteoporosis and/or obesity). Nutrition for vulnerable groups (for example infants and elderly) and health inequality issues. Research requirements.

7. Eatwell Plate – shows main food groups and related recommended portions visually 'on a plate'.

8. Fruit and vegetables; potatoes, bread, rice, pasta and other starchy foods; milk and dairy foods; meat, fish, eggs, beans and other non-dairy sources of protein; foods and drinks high in fat or sugar.

9. World Health Organization advises eating minimum 400 g (5 × 80 g) fruit and vegetable daily to lower risk of serious health problems (heart disease, stroke, type 2 diabetes and obesity). Almost all fruit and vegetables count towards 5 A DAY (including frozen, canned and dried).

10. Dietary fibre or roughage – it is a non-nutrient but necessary dietary item as provides 'bulk' to aid the transit of faeces through the digestive system.

11. Proteins, Carbohydrates, Fats, Vitamins, Mineral salts, Roughage, Water.

12. Vitamin A (fat soluble) – cheese, eggs, milk, fortified low-fat spreads. Vitamin B Complex – Thiamine (B1), Riboflavin (B2), Niacin (B3), Vitamin B6 and B12 plus Pantothenic and Folic Acids (water soluble) – seeds, grains, pulses. Vitamin C (water soluble) – fruit and vegetables. Vitamin D (fat soluble) – most from exposure of sunlight on skin, also oily fish (salmon, sardines, mackerel), eggs, fortified fat spreads, fortified breakfast cereals, powdered milk. Vitamin E (fat soluble) – plant oils (soya, corn, olive), nuts/seeds, egg yolk, wheat germ/cereals. Vitamin K (fat soluble) – leafy green vegetables (broccoli/spinach), vegetable oils, cereals.

13. Calcium, Sodium, Potassium, Phosphorus, Magnesium, Iron, Chloride, Iodine, Fluoride.

14. Phenylketonuria (PKU) – a rare inherited condition causing build-up of phenylalanine in the body. Phenylalanine is a natural substance. It is a 'building block of protein' that cannot be broken down into other elements that are needed by the body so can build up in bloodstream. Newborns are tested (heel prick test) after having ingested dietary protein for 24–48 hours (this applies to both breastfed and bottle-fed babies). If found to have Phenylketonuria, high-protein foods (meat, cheese, poultry, eggs and milk) are not permitted and diet will be supplemented with artificial protein.

15. Ingredients listed in descending order of weight at the time of manufacture. Amounts do not have to be listed.

16. Contact details for manufacturer and information on processing procedure as could involve processing of other items, for example, nuts (important for people who may have an allergy to these). Advise Best Before and Use By dates. List of food additives (preservatives, flavourings). Nutritional information – amounts of carbohydrate, protein, fat. May show Guided Daily Allowance (GDA) via traffic light system. Storage and Preparation instructions. Suitability for Vegetarians or those on Gluten-Free diet.

17. Best Before – although not in peak condition, safe to eat after date. Use By – product must be eaten by date advised otherwise will not be safe.

18. Items for rapid consumption such as fresh fruit and non-packaged goods.

19. Letter 'E' signifies a permitted additive number. Indicates additive tested and passed for use.

Dental recalls – NICE

1. NICE – National Institute for Health and Care Excellence.

2. NICE produces guidance in three areas of health: Public health – guidance on promotion of good health and prevention on ill health for those working in NHS, local authorities and wider public and voluntary sectors. Health technologies – guidance on the use of new and existing medicines, treatments and procedures within NHS. Clinical practice – guidance on appropriate treatment and care of people with specific diseases and conditions within NHS.

3. Recall periods can be set anywhere between 3 and 12 months (maximum) for Children. For Adults, the period is between 3 and 24 months (maximum). NICE Clinical Guideline (19) Dental Recall: Recall interval between routine dental examinations – October 2004.

4. Oral Health Assessment – includes information in relation to both present and previous dental treatment, medical history, social history, lifestyle risk factors, caries and periodontal risk.

5. NICE Guideline (19) Dental Recall Intervals. Delivering Better Oral Health, 3rd Ed 2014. Scientific Basis of Oral Health Education, 7th Ed. Smokefree and Smiling: Helping Dental Patients to Quit Tobacco, 2nd Ed, March 2014. SACN Carbohydrates and Health report – July 2015

CHAPTER 3

Dental sedation nursing

Post Registration Qualifications for Dental Care Professionals: Questions and Answers, First Edition.
Nicola Rogers, Rebecca Davies, Wendy Lee, Dominic O'Sullivan and Frances Marriott.
© 2016 John Wiley & Sons, Ltd. Published 2016 by John Wiley & Sons, Ltd.
Companion Website: www.wiley.com/go/rogers/post-registration-dental-care-questions

SECTION I Questions: Reasons for the provision of sedation

LEARNING OUTCOMES

At the end of this section, you should be able to identify any gaps in your personal knowledge associated with:

• Why dental sedation is used

Anxiety

1. Explain anxiety.

2. What might cause a patient to be anxious?

3. What feelings and experiences might a patient exhibit when anxious?

4. List two things that a patient's fear can be associated with?

5. When patients are anxious in a dental surgery setting they have a raised heart rate. What is the reason for this?

Phobia

1. Explain phobia.

2. If a patient became dentally phobic when would this commonly start in his/her life?

3. State the reasons/causes why a patient may be dental phobic.

4. If a dental phobic patient attended the dental surgery, how might they respond?

5. State one thing a dental phobic patient in particular is concerned about at the dental surgery.

Miscellaneous

1. What are the two main reasons for patients not attending the dentist?

2. State one other reason why a patient would not attend the dentist.

3. How does the provision of a form of dental sedation aid patients?

4. State the current definition of sedation.

5. State the three core reasons why a form of conscious sedation may be offered to patients.

6. Are patients who are anxious or phobic more likely to attend the dental surgery for treatment?

7. Is anxiety or phobia deemed a normal feeling to experience when attending the dental surgery?

8. Explain why patients are offered a form of sedation for humanitarian reasons.

9. Explain why patients are offered a form of sedation for physiological reasons.

10. Explain why patients are offered a form of sedation for complex dental treatment.

SECTION II Questions: Medico-legal aspects of dental sedation

> **LEARNING OUTCOMES**
>
> At the end of this section, you should be able to identify any gaps in your personal knowledge associated with:
>
> - Current legislation associated with the provision of dental sedation
> - Medico-legal considerations when providing dental sedation
> - Consent and its importance in the provision of dental sedation

Current legislation

1. Discuss the current recommendation in place for the provision of conscious sedation in relation to patient selection.

2. Discuss the current recommendation in place for the provision of conscious sedation in relation to the use of sedation in the form of oral, intranasal and transmucosal sedation.

3. Discuss the current recommendation in place for the provision of conscious sedation in relation to staff training in sedation techniques.

4. Discuss the current recommendation in place for the provision of conscious sedation in relation to the ergonomics of the dental surgery.

5. Discuss the current recommendation in place for the provision of conscious sedation in relation to medical emergency and resuscitation training.

6. Discuss the current recommendation in place for the provision of conscious sedation in relation to inhalation sedation.

7. Discuss the current recommendation in place for the provision of conscious sedation in relation to intravenous sedation.

8. Discuss the current recommendation in place for the provision of conscious sedation in relation to oral sedation.

9. Discuss the current recommendation in place for the provision of conscious sedation in relation to pre- and post-operative instructions provided to patients.

10. Discuss the current recommendation in place for the provision of conscious sedation in relation to the recovery phase of a patient's treatment.

11. Discuss the current recommendation in place for the provision of conscious sedation in relation to record-keeping.

12. Discuss the current recommendation in place for the provision of conscious sedation in relation to referring patients for conscious sedation.

13. Discuss the current recommendation in place for the provision of conscious sedation in relation to monitoring a patient's vital signs during treatment.

14. Discuss the current recommendation in place for the provision of conscious sedation in relation to sedation and paediatric patients.

Medico-legal considerations when providing dental sedation

1. State two medico-legal aspects that must be considered before providing dental sedation.

Consent

1. Define consent.

2. Explain the process of obtaining consent.

3. Why is it more important to gain a patient's consent when he or she is receiving treatment with intravenous sedation as opposed to local anaesthetic?

4. What forms can consent take?

5. State the types of consent.

6. Explain each type of consent.

7. Which type of consent is most common in a dental surgery setting?

8. Which type of consent should be taken when patients receive dental treatment with sedation?

9. For consent to be valid, what fundamental aspects of treatment must a patient be advised of?

10. Give two reasons why consent is required.

11. State four treatments/situations within the dental surgery that consent would be required.

12. What salient aspects of the consent process would mean that the consent is valid?

13. Who can take consent?

14. Who can give consent?

15. Who decides that patients have the capacity to give consent?

16. Where and when should consent be taken for a patient who is to receive treatment with sedation?

17. What would be the implications of treatment being undertaken where consent has not been obtained?

18. What would written consent provide if a patient complained about treatment received?

19. What is meant by a competent person within the process of consent?

20. Explain Gillick competent.

21. Who decides if a patient younger than age 16 is Gillick competent?

Confidentiality

1. Which staff members have a responsibility to maintain a patient's confidentiality?

2. If a staff member wished to share information with another colleague about a patient, what would be required from that patient?

3. When patients provide any information to the dental team, how should it be used?

4. In what situations/circumstances can information relating to a patient be disclosed?

5. If a court of law requested information about a patient how much should be provided?

6. Explain how patient information can be kept confidential.

Assault

1. When patients receive sedation for dental treatment, what measures can the dental team put into place to prevent allegations of assault?

2. Why is a patient more likely to make an allegation of assault when they have received intravenous sedation using midazolam?

Negligence

1. What would constitute negligence in the dental surgery?

2. What measures can be put into place to avoid any acts of negligence occurring?

Miscellaneous

1. Which organisation governs the practice of dentistry?

2. What information would you expect to be recorded in a patient's notes when receiving dental treatment with sedation?

3. State the titles of the booklets published by the organisation that the dental profession are registered with that address the legal and ethical issues that the dental team face every day?

4. In what year was the conscious decision published?

5. Conscious sedation in the provision of dental care published by The Standing Dental Advisory Committee who are recognised experts within the field of dental sedation was published in which year?

6. In what year was "The Standards for Conscious Sedation in the provision of Dental Care" a report of the intercollegiate committee for sedation in dentistry published?

7. How many continued professional development hours must the sedation team undertake in a five year cycle?

8. What was the sedation nurse historically known as?

SECTION III Questions: Role of the sedation nurse

LEARNING OUTCOMES

At the end of this section, you should be able to identify any gaps in your personal knowledge associated with:

- The role of the sedation nurse during the provision of any form of sedation

---

Role of the sedation nurse when a patient is receiving treatment with conscious sedation

1. Why must an appropriately trained person be available in the dental surgery when any form of conscious sedation is provided?

2. Which members of the dental team are normally present when any form of conscious sedation is provided?

3. Through what routes can a dental nurse obtain the necessary knowledge and skills that would make them suitable to act as the sedation nurse when conscious sedation is provided?

4. Why is it important for the sedation nurse to seek further training in conscious sedation techniques?

5. Why is it important for the sedation nurse to prepare all items required for the treatment session prior to the patient's appointment?

6. Explain how the dental surgery should be prepared in readiness for a patient attending who is to receive dental treatment with a form of conscious sedation.

7. State the equipment that the sedation nurse would prepare when a patient is receiving dental treatment with intravenous sedation.

8. State the equipment that the sedation nurse would prepare when a patient is receiving dental treatment with inhalation sedation.

9. State the equipment that the sedation nurse would prepare when a patient is receiving dental treatment with oral sedation.

10. State the equipment that the sedation nurse would prepare when a patient is receiving dental treatment with transmucosal/off-licence sedation.

Role of the sedation nurse during patient treatment

1. Discuss the generic role of the sedation nurse when any form of conscious sedation is provided.

2. State the role of the sedation nurse during a patient's treatment when intravenous sedation is provided.

3. Discuss how the sedation nurse will support both the clinician and patient when cannulation takes place and administration of the sedation drug midazolam.

4. Discuss the role of the sedation nurse during a patient's treatment when inhalation sedation is provided.

5. State the role of the sedation nurse during a patient's treatment when oral sedation is provided.

6. Discuss the role of the sedation nurse during a patient's treatment when transmucosal/off-licence sedation is provided.

Role of the sedation nurse during the patient's recovery period

1. Explain the role of the sedation nurse while a patient recovers after receiving intravenous sedation.

2. Explain the role of the sedation nurse while a patient recovers after receiving inhalation sedation.

3. Explain the role of the sedation nurse while a patient recovers after receiving oral sedation.

4. Explain the role of the sedation nurse while a patient recovers after receiving transmucosal/off-licence sedation.

SECTION IV Questions: Monitoring and equipment used

LEARNING OUTCOMES

At the end of this section, you should be able to identify any gaps in your personal knowledge associated with:

- Monitoring a patient's vital signs
- Recognition of normal and abnormal readings
- Monitoring equipment used during the provision of all forms of sedation

Monitoring a patient's vital signs by observation

1. Why are patients' vital signs taken and recorded when they receive dental treatment with a form of conscious sedation?

2. State the vital signs that should be monitored when a patient receives dental treatment with a form of conscious sedation.

3. When should a patient's vital signs be observed?

4. When should clinical monitoring commence?

5. Why are patients' vital signs re-taken on the day of treatment as well as at the assessment appointment?

Pulse rate

1. Define a pulse.

2. Why is a pulse taken from a patient when conscious sedation is being provided?

3. State where four pulses can be found on the body.

4. Explain how to take a manual pulse.

5. Which pulse would be taken during a patient's treatment pathway with conscious sedation?

6. What information does a pulse provide?

7. What is the abbreviation for beats per minute?

8. What is the normal pulse rate for an adult at rest?

9. What is the normal pulse range for a newborn baby?

10. What is the normal pulse range for an infant?

11. What is the normal pulse range for a child aged 2–6 years?

12. What is the normal pulse range for a child aged 6–12 years?

13. What is the normal pulse range for an adolescent to adult patient?

14. State one piece of electrical monitoring equipment that would provide a patient's pulse rate.

15. Where can the radial pulse be found?

16. State the medical terminology for a slow pulse rate.

17. State the medical terminology for a fast pulse rate.

Respiratory rate

1. Define the respiratory rate.

2. Why is it important to take the respiratory rate of a patient when conscious sedation is being provided?

3. Explain how to take the respiratory rate.

4. What is a cycle of respiration?

5. What information does the respiratory rate provide?

6. What is the abbreviation for respirations per minute?

7. What is the normal respiratory rate for a newborn baby?

8. What is the normal respiratory rate for patients aged 2–12 years?

9. What is the normal respiratory rate for a teenage patient?

10. What is the normal respiratory rate for an adult patient?

11. State the medical terminology for slow breathing.

12. State the medical terminology for fast breathing.

Level of consciousness

1. Why is it important to monitor a patient's level of consciousness when receiving a form of conscious sedation?

2. What factors would be monitored to establish a patient's level of consciousness?

3. State the equipment required to monitor a patient's level of consciousness.

Skin tone/complexion

1. Why is it important to monitor a patient's skin tone/complexion when receiving a form of conscious sedation?

2. At what point during a patient's appointment should the skin tone/complexion be noted?

3. Besides the answer to question 2, when else should a patient's skin tone/complexion be monitored?

Height/weight

1. What are the reasons for measuring a patient's height and weight?

2. Do all clinicians providing patients' dental treatment with a form of conscious sedation measure the patients' height and weight?

3. What equipment is required to measure a patient's height and weight?

4. What is the reference tool used to establish if a patient is underweight, a healthy weight, overweight or obese?

5. At what weight might a clinician refuse to treat a patient by using conscious sedation?

6. What is the reason a clinician would refuse to treat a patient who was overweight.

Temperature

1. Why might a clinician require a patient's temperature to be taken when receiving dental treatment with a form of conscious sedation?

2. What is deemed as a normal body temperature?

3. What equipment is required to take a temperature?

4. Considering the answer to question 3, state the types available.

5. Where can a temperature be taken?

6. Explain how a patient's temperature will be taken.

7. What instructions should a patient adhere to when having a temperature taken to ensure an accurate reading?

Equipment used to monitor a patient's vital signs

Pulse oximetry

1. What is pulse oximetry?

2. Who developed pulse oximeters?

3. In which decade were pulse oximeters developed?

4. What is the purpose of using a pulse oximeter?

5. What equipment checks are carried out on pulse oximeters prior to use with patients?

6. What information does a pulse oximeter provide?

7. When a pulse oximeter is used why doesn't the clinical team require the display in view to know the current status of a patient?

8. How should a sedation nurse use a pulse oximeter to monitor a patient's level of saturated oxygen?

9. At what point should a pulse oximeter probe be placed on a patient's finger when receiving intravenous sedation?

10. State two advantages of using a pulse oximeter.

11. State two disadvantages of using a pulse oximeter.

12. Explain how a pulse oximeter works.

13. Should pulse oximeters be relied upon to provide accurate information?

14. When should pulse oximeters be used?

15. State four factors that can affect/interfere with pulse oximeter readings.

16. Why is it important to set the integral alarms on a pulse oximeter?

17. What integral alarms are present in a pulse oximeter?

18. At what levels should the integral alarms be set on a pulse oximeter?

19. Is there any occasion when the integral alarms might be set differently to the recommended levels? Explain your answer.

20. Approximately how long does it take for the pulse oximeter to display any recordings after the finger probe has been placed?

21. What time lag does the pulse oximeter have?

22. What relevance is the oxygen disassociation curve within pulse oximetry?

23. What shape is the curve on the oxygen disassociation curve?

24. If the integral alarms were to activate, what action would be taken?

25. Why is it not mandatory to use a pulse oximeter while a patient receives dental treatment with inhalation sedation?

26. Which colour nail varnish does not affect the pulse oximeter readings?

27. Why are patients asked to remove nail varnish when pulse oximeters are used?

28. What is hypoxia?

29. What is meant by oxygen saturation?

30. What is the abbreviation for oxygen saturation?

31. What is meant by optical spectrophotometry?

32. What is meant by optical plethysmograph?

33. Apart from a pulse oximeter being used during conscious sedation sessions, when else might one be used within the dental practice?

Blood pressure

1. Define arterial blood pressure.

2. What factors determine a patient's blood pressure?

3. How does the body adjust a patient's blood pressure?

4. What does the blood pressure measure?

5. What happens within the heart to achieve a patient's blood pressure?

6. What does the blood pressure tell us?

7. How is blood pressure recorded?

8. What equipment is required to take a manual blood pressure?

9. When should blood pressure be taken when a patient is to receive dental treatment with conscious sedation?

10. Can a blood pressure vary from appointment to appointment?

11. Explain how a manual blood pressure is taken?

12. Why is an estimated reading taken when taking a manual blood pressure?

13. Why are 25–30 seconds allowed to elapse before taking the blood pressure after taking an estimated reading?

14. When taking a manual blood pressure what are you expecting to hear?

15. Which arteries are felt for when taking a manual blood pressure?

16. When taking a manual blood pressure which nearest number of mmHg should be recorded?

17. What is normal blood pressure?

18. Which of the two figures recorded are of concern if elevated? Explain why.

19. If a patient's blood pressure was raised dramatically, what action would be taken?

20. Why do we wait before taking another blood pressure from a patient whose blood pressure is elevated?

21. Why should patients not eat, drink, exercise or smoke for a minimum of 15 minutes before having their blood pressure taken?

22. Why must the patient's arm be supported when taking their blood pressure?

23. Hypnovel lowers the blood pressure and in turn raises the pulse. Explain why the pulse rate rises.

24. Name one medication a patient might be taking if they suffer from high blood pressure.

25. Explain how medication for high blood pressure acts on the body.

Miscellaneous

1. Is clinical monitoring mandatory when a patient receives dental treatment with conscious sedation?

2. When monitoring a patient's vital signs should the sedation nurse's observations or that of the monitoring equipment be relied upon?

3. State the monitoring equipment used during intravenous sedation.

4. State the monitoring equipment used during inhalation sedation.

5. State the monitoring equipment used during oral sedation.

6. State the monitoring equipment used during transmucosal (off-licence) sedation.

7. Why is it important to monitor a patient's skin tone when receiving conscious sedation?

8. Why is it important to monitor a patient's heart rate when receiving conscious sedation?

9. Why is it important to monitor a patient's respiratory rate when receiving conscious sedation?

10. Why is it important to monitor a patient's blood pressure when receiving conscious sedation?

11. Why it is important to monitor a patient's saturated oxygen levels when receiving conscious sedation?

12. Why is it important to monitor a patient's level of consciousness when receiving conscious sedation?

13. Why is it important to monitor a patient's height and weight when receiving conscious sedation?

14. Why is it important to monitor a patient's temperature when receiving conscious sedation?

15. When undertaking medical checks at the assessment appointment, are all of them always carried out? Explain your answer.

Equipment used for intravenous sedation

1. State the equipment that would be prepared for intravenous sedation.

Equipment used for cannulation

1. State the function of a tourniquet.

2. Why is a disinfectant surface medi-wipe used?

3. What is the function of a cannula, either a 22-gauge Venflon or Y can.

4. Explain why 22-gauge Venflon cannulas are best practice as opposed to a 23-gauge butterfly needle.

5. What is the purpose of a Luer lock on a 22-gauge Venflon?

6. Why are two 23-gauge drawing up needles required?

7. Why are filter needles used to draw up drugs?

8. Explain why a 5 ml sodium chloride flush is used?

9. What is the purpose of having a 2 ml sterile syringe with a sodium chloride label previously placed?

10. What is the purpose of having a 5 ml sterile syringe with a drug label (midazolam) previously placed?

11. Explain the function of the sedation drug to be used (midazolam).

12. Explain the need for flumazenil to be present when intravenous sedation has been administered.

Equipment used for inhalation sedation

1. State the equipment that would be prepared for inhalation sedation.

Equipment used for oral sedation

1. State the equipment that would be prepared for oral sedation.

Equipment used for transmucosal/off-licence sedation

1. State the equipment that would be prepared for transmucosal/off-licence sedation.

SECTION V Questions: Patient selection

LEARNING OUTCOMES

At the end of this section, you should be able to identify any gaps in your personal knowledge associated with:

- The process of patient selection

The assessment appointment

1. What is the purpose of a patient attending an assessment appointment prior to attending the dental surgery for treatment involving the provision of conscious sedation?

2. Why is an assessment appointment good practice?

3. At the assessment appointment, what factors must the clinician take into account prior to providing a patient with an appointment for dental treatment where conscious sedation is to be provided?

4. At the assessment appointment, what must the clinician ensure is undertaken before deciding to proceed with dental treatment with conscious sedation?

5. Is a separate assessment appointment always possible?

6. Explain the answer given in question 5.

7. What medical equipment could be used as part of the assessment process?

8. When preparing the dental surgery for an assessment appointment, what documentation should be sourced?

Medical history

1. What is the purpose of undertaking a medical history and physical examination?

2. Once a medical history and physical examination have taken place, what reference tool is available for the clinician to refer to in deciding what medical risk the patient might pose while being treated?

3. When clinicians take medical histories from patients, the conditions patients may suffer from are grouped into specific categories. State these categories.

4. State two medical conditions that would fall under the auspices of central nervous system conditions.

5. State two medical conditions that would fall under the auspices of cardiovascular system conditions.

6. State two medical conditions that would fall under the auspices of respiratory system conditions.

7. State two medical conditions that would fall under the auspices of gastrointestinal conditions.

8. State two medical conditions that would fall under the auspices of gastrourinary conditions.

9. State two medical conditions that would fall under the auspices of locomotor conditions.

10. What additional questions are asked when taking a medical history?

11. Why would clinicians ask patients if they have previously had any treatments involving conscious sedation or a general anaesthetic?

12. Why would clinicians ask patients if they currently take recreational drugs or drink alcohol?

The ASA physical status classification

1. What does the ASA stand for within the Physical Status Classification?

2. How many classifications are there within the ASA Physical Status Classification?

3. Define each patient group under each ASA Physical Status Classification and where applicable give two examples of each.

4. If a patient's blood pressure was 200/115 mm Hg, what ASA would they be classified as?

5. If a patient suffered with epilepsy and had several seizures per year, what ASA classification would they be?

6. If a patient was a diabetic and well-controlled with insulin, what ASA classification would they be?

7. If a patient suffered with unstable angina, what ASA classification would they be?

8. Which ASA classification would a patient aged 67 fit into?

9. Which ASA classification would a patient who had a terminal condition and was not expected to survive fit into?

10. If a patient had a blood pressure of 140–159/90–94 mm Hg, what ASA classification would they be?

11. If a patient was unable to walk up stairs or very far along the street, what ASA classification would they be?

12. If a patient is able to walk up stairs easily, what ASA classification are they?

13. If a patient was an ASA III, what would the current recommendation according to the ASA classification be for providing treatment?

14. If a patient was an ASA IV, what would the current recommendation according to the ASA classification be for providing treatment?

Miscellaneous

1. What is the purpose of obtaining a dental history?

2. What is the purpose of obtaining a social history?

3. What resource is available to establish a patient's level of anxiety and whether they are suitable to be treated within a dental surgery setting?

4. If a patient had no family or friend support and required a form of sedation for treatment, what options would be available to them?

5. Explain the rationale for the answer in question 4.

SECTION VI Questions: Types of sedation

LEARNING OUTCOMES

At the end of this section, you should be able to identify any gaps in your personal knowledge associated with:

- The forms of sedation offered to patients
- The route of administration for each type of sedation and their action on the body
- The advantages, disadvantages, indications and contraindications of usage

---

Intravenous sedation

Midazolam

1. State the class/family of drugs to which the most commonly used intravenous sedation agent belongs.

2. Is midazolam a trade or generic name?

3. What other name is midazolam known by?

4. For answer 3, is this name a trade or generic one?

5. In what year, was midazolam available in the United Kingdom?

6. State the half-life of midazolam.

7. What schedule of controlled drug is midazolam classified as?

8. Midazolam is available in what presentations?

9. From the presentations that midazolam are available in which one should be used for best practice?

10. What does the blue dot stamped on the ampoule represent?

11. What colour is midazolam?

12. How should midazolam be stored when not in use?

13. What are the routes of administration for midazolam?

14. What is the pH of midazolam?

15. State five advantages of providing a patient with intravenous sedation using midazolam.

16. State five disadvantages of providing a patient with intravenous sedation using midazolam.

17. If a patient had an allergic reaction to midazolam, how would the reaction be managed?

18. What information can be found stamped on an ampoule of midazolam?

19. What is the recommended titration of midazolam to a patient who is deemed an American Society of Anaesthesiologist medical fitness classification 1 (ASA1)?

20. How is the amount of midazolam administered to a patient calculated?

21. What is the recommended titration of midazolam to an elderly patient?

22. Why are the titrations of midazolam less and periods of observation longer for an elderly patient?

23. What is the approximate onset of action time for midazolam?

24. How does midazolam sedate a patient?

25. What test can be undertaken to establish if a patient is sedated?

26. What are the clinical signs of sedation using midazolam?

27. What are the clinical signs of over-sedation using midazolam?

28. If a patient was over-sedated, how would they be managed?

29. How is midazolam metabolised within the body?

30. Once midazolam is broken down, how is it excreted from the body?

31. What are clinical effects of midazolam?

32. State four side effects of midazolam.

33. State four contraindications for the use of midazolam.

34. List as many complications as you can that could occur when providing intravenous sedation to patients.

35. If midazolam is used in conjunction with an opiate, which would be administered first?

Anexate

1. State the class/family of drugs to which the reversal agent Anexate belongs to.

2. Is Anexate a trade or generic name?

3. What other name is Anexate known by?

4. For answer 3, is this name a trade or generic one?

5. State the half-life of Anexate.

6. What is meant by an immunobenzodiazepine?

7. What schedule of controlled drug is Anexate classified as?

8. State the presentation Anexate is available in.

9. What colour is Anexate?

10. What information can be found stamped on an ampoule of Anexate?

11. How should Anexate be stored when not in use?

12. When would Anexate be administered?

13. If a patient was over-sedated, what would be the recommended titration of Anexate?

14. How does Anexate reverse the effects of midazolam?

15. What side effects might a patient experience after Anexate has been administered?

16. Would it be possible for a patient to re-sedate if the sedative agent used was midazolam? Explain your answer.

17. How is Anexate metabolised?

18. Once Anexate has been broken down, how is it excreted from the body?

19. State two contraindications for the use of Anexate.

Propofol

1. State the class/family of drugs that propofol belongs to?

2. Is propofol a trade or generic name?

3. What other name is propofol known by?

4. For answer 3, is this name a trade or generic one?

5. State the half-life of propofol.

6. What schedule of controlled drug is propofol classified as?

7. How should propofol be stored when not in use?

8. Propofol is available in what presentation?

9. What colour is propofol?

10. What information can be found stamped on an ampoule of propofol?

11. Why is propofol known as the milk of amnesia?

12. How is propofol administered to a patient when used for conscious sedation?

13. Propofol causes pain on administration. How can this be overcome?

14. Who can administer propofol for dental sedation?

15. How does propofol sedate a patient?

16. What is the approximate onset of action time for propofol?

17. What are the clinical effects of propofol?

18. State two contraindications for the use of propofol.

19. State two adverse effects that can occur from the use of propofol for dental sedation.

20. How is propofol metabolised within the body?

21. Once broken down, how is propofol eliminated from the body?

22. If a patient had this recorded on their medical history they would not be able to have propofol administered. What would the patient be allergic to?

Miscellaneous

1. When a patient leaves the surgery after receiving intravenous midazolam, are they fit and well? If the answer is yes, discuss why and if the answer is no, discuss why not?

2. What is meant by a half-life?

3. What is meant by a trade name?

4. What is meant by a generic name?

5. What does titrated mean?

6. What is meant by a controlled drug?

7. State the year of the Misuse of Drugs Act.

8. State the year of the Medicines Act.

9. Which benzodiazepines were used before midazolam came onto the market?

10. Discuss in detail the phases of sedation.

11. What is meant by the arm brain time?

12. What is meant by drug metabolism?

13. What is meant by drug excretion?

14. What is meant by a metabolite?

15. State two substances that can affect patient treatment when receiving midazolam.

16. List the pre- and post-operative instructions attracted to intravenous sedation.

17. List the medical checks that would be undertaken when a patient is to receive intravenous sedation.

18. During intravenous sedation, what clinical and electrical monitoring takes place?

19. What questions would patients be asked prior to receiving intravenous sedation?

20. List the things that should be contained within patient notes when intravenous sedation takes place.

21. Why is contemporaneous note-keeping important when intravenous sedation is provided?

22. What medical emergency is midazolam used to manage?

23. What does pharmacokinetics mean?

24. Why might a patient require a numbing cream placed prior to cannulation?

25. State the name of one numbing cream available.

26. How long before the cannula is placed should a numbing cream be applied?

27. What are the contents of numbing creams?

28. What is the timeframe a patient should be kept in recovery before being discharged after receiving intravenous sedation?

29. List two complications that could occur in a patient's recovery phase.

30. When should a cannula be removed following dental treatment?

31. How should a patient be assessed for discharge?

32. What is meant by polypharmacy?

33. State the name of an opiate that can be used with midazolam as it does not require any further precautions to store it.

34. State the name of the reversal drug for question 33.

35. What is the purpose of using an opiate in conjunction with midazolam?

36. What is the common side effect of using an opiate?

37. What does mgs stand for?

38. What does mcgs stand for?

Oral sedation

Temazepam

1. State the class/family of drugs that temazepam belongs to.

2. What forms does temazepam come in?

3. What dosages do the current recommended forms of temazepam come in that are used for dental sedation?

4. What colour are the forms of temazepam currently recommended for use within dentistry for conscious sedation?

5. What is the usual dose of temazepam prescribed for an adult?

6. What is the usual dose of temazepam prescribed for a paediatric patient?

7. What is the usual dose of temazepam prescribed for an elderly patient?

8. How is the amount of temazepam administered to a patient calculated?

9. What are the clinical effects of temazepam?

10. What schedule of controlled drug is temazepam classified as?

11. How should temazepam be stored if held within a dental practice?

12. State two contraindications for the use of temazepam.

13. State three advantages of providing temazepam to patients.

14. State three disadvantages of providing temazepam to patients.

15. What is the half-life of temazepam?

16. What factors would the dentist consider before prescribing temazepam?

17. Why is temazepam the ideal choice for a premedication?

18. If temazepam were to be used as a premedication for a patient who is to receive intravenous midazolam, what factors would the dentist have to consider?

19. How would a patient be treated if they became over-sedated after being administered temazepam?

Diazepam (Valium)

1. State the class/family of drugs that diazepam belongs to.

2. What forms does diazepam come in?

3. What dosages do the current recommended forms of diazepam come in that are used for dental sedation?

4. What colour are the forms of diazepam currently recommended for use within dentistry for conscious sedation?

5. What is the usual dose of diazepam prescribed for an adult?

6. What is the usual dose of diazepam prescribed for a paediatric patient?

7. What is the usual dose of diazepam prescribed for an elderly patient?

8. How is the amount of diazepam administered to a patient calculated?

9. What are clinical effects of diazepam?

10. What schedule of controlled drug is diazepam classified as?

11. How should diazepam be stored if held within a dental practice?

12. State two contraindications for the use of diazepam.

13. State three advantages of providing diazepam to patients.

14. State three disadvantages of providing diazepam to patients.

15. What is the half-life of diazepam?

16. What factors would the dentist consider before prescribing diazepam?

17. Why is temazepam the ideal choice for a premedication as opposed to diazepam?

18. If diazepam were to be used as a premedication for a patient who is to receive intravenous midazolam, what factors would the dentist have to consider?

19. How would a patient be treated if they became over-sedated after being administered diazepam?

Miscellaneous

1. When a patient leaves the surgery after receiving oral sedation, are they fit and well? If the answer is yes, discuss why, and if the answer is, no explain.

2. When a patient is sedated using oral sedation what clinical signs would they exhibit?

3. If a patient was over-sedated using oral sedation, what clinical signs would they exhibit?

4. List the pre- and post-operative instructions attracted to oral sedation.

5. List the things that should be contained within patient notes when oral sedation is provided.

6. During oral sedation what clinical and electrical monitoring takes place?

7. Why is contemporaneous note-keeping important when oral sedation is provided?

8. Why is oral sedation used?

9. Which oral sedation is the cheaper one?

10. What is the timescale for a prescription for oral sedation validity?

11. What is the difference between oral pre-medication and oral sedation?

Inhalation sedation

1. What is inhalation sedation?

2. What is another name for inhalation sedation?

3. What is the aim of providing inhalation sedation to patients?

4. State the name of the gases used for inhalation sedation.

5. State three advantages of providing inhalation sedation to patients.

6. State three disadvantages of providing inhalation sedation to patients.

7. State two contraindications of the use of inhalation sedation.

8. For which group of patients is inhalation sedation the first choice of conscious sedation?

9. How does a patient become sedated using inhalation sedation?

10. What is the approximate onset of action time for primary saturation of nitrous oxide?

11. What is the approximate onset of action time for any additional percentages of nitrous oxide?

12. What is the approximate onset of action time for fat, muscle and connective tissues?

13. What action does inhalation sedation have on the body?

14. What are the signs of over-sedation?

15. How are the gases used for inhalation sedation eliminated from the body?

16. What is the purpose of providing a patient with 100% oxygen at the end of the dental procedure?

17. How long should 100% oxygen be administered to a patient on completion of dental treatment?

18. Discuss the stages and planes of anaesthesia.

19. What is the purpose of an acclimatisation appointment?

20. Where does inhalation sedation exist in relationship to the stages and planes of anaesthesia?

21. Discuss the subjective experiences a patient feels when being provided with inhalation sedation.

22. Why must a patient be able to breathe through their nose when receiving inhalation sedation?

23. List the pre- and post-operative instructions provided to patients who will receive inhalation sedation.

24. What is the importance of not placing a mouth prop in a patient's mouth during the delivery of inhalation sedation?

25. Why has inhalation sedation been described as the best clinical form of sedation?

26. When a patient receives inhalation sedation, is it mandatory for an escort to be present?

27. State two categories of patients unsuitable to receive inhalation sedation?

28. What medical pre-checks would be carried out upon patients prior to dental treatment with inhalation sedation?

29. What questions are patients asked prior to receiving inhalation sedation?

30. State the surgery checks that would be carried out prior to a patient attending for inhalation sedation.

31. What action would be taken if a patient was over-sedated?

32. How would a patient feel if the nitrous oxide were to stop delivery during a patient's treatment?

Nitrous oxide

1. What colour is a nitrous oxide cylinder?

2. Does nitrous oxide have a specific smell?

3. What pressure is nitrous oxygen stored under in an E size cylinder?

4. Is nitrous oxide a gas?

5. What substance is heated to produce nitrous oxide and water?

6. What is the minimum alveolar concentration for nitrous oxide?

7. What is meant by the minimum alveolar concentration?

8. How can the amount of nitrous oxide in a cylinder be gauged?

9. Is the reading on the gauges/dials advising the amount of nitrous oxide in the cylinder accurate?

10. How can it be determined how much nitrous oxide is in the cylinder if it is a liquid under pressure?

11. What information is stamped on a nitrous oxide cylinder?

12. Why does nitrous oxide maintain its toxicity even though it has been inhaled and exhaled by a patient?

13. What effects can nitrous oxide cause if prolonged volumes are used?

14. Are there any recommended guidelines associated with inhalation sedation?

15. The Health and Safety Commission has established Workplace Exposure Limits (WELs). What is the purpose of these limits?

16. Why do these limits extend to a 24-hour period?

17. What measures can be put into place to ensure staff working with nitrous oxide do not exceed the Workplace Exposure Limits?

18. In what year was nitrous oxide produced?

19. What is the name of the person who produced nitrous oxide?

20. In what year were the effects of nitrous oxide established?

21. What is the name of the person who discovered the effects of nitrous oxide?

Oxygen

1. What colour is an oxygen cylinder?

2. Does oxygen have a specific smell?

3. What information is stamped on oxygen cylinders?

4. What pressure is oxygen stored under in an E size cylinder?

5. Why is it important not to lubricate any of the connections, valves or fitments with oil or grease?

6. Is oxygen flammable?

7. What is the minimum amount of oxygen delivered to a patient at all times when providing inhalation sedation?

8. Why must oxygen be provided in conjunction with nitrous oxide when providing inhalation sedation?

9. Why is it important to provide 3–5 minutes of 100% oxygen at the end of the dental procedure before switching off the inhalation sedation machine?

10. How many litres of oxygen would be administered to a patient if the oxygen flush button was pressed?

The machine

1. What is the purpose of checking inhalation sedation machines prior to use?

2. Explain how a mobile inhalation sedation machine should be checked prior to use.

3. Explain how a piped inhalation sedation machine should be checked prior to use.

4. Whose responsibility is it to ensure that an inhalation sedation machine is safe for use with patients?

5. State five safety features of an inhalation sedation machine.

6. Besides a scavenging system, is there any other way of reducing the amount of nitrous oxide in the air?

7. What is the purpose of scavenging systems?

8. Discuss the types of scavenging systems available.

9. When checking a mobile inhalation sedation machine, how much oxygen would be stored in a full cylinder?

10. When checking a mobile inhalation sedation machine, how much oxygen would be stored in a cylinder that indicates it is a quarter full?

11. When should an oxygen cylinder be changed on a mobile inhalation sedation machine?

12. When checking a mobile inhalation sedation machine, how can the amount of nitrous oxide in a cylinder be determined?

13. What pressure is oxygen stored under within its cylinder on a mobile inhalation sedation machine?

14. What pressure is nitrous oxide stored under within its cylinder on a mobile inhalation sedation machine?

15. To what pressure do reducing valves reduce gases supplied to a patient?

16. How many litres per minute can the emergency flush deliver to a patient if pressed?

17. What is the size of a reservoir bag?

18. What functions does the air entrainment valve serve?

19. On mobile inhalation sedation machines, there is a pin index system. What is its function?

20. Where would you find a Bodok seal on a mobile inhalation sedation machine?

21. What function does a Bodok seal have?

22. If any of the cylinders were switched on and a screeching noise occurred, what would this indicate?

23. What is meant by calibration of the machine when undertaking the pre-checks?

24. Why is it important to ensure that the nitrous oxide safety cut-out feature is functional prior to using the machine?

25. How is the nitrous oxide safety cut-off feature checked?

26. At what point will the nitrous oxide dial provide an accurate reading on a mobile inhalation sedation machine?

Administration/delivery

1. How should the dental surgery be prepared in readiness for a patient who is to receive inhalation sedation?

2. Before dental treatment commences using inhalation sedation approximately what flow rate would be set (a) for an adult and (b) for a child.

3. If a more accurate flow rate was required for individual patients, how would the figure be calculated?

4. What percentage of oxygen should the inhalation sedation machine be set at prior to its provision?

5. Once a patient is sat in the dental chair explain how they would be prepared prior to inhalation sedation?

6. Once the nasal mask is in situ, what should be checked?

7. What would be the first thing to check on the inhalation sedation machine prior to the introduction of nitrous oxide?

8. Once a patient is settled, receiving oxygen only, how much nitrous oxide should initially be introduced?

9. If a reservoir bag was over-inflated, what action would be taken?

10. Why would a reservoir bag be over-inflated?

11. If a reservoir bag was under-inflated, what action would be taken?

12. Why would a reservoir bag be under-inflated?

13. How inflated would you expect a reservoir bag to be inflated during administration and why?

14. During the provision of inhalation sedation, how should a patient be spoken to?

15. If a patient is receiving 15% nitrous oxide, what plane of stage 1 anaesthesia would they be in?

16. If further increments of nitrous oxide are required to ensure a patient is nicely sedated, how much should be introduced at any one time?

17. If a patient is receiving 30% nitrous oxide, what plane of stage 1 if not stage 2 anaesthesia would they be in?

18. What feelings would a patient experience if receiving 20% nitrous oxide?

19. What feelings would a patient experience if receiving 35% nitrous oxide?

20. When the dental treatment is complete, what is the percentage of oxygen provided and for how long?

21. When treatment is complete, is the nitrous oxide percentage reduced slowly or switched off straightaway?

22. How long should a patient remain in the dental surgery prior to discharge after the inhalation sedation machine has been switched off?

23. During dental treatment with inhalation sedation what vital signs would be monitored?

Miscellaneous

1. Define diffusion hypoxia.

2. How can diffusion hypoxia be avoided?

3. What is the name given to a pre-mixed gas of 50% nitrous oxide and 50% oxygen?

4. What does the abbreviation COSHH stand for?

5. What does the abbreviation WELs stand for?

6. What does the abbreviation TWA stand for?

7. What does the abbreviation MAC stand for?

8. What does the abbreviation psi stand for?

9. Why is it not mandatory to use a pulse oximeter during the provision of inhalation sedation?

10. What relaxation methods could be used to support a patient during the administration of inhalation sedation?

11. What is the average tidal volume for a 70 kg adult?

SECTION VII Questions: Medical emergencies

> **LEARNING OUTCOMES**
>
> At the end of this section, you should be able to identify any gaps in your personal knowledge associated with:
>
> - The signs and symptoms of common medical emergencies that could occur in the dental surgery
> - Managing medical emergencies
> - Implementing ways to reduce the risk of a medical emergency occurring in the dental surgery

Faint

1. Define a faint.

2. State another name for a faint.

3. Explain why a faint is the most common cause of collapse in the dental surgery.

4. What causes a patient to faint?

5. What are the signs and symptoms of a faint?

6. Briefly state how a faint would be managed.

7. What is the purpose of placing a patient in the supine position?

8. What is meant by the supine position?

9. What would be provided to a patient who had fainted?

Cardiac arrest

1. Define cardiac arrest.

2. What is the aim of cardiopulmonary resuscitation?

3. What could cause a patient to go into cardiac arrest?

4. What are the signs and symptoms of cardiac arrest?

5. Briefly state how cardiac arrest would be managed in an adult patient.

6. Explain the different approach in management of a paediatric patient in cardiac arrest.

7. When would cardio pulmonary resuscitation be stopped?

8. What is the purpose of compressions?

9. What is the purpose of ventilations?

10. How many compressions to ventilations are administered to an adult patient in cardiac arrest?

11. How many compressions to ventilations are administered to a paediatric patient in cardiac arrest?

12. During the administration of compressions if the hands were too low what might occur?

13. Which structure of the heart should be compressed to ensure adequate circulation of the oxygenated blood?

14. In what manner should compressions be administered?

15. When a patient goes into cardiac arrest what is the timeframe for management before irreversible brain damage and death will occur?

16. What is the name of the equipment that gives an electric shock to the heart?

17. Explain how a patient in cardiac arrest would be managed if a pocket mask was not available.

Anaphylaxis

1. Define anaphylaxis.

2. State two things that could cause a patient to have an anaphylactic reaction.

3. What are the signs and symptoms of an anaphylactic shock?

4. Briefly state how anaphylaxis would be managed.

5. What additional drugs might the paramedics administer to patients experiencing an anaphylactic shock?

6. If a patient was suffering an allergic reaction and was exhibiting signs and symptoms such as wheezing or difficulty breathing, how would these conditions be treated?

7. Which drug is used to manage anaphylaxis?

8. Through which route would the emergency drug be given to manage anaphylaxis?

9. What is the recommended concentration of the emergency drug administered to manage anaphylaxis?

10. What concentration of the emergency drug would an autoinjector contain?

11. How does the emergency drug used to treat anaphylaxis work?

12. When the emergency drug used to manage anaphylaxis comes as an autoinjector, what is its name?

13. Why is it important not to administer too much adrenaline?

14. What is meant as the biphasic stage?

15. How quickly could a patient develop some signs and symptoms of an allergic reaction if exposed to something they are allergic to?

Adrenal insufficiency

1. Define adrenal insufficiency.

2. What are the signs and symptoms of adrenal insufficiency?

3. Briefly discuss the management of adrenal insufficiency.

4. State why a patient might experience an adrenal crisis.

Angina

1. Define angina.

2. What might angina also be known as?

3. Define ischemia.

4. State one factor that could cause a patient to have an angina attack.

5. What are the signs and symptoms of an angina attack?

6. Briefly state how an angina attack would be managed.

7. What is the reason for not laying a patient down when they suffer an angina attack?

8. What medication would a patient suffering from angina carry?

9. The medication carried by patients who suffer with angina comes in what forms?

10. How is the medication that relieves angina administered to patients who suffer with angina?

11. Why should patients not be administered too much of their medication?

12. How many administrations of medication can patients have before suspecting that the pain is not going to be relieved?

13. After the medication for angina has been administered for the recommended amounts and time and the pain had not been relieved, what condition would be suspected?

14. What action would be taken if the patient did not gain any relief from their medication when suffering an angina attack?

Asthma

1. Define asthma.

2. State one factor that could cause a patient to have an asthma attack.

3. What is the reason for not laying patients down when they suffer an asthma attack?

4. What medication would a patient suffering from an asthma attack carry?

5. Sometimes the medication that patients carry to relieve an asthma attack is known by another name. What is the alternative name?

6. What are the signs and symptoms of an asthma attack?

7. Briefly state how an asthma attack would be managed.

8. How does the medication carried by patients to relieve an asthma attack act?

9. During an activation of the medication used to relieve asthma, how many micrograms of the drug are administered?

10. If a patient was experiencing difficulty using the inhaler, what emergency aid could be provided?

11. Why are patients who suffer with asthma recommended to take a few activations of their medication before exercising?

12. State the name of a medication that patients who suffer with asthma would be taking to prevent an asthma attack.

Myocardial infarction

1. Define myocardial infarction.

2. What is another name for a myocardial infarction?

3. State why a patient might have a myocardial infarction.

4. What happens to the heart muscles after a myocardial infarction has occurred?

5. What are the signs and symptoms of a myocardial infarction?

6. Briefly state how a myocardial infarction would be managed.

7. What drug would be provided to patients suffering a myocardial infarction?

8. What action does the drug stated in question 7 have on the body?

9. Besides the drug stated in question 7 what additional medication could be administered to a patient suffering a myocardial infarction?

Respiratory arrest

1. Define respiratory arrest.

2. What could cause a patient to go into respiratory arrest?

3. What are the signs and symptoms of respiratory arrest?

4. Briefly state how respiratory arrest would be managed.

5. What will occur if respiratory arrest is prolonged?

Choking and aspiration

1. Define choking.

2. What causes a patient to choke?

3. What are the signs and symptoms of choking?

4. Briefly state how a choking patient would be managed.

5. How many back-slaps to abdominal thrusts are administered when managing a choking patient?

6. Define aspiration.

7. What are the signs and symptoms of aspiration?

8. Briefly discuss the management of aspiration.

9. If an item were to go into the lungs, which one is it more likely to enter and why?

Epilepsy

1. Define epilepsy.

2. State one factor that could trigger an epileptic seizure.

3. What are the signs and symptoms of epilepsy?

4. Briefly state how epilepsy would be managed.

5. What is meant by status epilepticus?

6. Which emergency drug would be used if a patient was diagnosed with status epilepticus?

7. Through which route is the emergency drug administered when a patient has been diagnosed with status epilepticus?

8. What drug is Epistatus?

9. When the emergency drug is administered to manage status epilepticus how many mgs of drug is in each ml?

Hypoglycaemia

1. If a patient had a hypoglycaemic episode in the dental surgery, what medical condition would be recorded in their medical notes?

2. What is hypoglycaemia?

3. Explain why a patient might experience a hypoglycaemic episode.

4. What are the signs and symptoms of the early stages of hypoglycaemia?

5. Briefly state how the early stages of hypoglycaemia would be managed.

6. What are the signs and symptoms of the later/severe stages of hypoglycaemia?

7. Briefly state how the later/severe stages of hypoglycaemia would be managed.

8. What emergency drug would be administered to a patient who suffering a severe hypoglycaemic episode?

9. Through which route would the drug named in question 8 be administered?

10. What emergency drug dosage is administered to a patient elder than the age of 8 when unconscious suffering from hypoglycaemia?

11. What emergency drug dosage is administered to an unconscious patient younger than the age of 8 suffering from hypoglycaemia?

12. Below what figure mmol/l would a patient be deemed as suffering hypoglycaemia?

Hyperventilation

1. Define hyperventilation.

2. Why might a patient hyperventilate in the dental surgery?

3. What happens to the body when a patient hyperventilates?

4. What are the signs and symptoms of hyperventilation?

5. Briefly explain the management of hyperventilation.

6. Discuss why oxygen is not used in the management of hyperventilation.

7. Why is a paper bag used during the management of hyperventilation?

Airway control and ventilation

Laerdal pocket mask

1. State two features of a pocket mask.

2. State one medical condition that a pocket mask would be used for.

3. What percentage of oxygen would a patient receive if a pocket mask was used without any supplementary oxygen being attached?

4. When attaching oxygen to a pocket mask what cylinder flow rate should be administered?

5. When providing supplementary oxygen through a pocket mask, what percentage of oxygen will the patient receive?

6. Why would the oxygen cylinder not be switched to maximum when attaching it to a pocket mask?

Hudson mask

1. State two features of a Hudson mask.

2. State two medical conditions that a Hudson mask would be used for.

3. State one other situation when a Hudson mask would be used.

4. When attaching oxygen to a Hudson mask what cylinder flow rate should the cylinder be administered?

Nasal cannulae

1. What is a nasal cannula?

2. State the benefit of using nasal cannulas to administer oxygen.

3. State one reason why nasal cannulas might be used.

4. When nasal cannulas are attached to oxygen, what cylinder flow rate should be administered?

Oropharyngeal airway

1. What is an oropharyngeal airway?

2. What is another name for an oropharyngeal airway?

3. What method is used to ensure the correct size airway is selected?

4. What size is commonly used for adults?

5. Briefly explain how an oropharyngeal airway is placed.

6. When the airway is inserted where does it sit anatomically?

7. What would happen if the airway was inserted incorrectly?

8. Can an oropharyngeal airway be used in a conscious patient?

9. What must be checked once an oropharyngeal airway has been placed?

Nasopharyngeal airway

1. What is a nasopharyngeal airway?

2. What method is used to ensure the correct size airway is selected?

3. What size is commonly used for adults?

4. Briefly explain how a nasopharyngeal airway is placed.

5. What might happen if the airway inserted was too long?

6. When the airway is inserted, where does it sit anatomically?

7. Can a nasopharyngeal airway be used in a conscious patient?

8. What must be checked once a nasopharyngeal airway has been placed?

Oxygen

1. Why is oxygen used during a medical emergency?

2. What is oxygen?

3. Is oxygen flammable?

4. In what size cylinders is oxygen provided?

5. What pressure is oxygen stored at?

6. What colour are oxygen cylinders?

7. What is stamped on the collar of an oxygen cylinder?

8. What colour is oxygen?

9. Does oxygen have a distinct smell?

10. How should oxygen cylinders be stored?

11. How should oxygen cylinders be transported?

12. Why shouldn't any of the connections, valves or fitments be lubricated, smoking avoided and hand cream be used when oxygen cylinders are present?

13. How often should piped oxygen hoses be changed?

Miscellaneous

1. State the common medical emergencies that could occur in the dental surgery.

2. Which medical emergency is the most common cause of collapse in the dental surgery?

3. Which medical emergencies are categorised as being conditions involving breathing difficulties and/or chest pains?

4. Which medical emergencies are categorised as conditions associated with fits?

5. Which medical emergencies are categorised as conditions involving the loss of consciousness?

6. State the mechanisms that can be put into place to reduce the risk of a medical emergency occurring in the dental surgery.

7. When dealing with a medical emergency what factors need to be considered?

8. If a patient were to have a medical emergency in the dental surgery, how would the situation be controlled?

9. State the drugs that should be held in an emergency drugs box within the dental surgery.

10. How should emergency drugs be stored in the dental surgery?

11. Thorough which routes can drugs be administered?

12. Through which preferred routes are drugs recommended to be administered within a dental surgery setting?

13. Which additional items that aid the management of a medical emergency should be held within the dental surgery?

14. When diagnosing a medical emergency we discuss the signs and symptoms to aid us. Explain what is meant by a sign.

15. When diagnosing a medical emergency we discuss the signs and symptoms to aid us. Explain what is meant by a symptom.

16. If a patient fainted and did not recover quickly, what medical condition might they be experiencing?

17. What item from the emergency kit would aid diagnosis of the answer to question 16?

18. What is another name for adrenaline?

19. If 50% nitrous oxide and 50% oxygen is premixed in a medical gas cylinder, what would the contents be known as?

20. If a patient were to have an epileptic seizure that lasted more than 5 minutes or the seizure stopped and then recurred quickly what would this be known as?

21. Which condition would a patient be suffering if he or she were to become pale sweaty and have a weak but rapid pulse?

22. Which condition would a patient be suffering if he or she were to become breathless, wheezing on expiration and panicking?

23. Which condition would a patient be suffering if they were to become truculent, gradually lose consciousness, have cold, clammy skin?

24. Which condition would a patient be suffering if they exhibited no signs of life and were not breathing?

25. If a patient had a dazed appearance, jerking movements and lose consciousness which condition would they suffering from?

26. If a patient was experiencing crushing chest pains, be vomiting and have a death-like appearance, which condition would they suffering from?

27. If a patient had a rash/skin irritation, oedema and lose consciousness, which condition would they be suffering from?

28. If a patient had a sharp pain down their left arm radiating into the neck with a regular pulse and be breathless, which condition would they suffering from?

29. When a patient hyperventilates, explain why they need to rebreathe carbon dioxide.

30. Which position is a patient placed in following a medical emergency?

31. What is another name for the answer to question 30?

32. Briefly explain how to place a patient in the position answered in questions 30 and 31.

33. State two airway adjuncts that could be used to provide oxygen when a patient experiences a medical emergency.

34. If a patient suffered a medical emergency where they were breathing for themselves, which airway adjunct would you provide?

35. If a patient suffered a medical emergency where they were not breathing for themselves, which adjunct would you provide?

36. If a patient required supplementary oxygen during treatment with intravenous sedation what adjunct would be provided?

37. What is the maximum flow rate of an oxygen cylinder?

38. State one sign or symptom that would indicate a patient has a blocked airway.

39. Briefly explain how to undertake a head, tilt and chin lift.

40. What is the purpose of undertaking a head, tilt and chin lift?

41. If a patient has a neck injury, why is a jaw thrust undertaken as opposed to a head, tilt and chin lift?

42. Briefly explain how to undertake a jaw thrust.

43. What should be ensured after either a head, tilt and chin lift or jaw thrust has been performed?

44. Of the two airways (oropharyngeal and nasopharyngeal), which is thought to be better tolerated by patients?

45. Why would a nasopharyngeal airway be used over an oropharyngeal?

SECTION VIII Questions: Essential anatomy

> **LEARNING OUTCOMES**
>
> At the end of this section, you should be able to identify any gaps in your personal knowledge associated with:
>
> - The heart, blood and circulation of the blood through the heart
> - The respiratory system
> - The sites for cannulation, associated veins and venepuncture complications

Heart

1. What is the average adult heart rate at rest?

2. What type of circulation is it when deoxygenated blood travels from the heart to the lungs?

3. If a thrombus blocked part of a vessel in the heart this could reduce the effectiveness of the pumping action and could cause what condition?

4. What structure of the heart divides the left and right sides?

5. Where does the deoxygenated blood originate to enter the superior vena cava to be transported to the heart?

6. Which type of blood is transported in the pulmonary vein?

7. Name three valves of the heart.

8. What is the function of the heart valves?

9. The aorta transports blood from the heart to the body. This is known as what type of circulation?

10. What is hypertension commonly known as?

11. What is hypotension commonly known as?

12. What is tachycardia commonly known as?

13. What is bradycardia commonly known as?

14. What is the name of the heart chamber that receives blood from the lungs?

15. Oxygenated blood leaves the heart via which structure?

16. Name the valve between the two left chambers.

17. Name the valve between the two right chambers.

18. Which is the only artery to carry deoxygenated blood?

19. Valves are a feature of which type of blood vessel?

20. Name the four chambers of the heart.

21. The tricuspid valve prevents the backflow of blood between which two chambers?

22. What type of blood does the aorta transport to the body?

23. What is the name of the artery that does not carry oxygenated blood?

Blood

Plasma
1. Plasma is described as what colour?

2. Plasma equates to what percentage of the blood volume?

3. What is the function of plasma?

4. List four substances that plasma carries around the body.

5. Of what is plasma mainly formed?

Red blood cells
1. What do red blood cells carry around the body?

2. Where are red blood cells formed?

3. What is the medical name for red blood cells?

4. What is the life span of a red blood cell?

5. Where are red blood cells destroyed?

6. What gives red blood cells their colour?

7. What is the percentage of the total number of red blood cells?

8. What is the function of red blood cells?

9. What shape are red blood cells?

10. Where are red blood cells stored in the body?

White blood cells

1. What is the medical name for white blood cells?

2. White blood cells are formed in bone marrow and where else?

3. What is the function of white blood cells?

4. What is the life span of a white blood cell?

5. Where are white blood cells stored in the body?

6. Where are white blood cells destroyed in the body?

Platelets

1. What is the life span of platelets?

2. What is the medical name given to platelets?

3. What is the function of platelets?

4. Where are platelets formed?

5. Where are platelets stored in the body?

6. What form/shape do platelets take?

7. Where are platelets destroyed in the body?

Diseases/conditions of the blood

1. What is a deficiency in haemoglobin called?

2. A malignant disease of white cells is called?

3. Patients with a low iron count may be suffering from?

4. Name a blood disorder that mainly affects Afro-Caribbeans.

5. What is the main characteristic of the blood disorder that affects some Afro-Caribbeans?

6. What drugs can affect the coagulation of blood?

7. What does INR stand for?

8. Name three diseases that are caused by a missing factor in the coagulation of the blood.

Miscellaneous

1. Blood cells are also known by which name?

2. What are the four main blood groups?

3. What is the most common blood group and universal recipient from all other groups?

4. Which blood cells possess a nucleus?

5. Which blood cells are biconcave in shape?

6. Human blood consists of plasma plus three other types of cells which are known as?

7. Approximately how many litres of blood does an adult have?

8. What is the pH of the blood?

9. Which blood cell is variable in shape?

10. Which blood cells are known as phagocytes?

11. What percentage of blood is water?

12. Which blood cell can form a clot without a severed vessel being present?

13. Which blood cells are responsible for coagulation?

14. Which blood cell transports oxygen around the body?

15. Which blood cell aids defence of the body?

16. What is the name of the transport medium of the blood?

17. Which blood cells live for approximately120 days?

18. Which blood cells live for approximately 13–21 days?

19. Which blood cells live for approximately 8–10 days?

20. What is meant by a phagocyte?

The respiratory system

The nose and the nasal cavity

1. What is the name of hair-like substances that line the nose?

2. What is the function of hair-like substances that line the nose?

3. What is the name given to the structure that separates the two chambers of the nose?

4. How are foreign bodies removed from the nose?

The pharynx

1. What is the pharynx also known as?

2. How long is the pharynx?

3. Which structures does the pharynx connect?

4. Once food has been masticated, through which structure does it pass into?

5. What anatomical structure protects the respiratory structure when eating, directing the food into the oesophagus?

The larynx

1. What is the larynx sometimes referred as?

2. Of what is the larynx made?

3. What does the larynx contain?

4. What is inflammation of the larynx known as?

5. What action does the larynx have?

6. What is the first section of the cartilage known as?

7. If a laryngeal blockage occurred and it was impossible to ventilate a patient by any other means, what emergency procedure would be carried out?

The trachea and the bronchial tree

1. What is the trachea lined with?

2. What is the function of the lining of the trachea?

3. What is the length of the trachea?

4. Of what is the trachea made?

5. What structure sits behind the trachea?

6. What are the branches known as where the trachea splits into two?

7. If an item was lost during dental treatment, which of the two branches at the bottom of the trachea is it more likely to enter?

8. What is the name given to the smaller tubes at the end of the second and tertiary branches?

9. What is the structure where the smaller tubes terminate?

10. What do the flattened epithelial cells line?

The lungs and the pleura

1. In which part of the lungs does oxygen exchange take place?

2. The lungs and heart are found in the chest cavity which is also known as?

3. Gaseous exchange occurs within which part of the lungs?

4. Through which structure does the deoxygenated blood enter the lungs?

5. Through which structure does the oxygenated blood leave the lungs?

6. Adult lungs contain approximately how many air-filled sacs?

7. Which lung is higher than the other?

8. Which lung is smaller than the other?

9. Which lung is shorter than the other?

10. How many lobes does the right lung have?

11. How many lobes does the left lung have?

12. What is the name of the lobes in the right lung?

13. What is the name of the lobes in the left lung?

14. When the lobes divide further into lobules, what shape are they?

15. What surrounds the lungs?

16. What is the function of the structure that surrounds the lungs?

17. What would cause the lungs to collapse?

18. If a patient has pleurisy when do they experience pain?

The diaphragm and the intercostal muscles

1. What is the function of the diaphragm?

2. Where are the intercostal muscles situated?

Respiration

1. What is the process of internal respiration?

2. What is the process of external respiration?

3. How much oxygen is present in the air we breathe?

4. Air breathed in consists of 20% oxygen plus what other gases?

5. List the three phases of breathing.

6. How much oxygen is delivered to a patient when a pocket mask is used without supplementary oxygen during cardiopulmonary resuscitation?

7. The frequency of breathing is directly related to the amount of carbon dioxide in the blood. However, which organ controls respiration?

8. What muscles are used during normal breathing?

9. If difficult breathing is experienced, which additional muscles aid the muscles used during normal breathing?

10. What can increase the rate and depth of respiration?

11. Through which structure in the respiratory system does gaseous exchange take place?

12. When gaseous exchange takes place what is this process known as?

13. Which gases are exchanged during respiration?

14. What percentage of oxygen is exchanged for carbon dioxide?

15. List the characteristics of gases.

16. Patients can sometimes increase their breathing voluntarily due to fear, which results in the level of carbon dioxide being reduced. This in turn results in their breathing stopping. If this happened, what name would be given to this state/condition?

17. If a patient voluntarily increased their breathing and as a result their breathing stopped, what action would be taken to restore their breathing?

Miscellaneous
1. Which organ initiates the cough reflex?

2. List the structures that make up the respiratory system.

3. What is pleurisy?

4. How much oxygen does expired air contain?

5. What is the name of the microscopic hairs that line the respiratory tract?

6. Through which structure does oxygenated blood leaves the lungs?

7. What are the main gases exchanged during respiration?

8. What is the name given to the sheet of muscle forming the base of the chest cavity?

9. Oxygen is carried around the body by what type of cells?

10. What is the correct name for the windpipe?

11. Of what is the windpipe made?

12. In the venous circulatory system what carries carbon dioxide?

13. Which arteries do not carry oxygenated blood?

14. What is the function of the microscopic hairs that line the majority of the respiratory tract?

15. What are the alveoli lined with?

16. What are the alveoli surrounded by?

17. What separates the chest cavity and the abdominal cavity?

18. Which structures make up the upper respiratory tract?

19. Which structures make up the lower respiratory tract?

20. What makes us breathe?

21. What is the function of the respiratory system?

22. Oxygen is necessary for life, and when in combustion with food what does it produce for all cells?

23. What is commonly known as tachypnea?

24. What is commonly known as bradypnea?

The dorsum of the hand and the antecubital fossa

The dorsum of the hand

1. What is the dorsum of the hand also known as?

2. What is the name given to the veins in the dorsum of the hand?

3. Which veins drain into the dorsum of the hand?

4. What are the disadvantages of cannulation in the dorsum of the hand?

5. What are the advantages of cannulation in the dorsum of the hand?

The antecubital fossa

1. Where is the antecubital fossa?

2. When cannulation takes place in the antecubital fossa, what is the name of the common veins used?

3. When cannulation takes place in the antecubital fossa, which artery must carefully be avoided?

4. What are the disadvantages of cannulation in the antecubital fossa?

5. What are the advantages of cannulation in the antecubital fossa?

Miscellaneous

1. Which vein connects the cephalic and basilica veins?

2. Anatomically, where does the basilica vein run?

3. Anatomically, where does the cephalic vein run?

4. How can veins be engorged prior to cannulation?

SECTION I Answers: Reasons for the provision of sedation

Anxiety

1. Anxiety is a state of unease that patients can often relate to as they remember whatever is causing them to feel anxious. Their memories may be something that they experienced or it may have been a translated experience from others. As many patients can explain and relate to the specific cause or occasion in their life that resulted in their feelings of anxiousness when faced with a similar situation/experience, they can cope with it. This means that they are amenable patients.

2. Being worried, frightened or concerned about dental treatment.

3. Sweaty palms, a raised heart rate and a fluttering sensation in their stomachs.

4. Pain. Fear of the unknown. Surrendering themselves into the total care of another. Bodily change and disfigurement and feelings of claustrophobia.

5. When pain or anxiety is experienced, it can lead to the sympathetic nervous system over-reacting. This can lead to a raised heart rate and blood pressure.

Phobia

1. Phobias are abnormal, deep-rooted, long-lasting fears of something that rarely goes away. This makes it very difficult to manage and treat someone who experiences this in the dental surgery.

This condition is very hard to overcome or to alter the way in which the patient thinks and feels. The cause of the phobia is usually deep rooted and is often initiated from a previous experience that they cannot recall that is now embedded in their subconscious. The patient has no control over it and quite often cannot explain its origin or why they are phobic about a specific thing, which means they are very difficult to treat.

2. In childhood or during adolescence.

3. The fears of their parents, as their phobias/fears can be transferred to the child by observation and the way a parent responds to and talks about the dentist. It may also be associated with the fear of blood, injury or hospitals, due to a personal experience. Some phobias can occur on their own without having a rational explanation.

4. They would tense their muscles and could become un-cooperative.

5. Dental injections and handpiece.

Miscellaneous

1. Fear and the cost of dental treatments.

2. Lack of a dentist in the patient's area. Not being able to register with a dentist or suffering ill health, resulting in mobility problems.

3. It allows them to accept dental treatment and therefore maintain a healthy mouth.

4. Conscious sedation is defined as 'a technique in which the use of a drug or drugs produces a state of depression of the central nervous system enabling treatment to be carried out, but during which verbal contact with the patient is maintained throughout the period of sedation. The drugs and techniques used to provide conscious sedation for dental treatment should carry a margin of safety wide enough to render loss of consciousness unlikely'.

5. Humanitarian (anxious and dental phobic patients) reasons, physiological factors and complex dental treatment.

6. Patients who are anxious. As anxiety is controllable to some degree, many patients will attend the dentist for treatment and with good patient management will undergo treatment with or without the aid of sedation, depending on their treatment plan.

7. Anxiety.

8. For patients who suffer feelings of anxiety and phobia regarding dental treatment, sedation can help them to accept it.

9. When a person experiences pain or is anxious, it can have an adverse effect on their myocardium resulting in a raised heart rate and high blood pressure. By providing a form of conscious sedation to patients more susceptible, that is middle-aged people, pre-existing hypertension and coronary artery disease, it allows them to receive treatment without unnecessary strain being placed on their myocardium.

10. Most patients will attend the dentist for routine treatment without the aid of conscious sedation. However, on occasions they may require an unusual procedure such as minor oral surgery. This can be more stressful, more complex and may take longer than routine treatment. A form of conscious sedation will make a complex treatment easier to cope with as it will be less stressful for them.

SECTION II Answers: Medico-legal aspects of dental sedation

Current legislation

1. Clinicians have to justify each provision of sedation, ensuring that the technique provided reflects the patient's medical, dental and social history and that the dental procedure to be undertaken reduces the patient's anxiety levels without being too invasive. Clinicians establish this through a thorough patient assessment being carried out with consent being taken.

2. These modes of sedation are not recommended for routine use in the dental surgery. If practiced, they must be administered by a clinician in appropriate circumstances and setting. They should only be used when no other titratable technique is appropriate.

3. For sedation to be offered, all members of the team must have undergone suitable practical and theoretical training, with staff members in training being adequately supervised. Training must encompass the drugs and equipment used. Any training received must be documented and can either be through attendance at a formal course or in-house. If in-house the course must be accredited. Anyone organising training for staff must ensure that the training received is delivered by appropriate instructors and in suitable settings. Continuing professional development should also take place. The sedation team must undertake 12 hours of sedation training within a five year period.

4. The surgery must be suitable for the provision of sedation, with both the treatment and recovery areas being large enough for the team to undertake treatment. The chair's equipment should allow for the head down tilt position to manage an emergency should one occur.

5. All members of the dental team must be familiar with emergency procedures. They must receive training and updates on a regular basis. Simulations should take place within the practice. All emergency drugs must be available, kept secure and re-stocked when required, coupled with a means of administering them to patients. They should be checked on a daily basis to ensure they are in date, with equipment serviced and maintained according to the manufacturer's guidelines. A means of securing a patent airway and administering oxygen must be available. Risk assessments must be undertaken in order to control the provision of sedation and to reduce the risk of accidents or mishaps. Dental practices should undertake audits to police the quality of care provided, thereby ensuring best practice.

6. Only dedicated machines for dental use should be used that conform to British Standards. They must be regularly serviced and looked after as per the manufacturer's guidelines. All documentation relating to the inhalation sedation machine must be kept. All oxygen and nitrous oxide cylinders must be stored securely. Colour-coded pipes on piped machines must only fit into their respective outlets. Inhalation sedation machines must comply with the set standards. To prevent a hypoxic mixture being administered fail-safe mechanisms must be installed. Scavenging systems should be used to remove the waste nitrous oxide from

the atmosphere. Nasal masks must be a good fit to avoid excess nitrous oxide being exhaled into the surgery.

7. The surgery must be stocked with all the required sedation and emergency equipment. All staff involved must have sufficient and suitable training, knowledge and skills. All electrical equipment used must be calibrated, serviced and maintained according to the manufacturer's guidelines with records of such being kept. Drugs and syringes must be labelled for correct identification. The administration of any drug should be according to accepted current guidelines and titrated against patient's responses.

8. The lowest possible dose of oral sedation should be prescribed. Patients must be advised that they will have to adhere to the same pre- and post-operative instructions as for intravenous sedation and therefore must be accompanied by a responsible escort.

9. Written and verbal pre- and post-operative instructions must be provided to both the patient and their escort. This must be in a format that reflects the patients age, maturity and understanding.

10. Patients must be supervised and monitored by an appropriate member of the team. The patient must be allowed time to recover and during this period the clinician must be available. Patients must be recovered in either the dental chair or a separate recovery area. Not in the waiting room. Patients must be assessed for discharge by ensuring they are able to walk without help and are steady on their feet. They will be discharged into the care of their responsible escort who will be provided with the post-operative instructions for both the sedation and the dental treatment. These instructions should also contain emergency telephone numbers.

11. Record-keeping must be excellent and reflect the patient's treatment pathway and consent to treatment.

12. Before referring patients for treatment with conscious sedation, the dentist must have explored all other avenues of pain and anxiety control. They must also be confident that the establishment to which they are referring their patient is practising treatment with sedation reflecting the guidelines.

13. Where clinical visual monitoring takes place and intravenous sedation is administered, it is mandatory to use electrical monitoring by using a pulse oximeter and blood pressure machine. The team providing sedation must be capable of monitoring a patient's skin tone, pulse, respiration, blood pressure, level of consciousness and anxiety, also ensuring the patient maintains a patent airway. Monitoring must take place at appropriate and regular intervals.

14. If children are uncooperative and difficult to manage, they may not be suitable for conscious sedation in which case a general anaesthetic may be considered as a treatment option. When assessing children for conscious sedation, it must be remembered that they are individuals with different levels of maturity and understanding. For children who will not accept dental treatment with local anaesthesia alone, inhalation sedation should be the first choice offered. Intravenous sedation is not ideal for children; however, on rare occasions if it is used then it will be administered by a clinician who specialises in paediatric sedation. When local anaesthetic is administered, a topical should be used to reduce any discomfort and if possible it

should also be applied on the cannulation site. Any information provided to a child must be age/maturity appropriate.

Medico-legal considerations when providing dental sedation

1. Taking and recording of consent, maintaining a patient's confidentiality, accusations of assault and negligence.

Consent

1. Consent is when one person gives another permission to undertake something such as dental treatment. It is granted once the person consenting is aware of what is going to happen and it can be withdrawn at any time.

2. Obtaining consent from patients for dental treatment is best practice. Many clinicians routinely take written consent for various dental procedures where complications could occur. There is not any recommended pro forma; however, whichever one is used it must contain both the patient's personal details and the practice details. It must be completed in ink without using abbreviations. It must be signed by both parties involved with the patient receiving a copy. Only a qualified clinician can take consent from patients and when doing so it should be in a quiet, private area in order to maintain the patient's confidentiality. Patients should be allowed to ask questions. If the patient is receiving sedation, consent should ideally be taken during a separate assessment appointment to allow a cooling-off period. Consent should never be taken under duress and it is not a one-off action but an ongoing process and it should be regularly checked and updated, especially if the course of treatment is lengthy involving several appointments.

3. With intravenous sedation, all eventualities must be discussed and recorded, allowing the patient to detail any treatments that he or she does not wish to undergo. This is because midazolam, the sedative drug used, produces anterograde amnesia, which means the patient may not be able to remember anything after the induction of the drug, including any conversations held. Therefore, if the treatment plan required changing the treatment would have to be stopped, the patient recovered and an appointment made for another day. This would be to discuss their options and further consent obtained, as they would not remember the conversation despite appearing to be alert.

4. Written, verbal or a compliant action.

5. Implied and expressed.

6. Implied consent is when a patient accepts treatment by a compliant action such as sitting in the dental chair and opening his/her mouth. Expressed is when a patient either verbally agrees or completes and signs a consent form to receive treatment.

7. Implied.

8. Expressed.

9. The patient must be provided with adequate information. Also be advised of the proposed treatment required, together with the mode of sedation being provided. They must be made aware of the advantages and disadvantages of any treatment proposed and the advantages and disadvantages of the mode of sedation. They must be made aware of any alternative treatments along with other forms of sedation that could be provided. All risks associated with the treatment that is higher than 0.5% must be discussed. Timescale of the appointment must be advised along with the patient being told that they must be able to make the necessary arrangements, to reflect the pre- and post-operative instructions for the mode of sedation they are to receive. The cost of treatment must be advised, coupled with the associated costs for the provision of sedation.

10. Patient education. Maximise patient cooperation. Improve clinician and patient communication and to protect the clinician from complaints, claims and charges.

11. For all sedation techniques. General anaesthetics. Clinical examination and treatment. When taking radiographs and photographs. Student observations. Research. Possible keeping of body parts.

12. The patient must be able to give consent, understand and retain the information being provided, consider it and come to a decision themselves, give their consent to treatment without feeling pressurised by anyone, so that it is given voluntarily.

13. The person who is capable of carrying out the procedure, that is, a qualified clinician. As dental nurses are not able to take consent, good practice would be for them to check that consent is in place before dental treatment commences.

14. Always – a competent adult. Persons between 16 and 18 years old. A legal guardian, appointed by a court, or by a parent taking parental responsibility for the child.
   Sometimes – adults considered incompetent in other aspects of life may be able to consent to simple treatments but not complex procedures where detailed information is provided. Children younger than 16 years of age who the clinician deems as Gillick competent refuses treatment, the person with parental responsibility can override that decision when a refusal is not in the patient's best interests, despite them being deemed Gillick competent.
   Never – the natural father if they are not married to the child's mother, unless his name is recorded on the child's birth certificate with the registration of the birth taking place before 1 December 2003. Friends and relatives.

15. The treating clinician.

16. It should ideally be taken during a separate assessment appointment, in a quiet place thus allowing the patient to ask questions whilst maintaining their confidentiality. This allows a cooling-off period. Consent should never be taken under duress. It is not a one-off action but an ongoing process. It should be regularly checked and updated, especially if the course of treatment is lengthy involving several appointments.

17. A patient could have cause to complain and possibly sue as this could constitute assault. Any treatment undertaken that was not documented could mean that the clinician was negligent and at fault.

18. Evidence of the agreement between the two parties as it would detail the discussions held and treatments the patient consented to.

19. Competent means that the person understands the treatment they require and the implications of receiving or declining it.

20. This is for patients younger than 16 years of age. The patient is assessed to establish if they have the maturity and capacity to understand, retain and make a decision based on the facts presented and fully understand the implications of receiving or not receiving treatment. It is only the clinician who can make the assessment of the patient's capacity to consent and when classed as Gillick competent they can consent to treatment without the person who holds parental responsibility being informed or giving their permission. The principle of Gillick competence is only used in exceptional circumstances.

21. The treating clinician.

Confidentiality

1. All.

2. Their consent to do so.

3. Only used for the purpose it was provided.

4. If it was of benefit to them, that is, their health was at risk. If it was in the interests of the general public or considered that a serious crime was imminent.

5. Only the minimum amount of information should be furnished.

6. Any information received must be treated as confidential. It should not be shared unless permission to do so has been provided. It must be stored safely. Any information being forwarded must be done under secure conditions and destroyed once dealt with. Dental records are to be stored away from others who have no need to access them. When discussing any patient's cases/history/treatment plans, the conversations should be held where conversations cannot be overheard. Screen savers and passwords should be used for computers. Any sensitive telephone calls/conversations must be held in private. All enquiries relating to another's appointments and so on or if a patient telephones for any results of treatment should be declined.

Assault

1. Consent to be obtained with written evidence provided of what was agreed. The dentist must only undertake dental procedures once the patient fully understands the treatment plan and is happy to proceed. The clinician must always be chaperoned.

2. Midazolam is a sedative that relaxes patients, reducing their anxiety whilst providing amnesic effects. Vivid dreams can be experienced by some patients who truly believe that they occurred.

Negligence

1. Any action where the dental team acts outside the law and/or will have provided dental treatment that is not acceptable.

2. Good communication with patients regarding treatment in order that they understand which treatments are to be undertaken and those that are not. Written consent being obtained. Contemporaneous record-keeping. Informing the patient of any lesions and so on, they are monitoring within their mouths. Well-trained staff. Recording any conversations held with patients over the telephone, ensuring the summary is factual. Recording any cancelled or failed appointments and non-payment for treatment. Providing a safe environment for all, ensuring all equipment is serviced at recommended intervals.

Miscellaneous

1. The General Dental Council (GDC).

2. Patient's medical, dental and social history, including any previous treatments, general anaesthetic and/or conscious sedation. Any change in the medical history/status.

   Details of the assessment appointment. The mode of sedation and the treatment being provided, the justification for its use and any patient preferences. Written consent and verbal and written pre- and post-operative instructions are provided. The patient is still happy to proceed with the planned treatment. They have adhered to all instructions, the responsible escort is in attendance and details of the mode of transport home. Details of the treatment appointment. All monitoring details, cannula site, drug used, batch number and expiry date, drug titrations and times administered.

   The recovery information and that the patient is assessed for discharge. Any complications and statements of how the patient responded to the mode of sedation used and/or reactions within the recovery phase.

3. Put patients' interest first. Communicate effectively with patients. Obtain valid consent. Maintain and protect patients' information. Have a clear and effective complaints procedure. Work with colleagues in a way that is in the patients' best interests. Maintain, develop and work within your professional knowledge and skills. Principles of confidentiality. Raise concerns if patients are at risk. Make your professional behaviour maintains patients' confidence in you and the dental profession.

4. 2000.

5. 2003.

6. 2015.

7. 12 hours.

8. Second appropriate person.

SECTION III Answers: Role of the sedation nurse

Role of the sedation nurse when a patient is receiving treatment with conscious sedation

1. To meet the General Dental Council (GDC) guidelines. If that person is a dental nurse, then the duties expected are extended beyond that of their primary training received. To ensure that every aspect runs as smoothly as possible. Ensure that the patient has followed all pre-operative instructions relevant for the type of sedation being provided. Act as a chaperone to both the patient and clinician, irrespective of gender. Assist the clinician in the clinical and electrical monitoring of a patient's vital signs, alerting the clinician to any changes and respond accordingly. Assist with the dental procedure. Provide reassurance to the patient throughout treatment. Respond and assist the clinician should an emergency arise. Assist with the recovery of the patient, although some clinicians may place this responsibility upon the sedation nurse. Assist when assessing the patient for discharge. Provide verbal post-operative instructions to the patient and the escort relevant to the mode of sedation provided, the procedure undertaken and to furnish the patient and escort with written instructions for reinforcement if the clinician requests them to. Possibly book a follow-up appointment and take payment for the treatment and the method of sedation provided. Practise excellent cross-infection control, ensuring the health and safety of all, maintaining the patient's diversity, dignity/rights and uphold the confidentiality of the patient.

2. The norm is a sedation nurse. In some clinical environments, it may be another clinician. In other dental surgeries where there are lots of staff members, there could be a clinician, a dental nurse to assist with the patient's treatment and a sedation nurse allocated to the conscious sedation aspect of the patient's appointment.

3. Many of the skills attained while training as a dental nurse and subsequently practised will be utilised. Further training can be acquired by accessing a recognised course in conscious sedation that leads to National Examining Board for Dental Nurses' qualification in dental sedation nursing. However, training can be sought via a short course that does not lead to a qualification, or accredited in-house training with the student being supervised and suitably assessed.

4. In order that the sedation nurse fully understands their role within the team, they do not work outside that remit and are able to recognise the areas of a patient's care for which they are responsible. For the patient to receive treatment with conscious sedation in a safe, relaxed and calm atmosphere.

5. To allow safe treatment to be received, everything required is available and checked that it is in working order and the clinician is not left unsupervised.

6. The surgery will be disinfected with primary and secondary zones identified. All instruments required for the procedure will be sterile. Any materials and medicaments required will be prepared. The appropriate equipment to reflect the type of sedation the patient is to receive will be prepared. Equipment required to carry out medical checks and monitoring equipment will be made ready. The patient's dental notes and radiographs will be available and the

sedation nurse will ensure that a signed consent form has been completed. At some point, the patient's notes will be read, especially the medical history. Previous treatments the patient has undergone with conscious sedation will be referenced along with the amount of sedation the patient received. Good contemporaneous notes being kept are vital in order that the team can refer to them. The medical emergency equipment will be present and functional and the drug expiry dates checked. If intravenous or oral sedation is being provided, the reversal drug flumazenil will be available. If inhalation sedation is being administered, the machine will be checked, the scavenging system attached and good ventilation present within the surgery.

7. Tourniquet, disinfectant surface medi-wipe, a cannula, either a 22-gauge Venflon or, a Y can, two 23-gauge drawing up needles, a 5 ml sodium chloride flush, a 2 ml sterile syringe with a sodium chloride label placed, a 5 ml sterile syringe with a drug label (midazolam) placed, ampoule of midazolam and the reversal drug flumazenil together with a 5 ml sterile syringe and a 23-gauge drawing up needle. The emergency drugs and equipment will also be available along with a blood pressure machine and pulse oximeter. In addition to this, the patient's notes, signed consent form and any radiographs will be made available.

8. A relative analgesia machine, whether it is a mobile machine or a piped system. It will be checked to ensure it is safe for use. A scavenging system will be attached and functional along with a range of nasal masks in case patients do not bring theirs. The emergency drugs and equipment will also be available along with the patient's notes, signed consent form and any radiographs with good ventilation being provided within the surgery.

9. Emergency drugs and equipment. A blood pressure machine and pulse oximeter. Cannulation equipment should also be present. Flumazenil will be prepared. If the patient is to receive intravenous midazolam, then ampoules will be available along with a blood pressure machine and pulse oximeter. In addition to this, the patient's notes, signed consent form and any radiographs will be made available.

10. Emergency drugs and equipment. A blood pressure machine and pulse oximeter. Cannulation equipment should also be present. Midazolam and flumazenil will be prepared. If per nasal sedation is being provided, a sterile syringe and nasal atomiser are available. If oral midazolam is being provided, either some cold tea or squash will be available. A log book outlining the transmucosal/off-licence sedation is being used along with drug amounts, patient and clinician details. In addition to this, the patient's notes, signed consent form and any radiographs will be made available.

Role of the sedation nurse during patient treatment

1. They will check that a consent form has been signed and that the patient's notes and radiographs, if required, are present. Prepare the surgery to reflect the form of sedation being administered. They will ensure that the patient has complied with all pre-operative instructions relevant to the type of sedation being administered, act as a chaperone to both the patient and clinician, aid the clinician in the clinical and electrical monitoring of a patient's vital signs and alert the clinician to any changes, responding accordingly. They will assist with the dental procedure, reassuring the patient throughout treatment. They will respond and assist the clinician should an emergency arise. They will assist with the recovery of the patient and if requested of by the clinician, recover the patient autonomously. They will assist when assessing the patient for discharge. They may provide verbal post-operative instructions to the patient

and escort relevant to the mode of sedation received, the procedure undertaken and to furnish the patient and the escort with written instructions for reinforcement. They may possibly book a follow-up appointment and take the payment for the treatment and the method of sedation provided. Throughout the appointment, they will employ excellent cross-infection control, ensuring the health and safety of all, maintain the patient's diversity, dignity/rights and uphold the confidentiality of the patient.

2. They will assist in accordance to the dental treatment being received. They will assist with cannulation. They will monitor the patient's vital signs and periodically observe the pulse oximeter, ensuring that the patient's percentage of saturated oxygen and pulse rate are still within the normal limits for that patient. If they recognise any changes in the patient's level of consciousness or are unhappy about vital signs of the patient, they must inform the clinician. They will continually praise and reassure the patient throughout the period of treatment. Document the administration times of drug titrated to the patient and if no more is given during treatment, record the patient's percentage of saturated oxygen and pulse rate periodically. If the patient experiences an emergency or becomes over-sedated, they will respond accordingly, assisting as directed by the clinician. They will record an overview of the patient's response to treatment with intravenous sedation. Once treatment has been completed, they will either assist or be asked to autonomously recover and assess the patient for discharge providing written and verbal post-operative instructions to both the patient and escort.

3. They will make sure that the patient is sitting comfortably and that the chair is placed in a high position, with the back semi-supine. They may be requested to help locate a suitable vein to place the cannula. If the patient has cold hands, provide a source of heat such as a jug of warm water. They will pass the tourniquet to the clinician. Some clinicians may request that the sedation nurse applies a tourniquet. If a clinician does not use a tourniquet, the sedation nurse may be requested to place both hands around the patient's arm to apply pressure. Once the veins are engorged, they will pass a medi-wipe to the clinician. Once it is used, they will accept it in exchange for the cannula. When the cannula is being inserted, they will make sure that the patient is as relaxed as possible by talking to them. They will remind the patient that they will feel a sharp scratch as the cannula is being inserted. Once a back flash of blood appears within the cannula, it will indicate that it has been inserted into the vein; however, it must be remembered that this indication is not a guarantee of successful cannulation. They will continue to make small talk to occupy the patient, taking his or her thoughts away from the placement. Once the cannula has been inserted, they may be requested to apply pressure at point of entry to restrict blood flow while the clinician removes the introducing needle. They will have a sharps bin ready for the clinician to place the used introducing needle. They may be requested to remove the tourniquet. The 2 ml sterile labelled syringe, previously drawn up by the clinician, containing the sodium chloride flush will be given to the clinician, stating the contents of the syringe. The batch number and the expiry date should have already been checked with the clinician and documented using the method of recording a patient's treatment pathway. They will watch the cannulation site as the sodium chloride flush is being administered for any swelling, somewhat like a fried egg, that might appear. The sedation nurse will inform the patient that he or she will experience a cold sensation travelling up his or her arm and that there should be no pain. They will record any failed cannulation in the documentation of the patient's treatment pathway, along with the successful cannulation, recording the size of the cannula and the site used. Once successful cannulation has been gained, they will secure the cannula with either non-allergenic tape or a Venflon dressing, taking care not to pull the cannula out of the vein wall. They will place the pulse oximeter probe onto the patient's finger, explaining the reason for its use and will have previously set the

pulse and oxygen saturation level warning alarms that are incorporated in the pulse oximeter to suit the physiology of the patient. Finally, they will give the 5 ml sterile, labelled syringe, containing the sedation drug to the clinician previously drawn up by him or her, stating its contents. Once again the batch number and the expiry date should have been checked with the clinician and documented, using the method of recording a patient's treatment pathway. During the administration of midazolam, they will continue talking to the patient asking him or her how he or she is feeling. They will continue to praise and reassure the patient. While midazolam is being administered, they will record, once again using the method of documenting the patient's treatment, the initial bolus and any incremental titrations of the drug given, making a note of the time. The patient's percentage of saturated oxygen and pulse must also be recorded, along with a brief statement of the patient's response.

4. The sedation nurse will provide the patient with a brief explanation of the equipment being used. Reassure and monitor the patient's vital signs throughout treatment. Assist the patient when placing the mask over his or her nose and ensure that it is a comfortable fit and not too big, checking for leaks. They will check the tubing attached to the mask is secure and will hold the mask in place throughout treatment. Continually monitor the patient's vital signs, ensuring they are within the normal limits for the patient and to ensure they are comfortable. They will record the time and the percentages of nitrous oxide and oxygen administered in the documentation used for the patient's treatment. They will monitor the reservoir bag, making sure it is not being sucked in or ballooning. They will continue to monitor the reservoir bag in conjunction with the patient's breathing. At the clinician's request, they will speak to the patient and constantly praise and reassure them. They will encourage the patient to breathe through the nose and not the mouth. They will record any changes to the percentage of nitrous oxide and oxygen administered in the documentation used for the patient's treatment. If the patient experiences an emergency or becomes over-sedated, they will respond accordingly, assisting as directed by the clinician. They will record an overview of the patient's response to treatment with inhalation sedation. They will document that 100% oxygen for 3–5 minutes was administered. Once the mask has been removed from the patient's nose, the machine can be switched off. Finally, they will either assist or be asked to autonomously recover and assess the patient for discharge, providing written and verbal post-operative instructions to both the patient and the escort if one is in attendance.

5. They will welcome the patient and start to monitor his or her vital signs. Invite the escort to take a seat. Ask the patient the same questions and undertake the same medical checks as for intravenous sedation and ensure they have complied with the pre-operative instructions and can comply with the post-operative ones. Record all discussions held and the outcome of the patient's medical checks in the documentation used to record the patient's treatment. They will assist with cannulation if a cannula is being inserted. If an intravenous drug is used in conjunction with oral sedation, any amounts titrated must be written in the method used to record the patient's treatment, along with the patient's percentage of saturated oxygen and pulse rate. Continually reassure and praise the patient and monitor vital signs of the patient, recording the percentage of saturated oxygen and pulse rate periodically in the method of documenting the patient's treatment. Inform the clinician if any changes occur that are not within the normal limit for the patient. If the patient experiences an emergency or becomes over-sedated, they will respond accordingly, assisting as directed by the clinician. Finally, they will either assist or be asked to autonomously recover and assess the patient for discharge, providing written and verbal post-operative instructions to both the patient and the escort.

6. They will welcome the patient and start to monitor the vital signs. Invite the escort to take a seat. Ask the patient the same questions and undertake the same medical checks as for intravenous sedation and ensure they have complied with the pre-operative instructions and can comply with the post-operative ones. Record all discussions held and the outcome of the patient's medical checks in the documentation used to record the patient's treatment. If the route being used is the nasal method, they will prepare a syringe and atomiser; and if the route is oral, they will have prepared a cup of cold tea, orange or blackcurrant and either Epistatus or an ampoule of midazolam. They will ensure that the drug log used for transmucosal/off-licence sedation has been completed. They will assist with cannulation if a cannula is being inserted. If an intravenous drug is used in conjunction with transmucosal/off-licence sedation, any amounts titrated must be written in the method used to record the patient's treatment, along with the patient's percentage of saturated oxygen and pulse rate. Continually reassure and praise the patient and monitor the vital signs, record the percentage of saturated oxygen and pulse rate periodically in the method of documenting the patient's treatment. Inform the clinician if any changes occur that are not within the normal limit for the patient. If the patient experiences an emergency or becomes over-sedated, they will respond accordingly, assisting, as directed, by the clinician. Finally, they will either assist or be asked to autonomously recover and assess the patient for discharge, providing written and verbal post-operative instructions to both the patient and the escort.

Role of the sedation nurse during the patient's recovery period

1. They will transport all dental instruments to be sterilised and put away all materials, medicaments and equipment. They will place all sharps, once removed, into a sharps bin placing all clinical waste into appropriate bins. They will ensure that all documentation relating to the sodium chloride flush and drug used has been recorded before disposing of empty ampoules into the sharps bin or container for waste drugs. If any drug or flush is left in syringes, they will squirt the surplus sodium chloride and midazolam into a cotton wool ball/swab and place it into clinical waste. Alternatively drugs containers may be available to dispose of excess drugs. They will document the time the treatment finished and the total amount of drug the patient received. They will invite the escort into the surgery to sit with the patient and advise them how the treatment went. They will reassure the patient, answering any questions that the patient and/or the escort may have. Monitoring will continue with outcomes being documented. They will take post-operative blood pressure. They will, if requested to do so, provide written and verbal post-operative instructions for the dental treatment and sedation, including the telephone number of the dental surgery. They may assist or be requested by the clinician to autonomously assess the patient for discharge by taking the patient for a little walk establishing how steady the patient is on his or her feet. They may be requested to remove the cannula. They may be requested to assist the patient with the help of the escort to the car. They will ensure that the method of documenting the patient's treatment is complete by adding the time the patient was discharged, coupled with a statement of how the patient responded while recovering. Finally, they will undertake any unfinished cross-infection control measures, tidy up and put away items not required.

2. They will transport all dental instruments to be sterilised and put away all materials, medicaments and equipment. They will place all sharps, once removed, into a sharps bin placing all clinical waste into appropriate bins. They will continually reassure and monitor the patient's

vital signs. If an escort is present, they will invite them into the dental surgery to sit with the patient. They will inform both the patient and escort how the treatment progressed. If requested by the clinician, they will give written and verbal post-operative instructions for the treatment and sedation, including the telephone number of the dental surgery. They will assist or, if requested by the clinician, will autonomously assess the patient for discharge. They should ensure the patient is kept for twenty minutes after treatment has been completed They will record the time of discharge, write a statement of the patient's response to inhalation sedation including whether the recovery stage was uneventful and record the patient's demeanour when leaving the building. Finally, they will undertake any unfinished cross-infection control measures, tidy up and put away items not required.

3. They will transport all dental instruments to be sterilised and put away all materials, medicaments and equipment. They will place all sharps, once removed, into a sharps bin placing all clinical waste into appropriate bins. They will continually reassure and monitor the patient's vital signs. If intravenous midazolam has been used in conjunction with oral sedation, they will ensure that all documentation relevant to the sodium chloride flush and drug used has been recorded before disposing of empty ampoules into the sharps bin or container for waste drugs. If an intravenous drug was used in conjunction with oral sedation, they will dispose of any drug or flush left in syringes by squirting the surplus sodium chloride and midazolam into a cotton wool ball/swab and place it into clinical waste. Alternatively drugs containers may be available to dispose of excess drugs. They will document the time the treatment finished and the total amount of drug the patient received. They will record the time the treatment finished in the method of documenting the patient's treatment and document the total amount of drug the patient received. They will invite the patient's escort into the dental surgery to sit with them and advise them how the treatment went. They will reassure the patient, answering any questions that the patient and the escort may have. They will continually monitor the patient's percentage of saturated oxygen and pulse rate and record in the method of documenting the patient's treatment. They will take post-operative blood pressure. They will, if requested, provide written and verbal post-operative instructions for the dental treatment and sedation, including the telephone number of the dental surgery. They may assist or be requested by the clinician to autonomously assess the patient for discharge by taking the patient for a little walk, establishing how steady the patient is on his or her feet. They may be requested to remove the cannula. They may be requested to assist the patient with the help of the escort to the car. They will ensure that the method of documenting the patient's treatment is complete by adding the time the patient was discharged, coupled with a statement of how the patient responded while recovering. Finally, they will undertake any unfinished cross-infection control measures, tidy up and put away items not required.

4. They will transport all dental instruments to be sterilised and put away all materials, medicaments and equipment. They will place all sharps, once removed, into a sharps bin placing all clinical waste into appropriate bins. If intravenous midazolam was used in conjunction with transmucosal/off-licence sedation, they will ensure that all documentation relevant to the sodium chloride flush and drug used has been recorded before disposing of empty ampoules into the sharps bin or container for waste drugs. If any drug or flush is left in syringes, they will squirt the surplus sodium chloride and midazolam into a cotton wool ball/swab and place it into clinical waste. Alternatively drugs containers may be available to dispose of excess drugs. They will document the time the treatment finished and the total amount of drug the patient received. They will invite the escort into the surgery to sit with the patient and explain them

how the treatment went. They will reassure the patient, answering any questions that the patient and/or escort may have. Monitoring will continue with outcomes being documented. They will take post-operative blood pressure. They will, if requested, provide written and verbal post-operative instructions for the dental treatment and sedation, including the telephone number of the dental surgery. They may assist or be requested by the clinician to autonomously assess the patient for discharge by taking the patient for a little walk, establishing how steady the patient is on his or her feet. They may be requested to remove the cannula. They may be requested to assist the patient with the help of the escort to the car. They will ensure that the method of documenting the patient's treatment is complete by adding the time the patient was discharged, coupled with a statement of how the patient responded while recovering. Finally, they will undertake any unfinished cross-infection control measures, tidy up and put away items not required.

SECTION IV Answers: Monitoring and equipment used

Monitoring a patient's vital signs by observation

1. To establish which form of sedation would be suitable for patients according to their medical, dental and social history. To establish if the patient is fit to receive a form of conscious sedation that day. For the clinician to decide if the patient should be referred to a specialist unit or treated by themselves and their dental team.

2. Pulse and respiratory rate, level of consciousness, skin tone, demeanour, temperature, saturated oxygen levels and height and weight.

3. At the assessment appointment, before, during and after treatment.

4. As soon as the patient walks through the dental surgery door by noting their skin tone and demeanour.

5. To ensure the patient is still fit and healthy enabling them to receive dental treatment using a form of conscious sedation. When monitoring a patient's vital signs the recordings are for that day only and are an aid to decide the most suitable form of sedation, according to the patient's medical fitness, expectations and required treatment. Current outcomes of medical checks provide up-to-date baseline figures/recordings, ensuring that the patient is treated and managed safely.

Pulse rate
1. A rhythmical throbbing of the arteries as blood is pumped through them.

2. It allows a comparison, should a complication arise, along with telling us what the heart is doing and how well it is performing.

3. Anywhere where an artery passes over a bone. A pulse is a wave of distension of the artery, which travels to the periphery. Temporal (ear region), facial (chin region), carotid – trachea region, brachial (anti-cubital fossa region), ulnar (baby finger side of wrist), radial (thumb side of wrist), femoral (groin region), popliteal (knee region), posterior tibial (ankle region), dorsalis (front of foot) and apical (heart region).

4. The area where the pulse is felt should be palpated using the middle and index fingers until its pulsation is found. The number of beats counted over 30 seconds is doubled.

5. The radial pulse.

6. Beats per minute, the strength and regularity of the pulse.

7. Bpm.

8. 72 bpm.

9. 100–180 bpm.

10. 80–150 bpm.

11. 75–120 bpm.

12. 70–100 bpm.

13. Between 60 and 80 bpm.

14. Pulse oximeter or blood pressure machine.

15. The inner wrist.

16. Bradycardia.

17. Tachycardia.

Respiratory rate

1. The rate at which a person inhales and exhales. It is usually measured to obtain a quick evaluation of a person's health.

2. It is extremely important, because the drug (midazolam) used for intravenous sedation has the ability to cause respiratory depression and this must be avoided. It also allows a comparison should a complication arise.

3. After taking a patient's pulse, the patient's wrist is held. Very discreetly the rise and fall of the chest is observed and counted for 30 seconds with the amount of cycles being doubled.

4. The rise, fall and brief pause of the chest.

5. The rate and depth of respirations.

6. Rpm.

7. 30–50 rpm.

8. 20–30 rpm.

9. 12–20 rpm.

10. 12–18 rpm.

11. Bradypnea.

12. Tachypnea.

Level of consciousness

1. The definition of conscious sedation states that it is a technique in which the use of a drug or drugs produces a state of depression of the central nervous system enabling treatment to be carried out, but during which verbal contact with the patient is maintained throughout the period of sedation. The drugs and techniques used to provide conscious sedation for dental treatment should carry a margin of safety wide enough to render loss of consciousness unlikely. Therefore, monitoring a patient's level of consciousness must be undertaken to reflect this statement and provide safe sedation.

2. Is the patient responding, their complexion/skin tone, pulse and respiratory rates, blood pressure and oxygen saturation levels.

3. Blood pressure machine and pulse oximeter.

Skin tone/complexion

1. In order that the dental team is aware that this is normal for the patient, whether it is pale or flushed thereby avoiding any unnecessary concerns.

2. As soon as the patient enters the dental surgery.

3. Throughout the appointment. From assessment to discharge.

Height/weight

1. To establish the risk posed and associated difficulties that may occur should they have to be moved at any point while sedated. To inform the paramedics, if called, for them to calculate the amount of emergency drug to be administered.

2. No, as it is entirely the clinician's choice to do so.

3. Visual, scales and a height chart.

4. Body Mass Index (BMI) Chart.

5. This is the clinician's decision as to what weight they would refuse to treat a patient; however, most would say over 26 stone or the weight that a dental chair would hold.

6. Undertaking cardio-pulmonary resuscitation (CPR) on an obese patient would prove a problem if the chair will not go back to the position required. Overweight patients are more difficult to cannulate and are at a respiratory risk.

Temperature

1. Some clinicians like to be aware of the patient's body temperature to ensure that it is normal. If elevated treatment could be deferred, because this is indicative of an underlying fever.

2. 37 °C.

3. A thermometer.

4. Digital, ones containing mercury and temperature strips.

5. Ear, under the arm or tongue and using the forehead.

6. If using a thermometer containing mercury, it should be shaken down and held in the mouth for 2–3 minutes. A digital thermometer will bleep when the temperature of the body has been reached.

7. They should avoid eating, smoking or drinking for the preceding 10 minutes.

Equipment used to monitor a patient's vital signs

Pulse oximetry

1. Pulse oximetry is measurement of transmitted light through a translucent measuring site to determine a patient's oxygen status non-invasively.

2. Takuo Aoyagi, a Japanese bioengineer.

3. Early 1970s.

4. To enable early detection of cerebral hypoxia, whereby any complications can be dealt with.

5. Make sure all leads are connected properly. Switch the machine on to ensure that it performs a self-calibration. Switch off the machine to test the battery. Set the alarms, if in situ. Place it in a position that it can be seen.

6. The pulse rate and the level of saturated oxygen bound to haemoglobin.

7. They have an audible bleep that mimics the pulse along with alarms incorporated, which will activate if a patient's physiological systems fall below or above what they have been set at.

8. Observe and reassure the patient. Listen to the bleep. Periodically observe the percentage of saturated oxygen displayed. If any concerns arise, inform the clinician immediately.

9. Once cannulation is successful and prior to midazolam being administered.

10. They under measure/indicate by 1–2%. Provide an instant reading, have very little delay as they update several times a second. Enable early detection of cerebral hypoxia. They have an audible bleep, alarms incorporated and a battery back-up.

11. The pulse oximeter readings can be affected by movement, cold hands, venous pulsation, external light source, nail varnish and false nails.

12. The probe placed over a vascular bed, that is, finger allows the pulse oximeter to pick up the change in the colour of the blood as it alters from dark red to a brighter red due to the haemoglobin shifting from de-oxygenated to oxygenated state. This occurs as two lights are projected through the vascular bed to a receptor on the other side of the probe. From this, a measurement is taken of the intensity of each light transmitted, allowing a comparison of the absorption of each wavelength, one against the other. The pulse oximeter then produces the percentage of saturated oxygen. This takes place due to the difference in the intensity of light absorption through the vascular bed. The difference is determined by the respective levels of oxygenated and deoxygenated blood present. The optical properties change as a consequence of oxygen saturation, which decreases the infrared transmission and increases the red light transmission.

13. No.

14. At the assessment appointment, prior to dental treatment, during dental treatment with conscious sedation and in the recovery stage.

15. Movement, cold hands, venous pulsation, external light source, nail varnish and false nails.

16. To alert the dental team to any complications.

17. Pulse and saturated oxygen levels.

18. Pulse – low 55 and high 140 beats per minute (bpm). Oxygen saturation levels – 90.

19. Yes. If a patient's vital signs were below the recommended alarm settings, that is, a pulse lower than 55 bpm.

20. Approximately a couple of minutes as it will have to read and work out the initial level of saturated oxygen present.

21. Approximately 30 seconds.

22. It aids in understanding of how the blood carries and releases oxygen. It is a graph that plots the amount of saturated haemoglobin on the vertical axis against the oxygen tension on the horizontal axis. The shape of the curve results from the interaction of the adjoined oxygen molecules to the haemoglobin with the incoming. The haemoglobin molecule can only carry four oxygen molecules. It is very difficult for the first molecule to join, but having done so it aids the adjoining of the second and third. Once the fourth molecule is adjoined, it is difficult to increase the level of oxygen due to overcrowding and oxygen's natural tendency to dissociate. The curve levels out as the haemoglobin becomes saturated with oxygen, giving the curve its sigmoidal or S-shape.

23. It is sigmoidal shape (non-linear or S-shaped).

24. Stop dental treatment. Look at the pulse oximeter display to see if this reflects the patient and their clinical diagnosis. Reassurance is provided and the patient asked to take a few deep breaths. The probe is adjusted in the hope that this will restore the oxygen saturation levels to a suitable percentage for the patient. However, if the pulse oximeter does not concur, the patient looks well and their level of consciousness is satisfactory, another cause, whether clinical or technical must be explored. If the clinical monitoring concurs with the pulse oximeter, the patient is asked to take a few more deep breaths. If the patient's vital signs do not improve, the airway must be checked for blockages. If this does not rectify the situation, a head tilt, chin lift must be undertaken and oxygen administered. At this point the use of flumazenil will be considered by the clinician, especially if the patient's level of consciousness is continuing to drop. If necessary, cardiopulmonary resuscitation must be performed with the emergency services called. At all times, the patient must be constantly monitored and reassured.

25. During inhalation sedation, the patient is provided with a minimum of 30% oxygen through the nasal mask. This means that the patient is perfused with oxygen (more than in atmospheric air); therefore, the pulse oximeter would reflect this.

26. Red.

27. As it will affect the readings.

28. Deficiency in the amount of oxygen reaching the tissues.

29. It is a measure of how much oxygen the blood is carrying as a percentage of the maximum it could carry.

30. SpO2.

31. Optical spectrophotometry utilises scientific technology by using various wavelengths of light, performing quantitative measurements of absorption through a given substance, that is, the blood, thus determining the percentage of saturation.

32. Optical plethysmography utilises technology by using light absorption to reproduce waveforms produced by the pulsatile blood known as plethysmographic waveforms.

33. During a medical emergency to establish whether the patient requires any supplementary oxygen.

Blood pressure

1. Blood pressure is the force per unit area exerted on the wall of a blood vessel by the blood.

2. Blood pressure is determined by the force that is used to push the blood through the veins every time the heart beats and rests. If the heart pumps more blood through the arteries, or they are narrowed and stiff, the arteries will resist the blood flow. This results in blood pressure being raised and if less blood is pumped through the arteries, or they are larger and more flexible, blood pressure will be lower.

3. By altering (i) the amount of blood pumped into the arteries, (ii) the volume and viscosity of the blood and (iii) whether or not the arteries will resist that blood flow, thereby regulating

it. It does this by nerve impulses being sent to the heart, arteries and kidneys so that they will in turn work together to make the necessary adjustments.

4. The heart at its highest (systolic) and lowest (diastolic) pressure.

5. The left ventricle pumps blood into the aorta. The aortic walls stretch to allow the increased volume of blood received and the heart is at its highest pressure to provide the systolic reading. The aortic walls start to recoil, pushing blood into the arteries ensuring an onward flow. The heart at this stage is between beats. The aortic valve then closes as the pressure exceeds that of the left ventricle to prevent a backflow of blood. As the aorta and artery walls return to normal, the pressure drops to its lowest, prior to the next beat, which provides the diastolic reading.

6. What the heart/body is doing and how well it is performing.

7. Systolic over diastolic.

8. Stethoscope and a sphygmomanometer.

9. At the assessment appointment, prior to treatment on the day of the appointment, periodically during treatment, after treatment and upon discharge.

10. Yes, as a person's blood pressure changes constantly to meet the demands of the body.

11. A sphygmomanometer and stethoscope are prepared ensuring that the stethoscope is switched on. The patient is invited to take their coat off and to sit down with their arm supported. The patient is asked if they have had their blood pressure taken before, whether they are aware of it being high or low and asked if they are taking any medication for their blood pressure. The procedure is briefly explained. A suitable size cuff is placed around the patient's upper arm approximately 2–3 cm above the anti-cubital fossa, ensuring that it is not too tight. The patient is advised that it will initially get tight, but that pressure will reduce quickly. An estimated reading is recorded by palpating the radial artery. The cuff is inflated while feeling for the disappearance of the radial pulse while taking a note of the sphygmomanometer level. The cuff is immediately released. The brachial artery is located and the head of the stethoscope is placed over the brachial artery, tucking it under the cuff. The cuff is reinflated so that that the sphygmomanometer level rises to 30 mmHg above the estimated reading or to a maximum of 160 mmHg. Slowly the cuff is deflated and the Korotkoff sounds are listened for, taking a note of the first sound and when it becomes inaudible. Once completed, the cuff is deflated and the outcome recorded.

12. To establish an auscultatory gap, which occurs when the Korotkoff (K) sounds disappear shortly after K5 and reappear 5–40 mmHg later. This can lead to underestimation of systolic blood pressure and/or an overestimation of diastolic blood pressure. Approximately 5% of patients have an auscultatory gap, usually those suffering with high blood pressure.

13. To allow venous emptying.

14. Korotkoff sounds. KI – audible sharp thud (systolic), K2 – blowing or swishing sound, K3 – thudding sound, K4 – muffled sound and K5 – blood flow is laminar (diastolic).

15. Radial and brachial arteries.

16. 2 mmHg.

17. 110/70 and 120/80.

18. The diastolic, as it reflects the heart at its lowest pressure. If a patient moves around this figure will increase and more strain will be placed on the heart. When a patient's blood pressure is taken they are sat still, consequently the heart is at rest.

19. It would be taken again after 2–3 minutes. If it is still elevated, then somebody else should be asked to take it. All three recordings would be taken to the clinician. They would make a decision whether to treat the patient or refer them to their doctor to investigate the underlying cardiovascular reason for the raised blood pressure.

20. To allow venous emptying.

21. An accurate reading will not be achieved as the body will be working to break down the food and drink, adjusting to accommodate the exercise undertaken.

22. To avoid muscle tension, which could raise the diastolic pressure.

23. To accommodate the low blood pressure, the heart rate (cardiac output) increases thereby increasing the blood volume, thereby raising the blood pressure due to more pressure being placed on the vessels through which the blood is travelling.

24. Atenolol (beta-blocker) and Ramipril (ACE inhibitor).

25. They act upon the blood vessels to widen them making it easier for blood to circulate without meeting resistance or they cause the heart to beat less forcefully.

Miscellaneous

1. Yes.

2. Sedation Nurse's observations.

3. Blood pressure machine and pulse oximeter.

4. Blood pressure machine, if required.

5. Blood pressure machine and pulse oximeter.

6. Blood pressure machine and pulse oximeter.

7. This must be noted as soon as the patient enters the dental surgery. The dental team is then aware of the skin tone, be it pale or flushed, and that this is normal for that patient on the day. This avoids any unnecessary concerns – if the patient's skin colour was not noted and the team noticed it was flushed it might be thought that they were suffering an allergic reaction, giving cause for concern. Whereas if the dental team were aware, they would know that the skin colour had not altered. Also if the patient was pale upon entry and this was noted, the team would not be alarmed.

8. To feel how strong or weak the patient's pulse is for future reference should the need arise for comparison.

9. Because the drug used for intravenous sedation has the ability to cause respiratory depression and this must be avoided. To observe the amount of breaths per minute in order to establish if the patient's breathing is within normal parameters. The depth of respirations will also be observed so that it is found to be normal for the patient.

10. To determine the patient's health/fitness to receive treatment with a form of conscious sedation.

11. To compare readings. Patients must be well oxygenated during sedative techniques, as the drug used causes respiratory depression and oxygen is vital for life.

12. To ensure that they can respond, that they are not over-sedated and in the case of intravenous sedation not experiencing respiratory depression.

13. Some clinicians will not use conscious sedation techniques for patients above a certain body mass index. To establish the risk that could occur and any associated difficulties that could arise should the patient have to be moved at any point while sedated. Establishing the patient's weight will prove invaluable in an emergency for the paramedics to calculate the amount of emergency drug to administer.

14. To establish if the patient's body temperature is normal and they do not have an underlying fever.

15. No, as some clinicians choose not to carry them out, that is, height and weight, as they do use a BMI as a reference tool. With children, medical checks such as blood pressure are not always carried out as they can be uncomfortable for the child.

Equipment used for intravenous sedation

1. Tourniquet, disinfectant surface medi-wipe, a cannula, either a 22-gauge Venflon or, a Y can, two 23-gauge drawing up needles, a 5 ml sodium chloride flush, a 2 ml sterile syringe with a sodium chloride label placed, a 5 ml sterile syringe with a drug label (midazolam) placed, ampoule of midazolam and the reversal drug flumazenil together with a 5 ml sterile syringe and a 23-gauge drawing up needle. The emergency drugs and equipment will also be available together with a blood pressure machine and pulse oximeter. In addition to this, the patient's notes, signed consent form and any radiographs will be made available.

Equipment used for cannulation

1. To restrict the venous return, thereby engorging the vein so that cannulation can take place.

2. To cleanse the selected cannulation site.

3. To gain access into the vein, which once sited is known as an indwelling cannula in order to administer the drug.

4. With a 23-gauge butterfly needle, a steel rigid needle is left in situ. This means that if used in the anti-cubital fossa region, an arm board would be required to stabilise the patient's arm movements thereby preventing extravasation of the cannula. With a 22-gauge Venflon despite there being an introducing needle all that is left in situ is a plastic Teflon tube, which prevents clots.

5. This will allow drugs to be provided to patients when attached to a drip.

6. One to draw the drug into a sterile syringe and the other to draw the flush into a sterile syringe.

7. As they will filter any potential minute particles of glass that may have dropped into the glass ampoule. This prevents them being drawn into the sterile syringe and being administered to the patient. The length of the needle means that it will reach the bottom of the glass ampoule drawing the entire drug into the syringe.

8. To administer when the cannula is in place after ensuring that it has been sited properly. Sodium chloride is used, because it is compatible with the body.

9. This is to contain the flush used to ensure the cannula is sited correctly.

10. This is to contain the drug prior to administration.

11. To relax and sedate the patient.

12. To reverse the effects of midazolam in the event that the patient becomes over-sedated.

Equipment used for inhalation sedation

1. A relative analgesia machine, whether it is a mobile machine or a piped system. It will be checked to ensure it is safe for use. A scavenging system will be attached and functional along with a range of nasal masks in case patients do not bring theirs. The emergency drugs and equipment will also be available along with the patient's notes, signed consent form and any radiographs plus good ventilation being provided within the surgery.

Equipment used for oral sedation

1. Emergency drugs and equipment. A blood pressure machine and pulse oximeter. Cannulation equipment should also be present. Flumazenil will be prepared. If the patient is to receive intravenous midazolam, then ampoules will be available along with a blood pressure machine and pulse oximeter. In addition to this, the patient's notes, signed consent form and any radiographs will be made available.

Equipment used for transmucosal/off-licence sedation

1. Emergency drugs and equipment. A blood pressure machine and pulse oximeter. Cannulation equipment should also be present. Midazolam and flumazenil will be prepared. If per nasal sedation is being provided, a sterile syringe and nasal atomiser. If oral midazolam is being provided, either some cold tea or squash will be available. A log book outlining the transmucosal/off-licence sedation being used along with drug amounts, patient and clinician details. In addition to this, the patient's notes, signed consent form and any radiographs will be made available.

SECTION V Answers: Patient selection

The assessment appointment

1. For the clinician to assess the patient's suitability for treatment with conscious sedation and the intended treatment thereby providing safe sedation.

2. It provides a clear picture of the patient's medical, dental and social history, thus ensuring safe sedation is provided. The patient can make suitable arrangements at their leisure, and it allows a cooling-off period once consent has been taken.

3. Knowledge, skills and experience of themselves and staff who will be involved in the patient's treatment. The patient's circumstances, wishes and expectations must be taken into account along with their medical, dental and social history.

4. Medical, dental and social history. The patient's wishes and circumstances. Take consent. Provide pre- and post-operative instructions. A physical examination in conjunction with the medical history comprises the following:
   • Heart rate.
   • Respiratory rate.
   • Blood pressure (BP).
   • Oxygen saturation.
   • Temperature.
   • Height.
   • Weight – BMI.

5. No.

6. A separate assessment appointment would not be carried out for a patient who attends an emergency appointment in pain, if assessed suitable for sedation and can comply with the instructions attracted to the form of sedation being provided.

7. Blood pressure machine, pulse oximeter, height and weight chart in conjunction with a BMI chart and a thermometer.

8. Patient notes, consent form, radiographs and pre- and post-operative instructions.

Medical history

1. To allow the clinician to assess the patient's suitability for treatment. To decide if the patient can be safely treated at the dental surgery. Whether the appointment would need extending or possibly the treatment being carried out over more than one appointment. If they need referring to a secondary care establishment, that is, the local dental hospital.

2. American Society of Anaesthesiologists (ASA) Physical Status Classification.

3. Respiratory, central nervous, cardiovascular, gastrointestinal, gastrourinary and locomotor conditions.

4. Epilepsy, convulsions, spastic, subnormal psychiatric problems and migraines. Drug, alcohol dependency, other neurological diseases.

5. Heart disease, hypertension, syncope, rheumatic fever, chorea, brucellosis. Bleeding disorder, anticoagulants and anaemia. Syncope.

6. Asthma, bronchitis, TB, smoking and any other chest diseases.

7. Gastric or duodenal ulcer, bleeding PR, other GI diseases, hepatitis and jaundice.

8. Renal, urinary tract or sexually transmitted disease. Menstrual problems and pregnancy.

9. Bone or joint disease. Diabetes or other endocrine disease. Skin disease. Any other disease including congenital abnormality.

10. Family relevant medical history. Allergies, for example, Penicillin. Recent or current drugs/medical treatment. Previous operations or serious illnesses. Recent travel abroad.

11. To ensure that the patient is treated safely, there are no contraindications to treatment and no drug interactions that could occur.

12. As they can both affect treatment by enhancing the effects of midazolam. With drug users, they can be difficult to cannulate along with being more difficult to sedate. If a patient was an alcoholic, midazolam could take longer to be broken down and eliminated from the body due to liver damage.

The ASA physical status classification

1. American Society of Anaesthesiologists (ASA) Physical Status Classification.

2. 6.

3.

Classification	Patient Group	Examples
ASA 1	Patients who are normal and healthy. Able to walk up a flight of stairs easily. Physiologically should present no difficulty in handling the proposed treatment. Is a candidate for any sedation technique.	
ASA II	Patients with mild systemic disease. Healthy, presenting extreme fear/anxiety towards dentistry. Older, that is, 60 years plus. Pregnant. Have to rest after mild exercise. Less stress tolerant but still represent a minimal risk during treatment. Proceed with caution.	Healthy patients, 60 years plus. Healthy but very phobic. Non-insulin controlled diabetic. Mildly raised BP: 140–159/90–94 mm Hg. History of atopic allergies.
ASA III	Patients with systemic disease that limits activity, but is not incapacitating. Not stressed at rest, but have to stop frequently during mild exercise such as walking or climbing stairs. Sedation procedure may need modifying/shortening or may be kept lighter.	Well-controlled insulin controlled diabetic. Myocardial infarction 6 months previously with no symptoms since. High BP: 160–190/95–114 mm Hg. Fragile asthmatic. Epileptic with several seizures a year.
ASA IV	Patients who have an incapacitating disease that is life threatening. Unable to walk upstairs or far along the street. Exhibit fatigue or shortness of breath while seated. Treatment should be avoided or carried out as conservatively as possible or referred to a suitable hospital department.	Unstable angina. Recent myocardial infarction. Poorly controlled diabetic. Very high BP: 200/115 mm Hg.
ASA V	Patients with a terminal condition and not expected to survive. Not suitable for treatment.	
ASA VI	Brain dead awaiting organ transplantation	

4. ASA IV.

5. ASA III.

6. ASA III.

7. ASA IV.

8. ASA II.

9. ASA V.

10. ASA II.

11. ASA IV.

12. ASA I.

13. The sedation procedure may need modifying/shortening or may be kept lighter.

14. Treatment should be avoided or carried out as conservatively as possible or referred to a suitable hospital department.

Miscellaneous

1. To establish any important factors that could be detrimental to effective management, along with the patient's expectations, motivation and attendance pattern.

2. A social history is as important as other histories taken as the clinician has a duty of care to ensure that patients are adequately cared for at home. They will establish how they will travel home and if they can afford the planned treatment.

3. Corah anxiety scale.

4. Inhalation sedation. Local anaesthetic could be an option with lots of reassurance and support. If the patient met the criteria and the clinician thought it justified a general anaesthetic could be offered.

5. The patient could not have intravenous sedation as he or she would not be able to comply with the pre- and post-operative instructions, that is, bring an escort. With inhalation sedation, there are no post-operative restraints apart from those attracted to the dental procedure. This is because 99% of the gases are eliminated straightaway with the remaining 1% being eliminated over the following 24 hours.

SECTION VI Answers: Types of sedation

Intravenous sedation

Midazolam

1. Benzodiazepines.

2. Trade.

3. Hypnovel.

4. Generic.

5. 1983.

6. 1–4 hours. Approximately 5 mgs of drug will be eliminated from the body within 5 hours.

7. Schedule III Controlled Substance.

8. Clear liquid: 10 mg in 5 mls. 10 mg in 2 mls. 5 mg in 5 mls.

9. 5 mg in 5 mls.

10. It signifies a place that should be held for ease of opening.

11. Clear liquid.

12. In a controlled drug cabinet, which is locked, made of metal and fixed to the wall. When required it should be signed in and out of the drug cabinet and by two members of staff who have authorisation to do so. An inventory/record of stock must be kept with documentation being held for 2 years.

13. Intravenously, per-nasal and buccally (transmucosal).

14. pH of 3.4.

15. Anxiolytic, hypnotic, anticonvulsant, muscle relaxant and anterograde amnesia. They produce sedation. It has a rapid onset with a pronounced effect and is short acting. It can be titrated to produce a desired effect to reflect individual patient's needs and are water soluble. As a patient's vein is continually maintained, drugs can be provided in the event of an emergency or the patient becomes over sedated. Patient recovery time is quicker than oral or intramuscular drugs. Nausea and vomiting rarely occur. It reduces the gag reflex slightly.

16. Venepuncture is mandatory. Training is necessary to undertake venepuncture and it requires great skill. Venepuncture sites can cause problems. A sedation nurse must be available at all times. Midazolam can cause respiratory depression and minimal cardiovascular depression. Due to the rapid onset of midazolam, its action and its more pronounced effects, the risk of potential complications is elevated. No analgesia is provided. Elderly and paediatric patients occasionally experience paradoxical effects. Appointment times must be longer to allow for the patient's recovery period. Consent must be taken, with patients complying with rigid pre- and post-operative instructions.

17. The administration of the midazolam would be stopped, the patient's airway maintained, oxygen provided and adrenaline administered. As the patient will have an indwelling cannula, the intravenous concentration of adrenaline can be provided, which is 0.5 mls 1:10,000. However, not all health-care settings will have adrenaline in that concentration therefore 0.5 mls 1:1000 intramuscular adrenaline will be provided. Alternatively, an EpiPen can be used.

18. Drug name, concentration, batch number and expiry date.

19. Initial bolus 2 mg over 30 seconds. Observe patient response for 2 minutes. After 2 minutes a further 0.5–1 mg is administered until the level of sedation required has been achieved. The usual dose is between 2.5 and 7.5 mg.

20. It is based on their age.

21. Initial bolus to be as low as 1–1.5 mg. The total amount may not need to exceed 3.5 mg. It is important to observe an elderly patient for longer after the first bolus before administering any more midazolam to avoid over-sedation.

22. Elderly patients are more sensitive to midazolam as the arm brain time is much slower than that of a younger patient. This means if midazolam was titrated in the same way, an elderly patient would be more likely to become over-sedated. This is because it takes longer for the initial bolus to reach the brain.

23. 1–3 minutes.

24. It produces conscious sedation by acting on the central nervous system, reducing the excitability of neurones in the mid brain. Benzodiazepine receptors are parallel to inhibitory neurotransmitters. When midazolam attaches to the benzodiazepine receptors, they enhance the effect of the inhibitory neurotransmitters. This occurs as a brain chemical that is naturally calming, enhancing the effects of the gamma-aminobutyric acid (GABA) resulting in either the slowing down or stopping of certain nerve signals within the brain.

25. Eve sign.

26. Conscious and able to converse. Slurred speech and impaired coordination.

27. Drowsiness, mental confusion, lethargy and muscle relaxation. They would not respond if they were asked a question or not rouse if tapped on the shoulder. More serious signs and symptoms would be hypotension, cardiorespiratory depression, apnoea and rarely, a coma.

28. Careful observation of the patient's vital signs is necessary along with airway maintenance and the provision of oxygen. The benzodiazepine antagonist flumazenil (Anexate) will be used to control the effects of over-sedation. If necessary cardiopulmonary resuscitation would be undertaken and the emergency services called.

29. Within the liver and gut.

30. In urine via the kidneys.

31. Anxiolytic to reduce a patient's anxiety levels. Hypnotic, anticonvulsant, muscle relaxant, anterograde amnesia. The blood pressure is lowered and in return the pulse rate is increased. They produce sedation and cause slurred speech and impaired coordination. They have a rapid onset with a pronounced effect and are short acting. Can be titrated to produce a desired effect to reflect individual patient's needs and are water soluble. As a patient's vein is continually maintained, drugs can be provided in the event of an emergency or the patient becomes over-sedated. Patient recovery time is quicker than oral or intramuscular drugs. That nausea and vomiting rarely occur. They reduce the gag reflex slightly.

32. Respiratory depression and minimal cardiovascular effects. Hiccoughs and coughing. Headaches and drowsiness. Nausea and vomiting. Loss of inhibition and restlessness.

Irritation at the cannula site. However, as midazolam is water soluble it is not common for patients to experience any irritation.

33. Pregnant and nursing mothers. Patients with kidney or liver impairment. Paediatric and elderly patients. Patients who are allergic to benzodiazepines suffer cardiorespiratory disorders. Alcoholic patients and drug users. Patients who take erythromycin and St. John's Wart.

34. Over-sedation. The wrong drug being administered. Out-of-date drug being used. An allergic reaction occurring. Venepuncture complication, that is, extravasation. Cannula becoming loose or venous access being lost. Inadequate post-sedation supervision resulting in an accident. The patient not being fit for discharge when they left the dental surgery or the escort did not attend or was unsuitable.

35. Opiate.

Anexate

1. Benzodiazepines.

2. Trade.

3. Flumazenil.

4. Generic.

5. 50 minutes.

6. Reverses the effects of a benzodiazepine. It is an antidote.

7. POM.

8. 500 mcgs in 5 mls/0.5 mg/5 mls.

9. Clear liquid.

10. Drug name, concentration, batch number and expiry date.

11. In a controlled drug cabinet, which is locked, made of metal and fixed to the wall. When required, it should be signed in and out of the drugs cabinet by two staff members who have authorisation to do so. An inventory/record of stock must be kept with documentation being held for 2 years.

12. When a patient is over-sedated and does not respond to verbal or physical commands.

13. 200 mcgs over 15 seconds. Wait for 60 seconds and if required further 100 mcgs are administered every 60 seconds until the level of consciousness required has been achieved. The usual dose is 300–600 mcgs. Maximum dose is 1 mg. which is two vials.

14. It is the antidote for an overdose of a benzodiazepine and is an imidazobenzodiazepine derivative, which antagonises the clinical actions of benzodiazepines on the central nervous system.

The pharmacology of flumazenil is that it competitively inhibits the activity at the benzodiazepine gamma-aminobutyric acid (GABA) receptors. This allows the neurones to return to their normal state of excitability, thus reversing the sedative effect.

15. Anxiety, disorientation, head pains, aggressiveness and agitation. If a patient is epileptic the drug is used to control their condition. Patients who suffer from epilepsy are prescribed medication that belongs to the benzodiazepine family. Therefore, when the action of midazolam is reversed so will their epileptic therapy, resulting in the patient experiencing convulsions.

16. As the half-life of Anexate is approximately 50 minutes and the half-life of midazolam being 1–4 hours, it is possible that when used to reverse the action of midazolam, the patient will initially be reversed, but could re-sedate as the action decreases. However, very little re-sedation will occur as both drugs will wear off together.

17. In the liver.

18. In urine via the kidneys.

19. Patients dependent on benzodiazepines, those allergic to benzodiazepines. Epileptic patients and patients who suffer heart conditions.

Propofol
1. Hypnotics or anaesthetics.

2. Generic.

3. Diprivan.

4. Trade.

5. Estimated between 2 and 24 minutes.

6. Schedule IV Controlled Substance.

7. In a controlled drug cabinet, which is locked, made of metal and fixed to the wall. When required, it should be signed in and out of the drug cabinet and by two staff members who have authorisation to do so. An inventory/record of stock must be kept with documentation being held for 2 years.

8. 200 mgs in 20 mls. 10 mgs per ml.

9. White milky liquid.

10. Drug name, concentration, batch number and expiry date.

11. Because of its milk-like appearance.

12. Propofol is used with a patient-controlled electronic infusion pump driver so that it can be continually administered. These drivers are similar to those used after general surgery for

post-operative pain relief in general hospitals. The pump driver is set up by the clinician or the anaesthetist by inputting the amount of drug a patient will receive each time they press a button and the interval period between activations. This means that the patient is in control, because they hold the button throughout treatment, which when pressed will administer a dose of propofol. Due to the data input, they would not receive a dose every time they pressed the button, because of the lock-out time. The initial bolus is approximately 1 mg/kg over 1–5 minutes followed by 1.5–4.5 mg/kg/hour.

13. By administering a local anaesthetic into the vein prior to the induction of propofol.

14. Anaesthetists and clinicians trained in intensive care procedures. It is normally provided in a hospital setting.

15. It works by enhancing the effect of the gamma aminobutyric acid (GABA) to depress the central nervous system without using the receptors directly.

16. 30–45 seconds.

17. Produces sedation and can cause unconsciousness. Causes a 30% fall in BP on induction. Apnoea can occur.

18. Respiratory depressants such as benzodiazepines, opiates, alcohol, heroin and morphine.

19. It is a respiratory depressant. Low blood pressure and apnoea. Pain on administration, mild myoclonic movements (muscle twitches) and euphoria. Some patients can experience profound sedation even with small doses of propofol. Patients allergic to eggs. Pregnant and nursing mothers.

20. In urine via the kidneys.

21. In the liver.

22. Eggs.

Miscellaneous
1. No. The patient will look fit, well and fully recovered but will not be as the drug will still be in his or her body and will have the beta phase (metabolism and excretion) of the half-life to go through.

2. The time it takes for the plasma level of the drug to drop to half. This is divided into two stages alpha and beta. Alpha is distribution and redistribution. Beta is metabolism and excretion.

3. A name given to a drug by the manufacturer.

4. A name given to a drug for prescriptions.

5. A drug given in increments against the patient's response. This means that patients can receive different amounts and patients receiving more than one treatment session can also receive varying amounts.

6. Controlled drugs (or controlled substances) are substances and medications that can only legally be obtained by getting a signed prescription from a registered medical practitioner.

7. 1971.

8. 1968.

9. Diazepam and diazemuls.

10. **Phase 1:** The midazolam within the blood at the site of the brain is at its maximum. This will result in sedation with the patient's coordination being impaired and their speech slurred. At this stage, the patient will be unaware of their surroundings. They will experience a period of almost total amnesia despite conversing normally.

    Phase II: The amount of midazolam within the blood will now start to decrease correspondingly so will the effects of sedation. This is attributed to the midazolam being redistributed to other tissues within the body (alpha half-life). As a result, the patient will experience an awareness of their surroundings as the amnesic effect decreases. This means that some patients may remember some of their treatment.

    Phase III: Patients will start to feel normal and will still appear to look relaxed. They will not be anxious as the anxiolytic effect of midazolam is still active.

    Phase IV: Patients will look and feel recovered. It must be remembered that the patient is not fully recovered at this stage as it is only the alpha half-life of distribution and redistribution has occurred. Midazolam has yet to undergo the beta half-life metabolism and excretion and is therefore still present within the body. The amnesic effects of midazolam must also not be forgotten. They can be profound enough to last until phase 4 of sedation, meaning that the post-operative instructions must be repeated and always provided in writing to both the patient and escort.

11. The time it takes for the drug to reach the brain.

12. Drug metabolism is the process by which the body breaks down and converts medication into active chemical substances.

13. Drugs and their metabolites are removed from the body.

14. Drug metabolites are what the liver breaks a drug down into within the bloodstream.

15. Porridge, alcohol, other benzodiazepines and antihistamines.

16. To be accompanied by a responsible adult to act as an escort. This person must remain at the surgery while treatment takes place and accompany the patient home by car. They must also be able to stay with the patient for the next 24 hours and be free of other responsibilities. Not to be in charge of other people on the day of sedation. Not to make any responsible decisions or sign any legal documents for the remainder of the day. Not to drive any vehicles, operate any machinery or climb ladders or scaffolding. Not eat or drink for 4 hours prior to the appointment time. Some clinicians do not request their patients to be starved of food and drink but advise a light meal a few hours prior. To wear loose clothing with sleeves that can easily be pulled above the elbow and not to wear high heel shoes. To remove any nail varnish, avoid alcohol on the day of sedation and ensure that their teeth and gums are clean.

17. Blood pressure, pulse and respiratory rate. Skin tone and colour of the mucous membranes. Levels of saturated oxygen. Height and weight (BMI) and possibly the body temperature. The patient's anxiety levels would also be noted.

18. Before, during and after treatment – blood pressure, pulse and respiratory rate. Level of consciousness and responsiveness. Skin tone and colour of the mucous membranes. Levels of saturated oxygen. Before – height and weight (BMI) and possibly the body temperature. The patient's anxiety levels would also be noted.

19. Escort in attendance, transport home and who will care for them after leaving the surgery. Last food and drink. Any alcohol consumed. Any change in medical history or medication. Taken routine medication and complied with any special pre-operative medications or changes to existing. Happy to proceed with treatment and do they have any questions or concerns.

20. Notes must contain patient's medical, dental and social history, including any previous treatments, general anaesthetic and/or conscious sedation. Any change in the medical history/status. Details of the assessment appointment. The form of sedation and treatment provided with the justification for its use and any patient preferences. Written consent and verbal and written pre- and post-operative instructions were provided. The patient is happy to go ahead with the planned treatment. All instructions have been adhered to and the name of a responsible escort in attendance and details of transport home. Details of the treatment appointment. All monitoring details, cannula site, drug used, batch number and expiry date, drug titrations and times administered. The recovery information and the patient is assessed for discharge. Any complications and statements of how the patient responded to the mode of sedation used and/or reactions within the recovery phase.

21. Excellent record-keeping is important and must reflect the patient's treatment pathway. They will provide evidence that the patient consented to treatment, they will prove valuable for future appointments with respect to the amount of drug the patient received, how they responded to treatment from start to finish, which aids future appointment planning and management of patients.

22. Epilepsy.

23. What the body does to the drug. It is divided into several areas including the extent and rate of absorption, distribution, metabolism and excretion. This is commonly known as ADME.

24. To make an area of the skin temporarily numb, resulting in less painful cannulation.

25. Ametop or EMLA.

26. Approximately 30 minutes prior to cannulation.

27. EMLA – lidocaine and prilocaine. Ametop – tetracaine, previously known as amethocaine.

28. A minimum of 1 hour after the last titration of drug and only when the patient has been deemed fit for discharge.

29. The cannula comes out or becomes loose, a medical emergency, patient injures themselves or falls. Prolonged recovery.

30. Just before they leave the surgery having been assessed for discharge and deemed fit.

31. Ensuring that the patient can stand and walk unaided, they feel okay and their vital signs are within the normal range for them.

32. The use of two drugs.

33. Nubain (Nalbuphine).

34. Narcan (Naloxone).

35. It enhances the effects of midazolam and provides additional pain relief.

36. Nausea and vomiting.

37. Milligrams.

38. Micrograms.

Oral sedation

Temazepam

1. Benzodiazepines.

2. Tablets and elixir.

3. 10 and 20 mg tablets. 10 mgs/5 mls elixir.

4. Tablets are white and elixir is green.

5. 10–30 mgs 1 hour prior to procedure.

6. Half the adult dose.

7. For elderly patients, half the adult dose is prescribed although some patients may require a higher dose than that of children.

8. Based on the patient's weight.

9. It produces sedation and a state of relaxation. It has anxiolytic, anticonvulsant, muscle relaxant properties and is considered to be a hypnotic drug.

10. Schedule III.

11. Exempt from safe custody requirements and can be stored on the open dispensary shelf. Best practice would be storing it in the same manner as a Schedule IV drug.

12. Paediatric and elderly patients. Patients prescribed antidepressants. Patients who are pregnant or alcoholics. Patients who suffer from myasthenia gravis and those who are allergic or have sensitivity to benzodiazepines.

13. Easy to administer, not expensive to provide, universally accepted and works well for most patients. Produces sedation, relaxes patients and provides some amnesic effects. A cannula is not always placed. Specialised training is not always required as with intravenous and inhalation sedation, as it is safe and easy to monitor. Decreased incidence and severity of adverse drug reactions.

14. If the patient has been given the medication for home use, they might not take it as directed. They might drive to the surgery and not bring an escort. The clinician is putting their trust in the patient to comply with these and other instructions. If a cannula is not placed, there is no venous access. Patients could attend their appointment over-sedated. Oral temazepam cannot be titrated against patients' response, it does not provide any analgesia, can take some time to take effect, stay in the body for a long time and the absorption and elimination of the drug can be erratic.

15. 8–10 hours.

16. The best environment for the patient to take the medication and the optimum time for it to be taken along with the dose to be prescribed.

17. Due to its more profound effect and shorter half-life.

18. When prescribing temazepam, the dentist will have to decide when the optimum time will be for the patient to take the prescribed amount, that is, at home or within the surgery. They also have to consider the amount they prescribe. The dentist would also have to take into account the effects of temazepam when administering midazolam. They will provide slow titrations and a reduced amount to avoid over-sedation.

19. Careful observation of the patient's vital signs would be necessary along with airway mainte-nance and the provision of oxygen. The benzodiazepine antagonist flumazenil (Anexate) will be used to control the effects of over-sedation. If necessary, cardiopulmonary resuscitation would be undertaken and the emergency services called.

Diazepam (Valium)

1. Benzodiazepines.

2. Tablets and syrup.

3. Tablets – 2, 5 and 10 mg. Syrup – 2 mgs/5 ml and 5 mgs/5 mls.

4. 2 mg white tablet, 5 mg yellow tablet and 10 mg blue tablet. Syrup – wintergreen.

5. For an adult, 10 mgs can be given 1 hour before the procedure or 5 mgs the night before, 5 mgs upon wakening and 5 mgs 2 hours prior to the procedure.

6. Half the adult dose.

7. For elderly patients, half the adult dose is prescribed although some patients may require a higher dose than that of children.

8. Based on the patient's weight.

9. It produces sedation and a state of relaxation. It has anxiolytic, anticonvulsant, muscle relaxant properties and is considered to be a hypnotic drug.

10. Schedule IV.

11. In a controlled drug cabinet, which is locked, made of metal and fixed to the wall. When required, it should be signed in and out of the drug cabinet by two staff members who have authorisation to do so. An inventory/record of stock must be kept with documentation being held for 2 years.

12. Paediatric and elderly patients. Patients prescribed antidepressants. Patients who are pregnant and alcoholics. Patients who suffer from myasthenia gravis and those who are allergic or have sensitivity to benzodiazepines.

13. Easy to administer, not expensive to provide, universally accepted and works well for most patients. Produces sedation, relaxes patients and provides some amnesic effects. A cannula is not always placed. Specialised training is not always required as with intravenous and inhalation sedation, as it is safe and easy to monitor. Decreased incidence and severity of adverse drug reactions.

14. If the patient has been given the medication for home use, they might not take it as directed, they may drive to the surgery and not bring an escort. The clinician is putting their trust in the patient to comply with these and other instructions. If a cannula not is placed, there is no venous access. Patients could attend their appointment over-sedated. Oral diazepam cannot be titrated against patients' response, it does not provide any analgesia, can take some time to take effect, can stay in the body for a long time with absorption and elimination of the drug can be erratic.

15. 36–57 hours.

16. The best environment for the patient to take the medication and the optimum time for it to be taken along with the dose to be prescribed.

17. It has a more profound effect and a shorter half-life.

18. When prescribing diazepam, the dentist will have to decide when the optimum time will be for the patient to take the prescribed amount, that is, at home or within the surgery. They will have to also consider the amount they prescribe. The dentist would also have to take

into account the effects of diazepam when administering midazolam. They will provide slow titrations and a reduced amount to avoid over-sedation.

19. Careful observation of the patient's vital signs would be necessary along with airway maintenance and the provision of oxygen. The benzodiazepine antagonist flumazenil (Anexate) will be used to control the effects of over-sedation. If necessary, cardiopulmonary resuscitation would be undertaken and the emergency services called.

Miscellaneous

1. No. They will look fit, well and fully recovered but will not be as the drug will still be in their bodies and will have the beta phase (metabolism and excretion) of the half-life to go through.

2. Anxiolytic, hypnotic, anticonvulsant, muscle relaxant and anterograde amnesia. They produce sedation. It has a rapid onset with a pronounced effect and is short acting. It can be titrated to produce a desired effect to reflect individual patients' needs and are water soluble. As a patient's vein is continually maintained, drugs can be provided in the event of an emergency or the patient becomes over-sedated. Patient recovery time is quicker than oral or intramuscular drugs. Nausea and vomiting rarely occur. It reduces the gag reflex slightly.

3. Drowsiness, mental confusion, lethargy and muscle relaxation. They would not respond if they were asked a question or not rouse if tapped on the shoulder. More serious signs and symptoms would be hypotension, cardiorespiratory depression, apnoea and rarely, a coma.

4. To be accompanied by a responsible adult to act as an escort. This person must remain at the surgery while treatment takes place and accompany the patient home by car. They must also be able to stay with the patient for the next 24 hours and be free of other responsibilities. Not to be in charge of other people on the day of sedation. Not to make any responsible decisions or sign any legal documents for the remainder of the day. Not to drive any vehicles, operate any machinery or climb ladders or scaffolding. Not eat or drink for 4 hours prior to the appointment time. Some clinicians do not request their patients to be starved of food and drink but advise a light meal a few hours prior. To wear loose clothing with sleeves that can easily be pulled above the elbow and not to wear high heel shoes. To remove any nail varnish, avoid alcohol on the day of sedation and ensure that their teeth and gums are clean.

5. Notes must contain patients' medical, dental and social history, including any previous treatments, general anaesthetic and/or conscious sedation. Any change in the medical history/status. Details of the assessment appointment. The form of sedation and treatment provided with the justification for its use and any patient preferences. Written consent and verbal and written pre- and post-operative instructions were provided. The patient is happy to go ahead with the planned treatment. All instructions have been adhered to and the name of a responsible escort in attendance and details of transport home. Details of the treatment appointment. All monitoring details, cannula site, drug used, batch number and expiry date, drug titrations and times administered. The recovery information and that the patient is assessed for discharge. Any complications and statements of how the patient responded to the mode of sedation used and/or reactions within the recovery phase.

6. Before, during and after treatment – blood pressure, pulse and respiratory rate. Level of consciousness and responsiveness. Skin tone and colour of the mucous membranes. Levels of

saturated oxygen. Before – height and weight (BMI) and possibly the body temperature. The patient's anxiety levels would also be noted.

7. Excellent record-keeping is important and must reflect the patient's treatment pathway. They will provide evidence that the patient consented to treatment, they will prove valuable for future appointments in respect of the amount of drug the patient received, how they responded to treatment from start to finish. This aids future appointment planning and management of patients.

8. It reduces the patient's level of anxiety. This means that the patient will attend the dental surgery.

9. Diazepam.

10. 28 days. It will only contain the required oral sedation for the next dental appointment.

11. Oral pre-medication is where the patient self administers a small amount of an oral sedative. Oral sedation is where a much larger dose of an oral sedative is given in the dental surgery.

Inhalation sedation

1. It is the appropriate use of nitrous oxide and oxygen being delivered to a patient through a nasal hood.

2. Relative analgesia.

3. To use as little nitrous oxide as possible combined with oxygen to sedate a patient.

4. Nitrous oxide and oxygen.

5. Its use is extremely safe as it is a non-invasive technique. There is no gastric absorption or any significant metabolism; therefore, there will not be any adverse effects on the liver, kidneys, brain, cardiovascular or respiratory system. There is minimal impairment of cough and swallowing reflexes so the patient's airway is not compromised. Patients recover very quickly and there are not any post-sedation restrictions so they can undertake any of their normal responsibilities/activities. A minimum of 30% oxygen is provided at all times. The patient will feel its effect within 20 seconds and within 3–5 minutes will experience its full effect. The length of the patient's appointment can reflect the treatment being undertaken. It is ideal for long or short procedures, and it can be provided for all ages with very few contraindications. It can be accurately delivered to patients with the amount of nitrous oxide and oxygen being altered to suit their needs. When altering the depth of sedation, it takes approximately 2–3 minutes for a change to be noticed. The nitrous oxide sedates whilst providing some analgesia and anterograde amnesia.

6. The team must provide psychological support to patients to achieve successful sedation. The depth of sedation can vary between patients and can even differ for the same patient at other appointments. If a patient has a cold or cannot breathe properly through his/her nose on the day of their appointment, they must cancel. Nitrous oxide is not very potent; therefore,

some patients will not achieve a suitable level of sedation for treatment to take place. The cost of providing this form of sedation is high as the equipment is expensive and requires ongoing servicing and maintenance, plus the continuous use of the gases. Whether a mobile machine or a piped system is used, they are awkward in shape. This makes space and storage an issue. If a mobile machine is used, the cylinders have to be stored securely so additional safe storage is required. Long-term exposure to nitrous oxide can cause harm to the team; therefore, control measures must be put in place, coupled with the use of a scavenging system to remove it, thereby limiting the risk of a harmful effect. It cannot be used without oxygen, with a minimum of 30% provided by the machine at all times to avoid the risk of death. Unfortunately, it is very accessible to the team, so there is a risk of recreational abuse.

7. Dental procedures where the mask might impair vision and access, for example, an anterior apicectomy. The common cold, flu or nasal obstruction. Claustrophobia. Tuberculosis and acute pulmonary conditions. Psychiatric and immunosuppressed patients. Pregnant patients in the first trimester. Myasthenia gravis. Pneumothorax, Middle Ear and Sinus Disease.

8. Paediatric.

9. Through the respiratory structure. A patient is provided with nitrous oxide and oxygen through a nasal mask by inhaling these gases into the respiratory system until they reach the alveoli sacs within the lungs. Nitrous oxide diffuses across the alveolar membrane and into the blood. It is then carried round the body with its action within the brain and blood being within 3–5 minutes. The same process occurs as it enters the fat, muscles and connective tissue.

10. 3–5 minutes.

11. 2–3 minutes.

12. 6–7 hours.

13. It results in a sedated patient whose cooperation is improved as their levels of anxiety are reduced. It provides analgesia and anterograde amnesia. The patient will feel detached and dissociated from their surroundings, they are floating; they may feel dreamy, euphoric and experience tingling of lips tongue and fingers.

14. Spontaneous closure of the mouth. Sweating of the upper lip and brow. Patient no longer communicating.

15. Via the respiratory structure. The nitrous oxide diffuses across the alveolar membrane from the blood into the lungs to be exhaled.

16. To avoid diffusion hypoxia.

17. 3–5 minutes.

18. **Stage 1 – Plane 1:** Moderate sedation and analgesia. The patient is administered between 5% and 25% nitrous oxide. Patients will be relaxed, which leads to the reduction of anxiety. Their perception to painful stimuli is reduced and they experience some tingling sensations in

their fingers, toes, lips and tongue. Minor amnesic effects may be felt due to nitrous oxide. At this stage, patients can be communicative, able to answer any questions and are responsive to requests.

Plane 2: Dissociation sedation and analgesia. The patient is administered between 25% and 55% nitrous oxide. Patients will be relaxed further and appear unperturbed by the dental environment. They will feel detached from their surroundings. Their fears and anxieties will disappear and their perception to painful stimuli will be further reduced. They feel as if they are floating, euphoric, lethargic and very contented. Nausea is rare. Their speech will be slow and their voice will be husky and sluggish. They are able to maintain an open mouth. The amnesic effect of nitrous oxide is slightly more at this stage.

Plane 3: Total amnesia. The patient is administered between 55% and 70% nitrous oxide. The patient's fears and anxieties are eliminated, as is their response to pain. Although the amnesic effect of nitrous oxide is obvious, the patient can become agitated and have a fixed stare with unpleasant hallucinatory dreams. Nausea may also be felt and their mouth may close.

Stage 2: Known as the excitement stage. The patient will lose consciousness and could experience uncontrolled movements, vomit and hold their breath. Their pupils may become dilated with their heart rate and breathing being irregular.

Stage 3: The surgical stage. The patient's muscles relax with their breathing returning to a regular rhythm. Their eye movements slow and then stop, becoming fixed with a central stare. This stage has been divided into four planes where the following will be observed – the patient's eyes roll and then become fixed; the corneal and laryngeal reflexes are lost. Reflexes are lost and the pupils dilate. The intercostal muscles are paralysed, abdominal respiration is shallow and the pupils dilate.

Stage 4: Also known as the overdose stage, as the patient will be administered too high a percentage of nitrous oxide, resulting in medullary depression. The patient's breathing stops and a potential cardiovascular collapse occurs.

19. To fit the patient with the correct size nasal mask, for the patient to observe the machine and experience the mask being worn with the introduction of a small amount of oxygen. To explain the next appointment pathway. All this will result in a more cooperative patient.

20. Plane 1 or 2 of stage 1.

21. Reduced anxiety levels, analgesia and anterograde amnesia. Detached and disassociated from their surroundings. They will feel as if they are floating; they may feel dreamy, euphoric and experience tingling of lips tongue and fingers.

22. The sedation will be ineffective as it will be impossible for the patient to inhale the gases into the lungs, thus allowing gaseous exchange to take place. Instead, it will be breathed into the atmosphere as the patient will be breathing by mouth. The gases that are under pressure and this positive pressure could push the infection further down into the respiratory structure. This could result in the patient leaving with a lower respiratory tract infection.

23. Pre-operative – to cancel appointment if they have a cold, cough or blocked nose. To bring the mask with them if one has previously been provided. If the patient is an adult and they wish to bring an escort to do so. Post-operative – to go home and take it easy for the rest of the day with the remaining instructions being dependent on the dental treatment received. There are no post-operative restrictions placed on patients with respect to daily activities.

24. If the patient could not maintain an open mouth and close it spontaneously, this is indicative of over-sedation.

25. There is no gastric absorption or any significant metabolism; therefore, there is not any adverse effect on the liver, kidneys, brain, cardiovascular or respiratory system. There is minimal impairment of cough and swallowing reflexes, so the patient's airway is not compromised. Patients recover very quickly and there are not any post-sedation restrictions so they can undertake any of their normal daily responsibilities/activities. One of the key factors that make it a safe form of sedation is that at all times a patient receives a minimum of 30% oxygen. There is no need for a cannula to be placed. An escort is not required.

26. No.

27. Dental procedures where the mask might impair vision and access, for example, an anterior apicectomy. The common cold, flu or nasal obstruction. Claustrophobia. Tuberculosis and acute pulmonary conditions. Psychiatric and immunosuppressed patients. Pregnant patients in the first trimester. Myasthenia gravis. Pneumothorax, Middle Ear and Sinus Disease.

28. The patient's breathing would be observed along with the colour of the patient's skin tone and demeanour.

29. Patients do not have a cold, cough or blocked nose. They are happy to proceed with treatment and if they have any questions. They have brought their mask with them if one was provided for them to take home.

30. All required dental instruments, material and medicaments are available along with the patient's notes, consent form and radiographs. The emergency equipment has been checked. Colleagues are informed that there should be no interruptions during the treatment session and telephone calls are diverted. Good ventilation. Staff have been rotated. Different size masks are available. Whether the machine being used is a piped system or a mobile system, it has been checked prior to use.

31. Reassure the patient, monitor and reduce the nitrous oxide percentage.

32. As they would no longer be sedated, they would be anxious.

Nitrous oxide
   1. Blue.

   2. It has a sweet odour and taste.

   3. 800 lb per square inch.

   4. No, it is a liquid under pressure.

   5. Ammonium sulphate.

   6. 50%.

7. This is a theory used to compare the strength or potency of anaesthetic vapours. It is defined as the concentration of a vapour in the lungs that is required to prevent movement (motor response) in 50% of subjects in response to surgical (pain) stimulus. For nitrous oxide, this is reached at 105% and is not compatible with life if sustained for anything other than short periods.

8. By tapping the cylinder on the basis of the principle that the duller the sound the less full or by weighing cylinders. If weighing, the principle used is that a full cylinder weighs approximately 8.8 kgs. An empty cylinder weighs approximately 5.4 kgs. Therefore, the gas contained within the cylinder would be approximately 3.4 kgs.

9. No, as the contents of the cylinder is a liquid under pressure.

10. By tapping the cylinder on the basis of the principle that the duller the sound the less full, or weighing the cylinders. If weighing, the principle used is that a full cylinder weighs approximately 8.8 kgs. An empty cylinder weighs approximately 5.4 kgs. Therefore, the gas contained within the cylinder would be approximately 3.4 kgs.

11. Stamped on a plastic collar on the top of a cylinder are the content, batch number, expiry date and approximate weight.

12. Because only a small amount of nitrous oxide is metabolised by the patient.

13. Decrease mental performance, affect manual dexterity and inhibit the bone marrow function. It can cause infertility in female workers and birth defects. It can lead to numbness in the peripheral extremities causing pins and needles sensations. It causes Vitamin B12 deficiency, which is required for the brain and nervous system to function normally and is also required for formation of blood. It can cause anaemia.

14. Yes. The Health and Safety Commission has established Workplace Exposure Limits (WELs), which are in place to prevent excessive exposure thus limiting risk to health.

15. Long-term exposure for nitrous oxide is a time-weighted average of 100 parts per million over an 8-hour period in any 24 hours.

16. To account for staff who work in operating theatres at night.

17. Anaesthetic gas scavenging systems. Servicing by a manufacturer or authorised personnel. Checking the machine prior to use for leaks. Using good fitting nasal masks. Good room ventilation. Any fans used must be placed at floor level. Limiting the amount of sessions per week and rotating staff. Encouraging the patient not to talk. Use of rubber dam and high volume aspiration to suction exhaled nitrous oxide. Air and personal nitrous oxide monitors can be used to ensure time-weighted averages are not exceeded.

18. 1772.

19. Joseph Priestley.

20. 1844.

21. Dr. Horace Wells, an American dentist.

Oxygen

1. White with a white shoulder.

2. No, it is odourless.

3. Stamped on a plastic collar on the top of a cylinder are the content, batch number, expiry date and approximate weight.

4. 2000 lb per square inch.

5. There would be a risk of an explosion occurring as oxygen is not flammable but will support combustion.

6. No, but it will support combustion.

7. 30%.

8. If oxygen is not provided, it will lead to unconsciousness as nitrous oxide is a weak anaesthetic.

9. To prevent diffusion hypoxia.

10. 30 l per minute.

The machine

1. To ensure it is safe for use, there are not any leaks, nitrous oxide stops delivery if oxygen fails and there are enough gases for the intended procedure.

2. All four cylinders (two nitrous oxide and two oxygen) should be switched off and firmly attached to the machine. One of each. The nitrous oxide and oxygen cylinders should be labelled in use and full. Blue piping is checked to ensure it is connected to the nitrous oxide cylinder and white piping to the oxygen cylinder. The full oxygen cylinder is checked first by turning the tap to ensure that the oxygen gauge/dial reads full. This equates to approximately 2000 lb per square inch. The tap is then turned off again. Depending on the top of the oxygen cylinder, the tap will either be opened by a key or by hand. The oxygen flush button is then pressed to release all oxygen from the system and to check that it is functional. The dial indicator should then return to zero. The reservoir bag will inflate and is checked for leaks or tears. The reservoir bag should be removed to check that the air entrainment valve is not blocked and then replaced. The in-use oxygen cylinder is then checked by turning the tap on, making sure that it is at least a quarter full. This equates to 500 lb per square inch. If the cylinder contains less than this, a new cylinder is fitted. As stock must be rotated, the existing full cylinder becomes the in-use one and the new cylinder then becomes the full one. When changing any cylinder, it is important to ensure that the Bodok seal, similar to a washer, is not worn and is in place. The in-use cylinder is left switched on. The full nitrous oxide cylinder is switched on and off. The nitrous oxide gauge/dial will, if not recently used, reach 800 lb per square inch. Nitrous oxide in some machines cannot be flushed out of the system; therefore, when switching on the in-use nitrous oxide cylinder, it is impossible to tell how much it contains as its gauge/dial will still give the reading of the full cylinder. A rough indication is to tap both cylinders while listening to the difference in sound. The duller the sound, the

less it contains. For more accuracy, the cylinders can be weighed – a full cylinder weighs approximately 8.8 kg. An empty cylinder weighs approximately 5.4 kg. The gas therefore equates to approximately 3.4 kg. The in-use nitrous oxide cylinder is left switched on. The automatic nitrous oxide safety cut-off valve is then checked by setting the flow meter to 8 l per minute of 100% oxygen, altering the percentage to 50%, which alters the flow of nitrous oxide and oxygen to 4 l per minute each. Calibration of the machine is checked at this point. The in-use oxygen cylinder is switched off. As oxygen supply failure has been simulated, nitrous oxide should automatically fail and both metal balls in the flow meters should drop to zero. There will be a slight delay in the metal balls dropping to zero as there will still be some oxygen present in the system. Once this check has been undertaken satisfactorily, the in-use oxygen cylinder is switched back on and the in-use nitrous oxide cylinder switched off. The dial is retuned to 100% and the oxygen cylinder is switched off. The oxygen flush button is then pressed to expel all oxygen from the machine and all tubing is inspected for holes and to ensure they have not perished.

3. The white oxygen pipe is placed into the oxygen outlet valve and the blue nitrous oxide pipe into the nitrous oxide outlet valve, making sure they are secure. The scavenging system is connected. The dial on the delivery head is turned to 100% oxygen. The on button turned until the metal ball in the oxygen flow meter reaches 8 l per minute. The oxygen flow is altered to 50%. This will automatically dial in 50% nitrous oxide and the metal ball in the nitrous oxide flow meter will rise to 4 l per minute. The metal ball in the oxygen flow meter will drop to 4. The calibration of the machine is checked. The nitrous oxide safety cut-out valve is checked by simulating oxygen failure by removing the oxygen piping from the outlet valve. If functional, nitrous oxide will stop delivery and both metal balls in the flow meters will drop to zero, the oxygen pipe is then replaced into the outlet valve with the flow meter being returned to 100% and the machine switched off. The oxygen flush button is pressed to ensure it is functional and inflates the reservoir bag. The reservoir bag once inflated is checked for any leaks or hole and is removed to check that the air entrainment valve is not blocked and then replaced. The last check is to inspect all tubing for holes and that they have not perished.

4. The clinician using the machine, however, the norm is the sedation nurse undertakes this role.

5. Both piped and mobile machines – nitrous oxide stops delivery if the oxygen supply fails. The reservoir bag allows monitoring of a patient's respiration. The air entrainment valve allows atmospheric air to be inhaled if both gases fail to deliver. Scavenging system allows the excess waste nitrous oxide to be removed from the atmosphere. Flush button can be pressed to provide additional oxygen. The machine will not allow any less than 30% oxygen to be delivered to a patient. Different colour pipes. Mobile only – different size connection nuts, which are stamped with either nitrous oxide or oxygen. In use, full and empty labels indicate the cylinder's status. 'E' size cylinders have unique pin indexing, making it impossible for the wrong cylinder to be connected to the machine. Bodok seals provide a tight fit between the cylinder and the machine to prevent leakage.

6. Yes. Servicing by a manufacturer or authorised personnel. Checking the machine prior to use for leaks. Using good fitting nasal masks. Good room ventilation. Any fans used must be placed at floor level. Limiting the amount of sessions per week and rotating staff. Encouraging patients not to talk. Use of rubber dam and high volume aspiration to suction exhaled nitrous

oxide. Air and personal nitrous oxide monitors can be used to ensure time-weighted averages are not exceeded.

7. To remove the waste nitrous oxide from the atmosphere.

8. There are two systems used: Active system, which pumps the gas away, and passive system, which has one entry and one exit for the gas.

9. 2000 lb per square inch.

10. 500 lb per square inch.

11. When it is a quarter full (500 lb per square inch).

12. By tapping the cylinder on the basis of the principle that the duller the sound, the less it contains or by weighing the cylinder. If weighing, the principle used is that a full cylinder weighs approximately 8.8 kg. An empty cylinder weighs approximately 5.4 kg; therefore, the gas contained within the cylinder would be approximately 3.4 kg.

13. 2000 lb per square inch.

14. 800 lb per square inch.

15. 45 lb per square inch.

16. 30 l per minute.

17. 2 l.

18. To allow atmospheric air to be inhaled if both gases fail to deliver.

19. They make it impossible for the wrong cylinder to be connected to the machine.

20. Fitted on prongs between the cylinder and the machine.

21. To provide a tight fit between the cylinder and the machine, thus preventing any gas leakage.

22. The Bodok seal was worn and would require replacement.

23. When the dial has been set at 50% nitrous oxide and oxygen, the metal balls in the flow metres are equal.

24. So that the patient does not receive pure nitrous oxide, which would render them unconscious.

25. By setting the flow rate to 8 l per minute and the dial to 50% nitrous oxide and oxygen so that the metal balls in the flow metres are equal at 4 l per minute each. Oxygen failure is simulated by cutting off the oxygen supply.

26. When nitrous oxide is running low, it will burn off as a gas; therefore, the dial reading will be accurate.

Administration/delivery

1. All required dental instruments, material and medicaments are available along with the patient's notes, consent form and radiographs. The emergency equipment has been checked. Colleagues are informed that there should be no interruptions during the treatment session and telephone calls are diverted. Good ventilation and staff have been rotated. Different size masks are available. Whether the machine being used is a piped system or a mobile system, it has been checked prior to use.

2. For an adult 8 l per minute and for a child 6 l per minute.

3. The patient's respiratory rate would be multiplied by the tidal volume for the age of the patient.

4. 100%.

5. The patient is asked to place the nasal mask over his or her nose and it is checked to ensure that it is seated correctly. The clinician briefly explains in a soft, quiet hypnotic voice the sensations/feelings that the patient may experience and the dental chair is slowly lowered into the supine position.

6. The patient can breathe through their nose, the mask is seated so that it is a good fit, the reservoir bag is inflating and the patient is happy.

7. The reservoir bag has filled and is inflating and deflating rhythmically to reflect the patient's respiratory rate. The nasal mask still has a good fit.

8. 15%.

9. The flow rate would be reduced.

10. The patient is not utilising the full amount of gas flow being provided.

11. The flow rate would be increased.

12. The patient requires more than the amount of gas flow being provided.

13. Approximately a quarter full as it corresponds to a patient's tidal volume.

14. In a soft, hypnotic voice using lots of reassurance and positive images.

15. Plane 1 – Moderate sedation and analgesia.

16. 5%.

17. Plane 2 – Dissociation sedation and analgesia.

18. They would be sedated and experience some analgesia, tingling feelings. They would feel relaxed and as if they are floating, slightly odd and giggly.

19. They would feel heavy, dissociated from the surroundings as if they are floating and spinning.

20. 100% oxygen for 3–5 minutes.

21. It is slowly reduced.

22. For as long as required until they are deemed fit for discharge after being assessed. Normally patients are fit to leave after approximately 20 minutes.

23. Level of consciousness, respiration, demeanour and skin tone.

Miscellaneous

1. Stopping of high-concentration nitrous oxide after delivery will result in its elimination from the blood very quickly. This will result in more carbon dioxide than usual being expelled together with nitrous oxide. This reduces the amount of carbon dioxide in the blood. The reason a breath is taken is attributed to the rising level of carbon dioxide in the blood. If the level is reduced, the patient will not breathe and will suffer respiratory depression. This is known as the second gas effect.

   When the inhalation sedation machine is switched off, nitrous oxide will leave the blood and flood into the lungs to be exhaled, because the concentration in the blood is higher than that in the lungs. This will result in a dilution of oxygen levels within the lungs and the patient will experience hypoxia, headaches, nausea and lethargy.

2. By providing 3–5 minutes of 100% oxygen at the end of the procedure.

3. Entonox.

4. Control of substances hazardous to health.

5. Workplace Exposure Limits.

6. Time-weighted average.

7. Minimum alveolar concentration.

8. Pound per square inch.

9. One of the safety features of inhalation sedation machines is that it always delivers a minimum of 30% oxygen. As pulse oximeters measure the amount of saturated oxygen a patient has bound to their haemoglobin the recorded reading will reflect this. A delivery of 30% oxygen is also more than in atmospheric air.

10. Speaking to the patient in a soft, calm reassuring manner. Boosting the patient's confidence by telling them how well they are doing. Using positive images, for example, the last holiday that the patient went on or something that they enjoy doing.

11. 500 mls.

SECTION VII Answers: Medical emergencies

Faint

1. A sudden and temporary loss of consciousness.

2. Vasovagal attack or syncope.

3. All of the following factors can contribute to a patient's fainting when attending the dental surgery: anxiety, pain, fatigue, not eating; having a high temperature and being hot. When patients experience these factors, they may faint. Patients might faint after the administration of a local anaesthetic. In most procedures, anaesthetics are given to relieve pain, but they can cause patients to faint.

4. It is either caused by hypotension or inadequate cerebral perfusion to the brain, therefore, less oxygen, any of which results in the patient losing consciousness.

5. Pallor (putty colour), dizziness, light headedness and feeling weak, blurred vision, nausea and vomiting, sweating, especially on the brow and upper lip. Patients may complain of being hot and thirsty and can yawn. The pulse will initially be slow and weak, then rapid due to low blood pressure. The patient may lose consciousness and become limp.

6. The patient's head should be lowered by laying them down with their legs raised. If the patient is pregnant or obese, they should be laid on their left side. Clothing should be loosened, especially round the neck and the patient should be advised of this action. The surgery should be ventilated and a cold compress placed on the patient's forehead. Upon recovery, the patient is provided with a glucose drink. If the patient does not recover within 2–3 minutes, re-diagnose the situation and if necessary call the emergency services, and in the absence of breathing, ignoring the occasional gasp, and signs of life, prepare to undertake cardiopulmonary resuscitation. Oxygen should be provided. At all times, the patient should be monitored and reassured.

7. This will improve the venous return and increases the oxygenated blood flow to the brain.

8. The patient's head is lower than their legs.

9. Glucose drink or dextrose tablet. If required oxygen would be administered.

Cardiac arrest

1. A sudden, sometimes temporary, cessation of function of the heart.

2. It is to sustain life by keeping the oxygenated blood circulating to perfuse the vital organs until emergency treatment can be administered.

3. Pre-existing coronary heart disease. Many cardiac arrests that cause sudden death occur when electrical impulses in the diseased heart become rapid (ventricular tachycardia) or chaotic

(ventricular fibrillation) or sometimes even both and the resulting irregular heart rhythm (arrhythmia) causes the heart to suddenly stop beating. Some cardiac arrests can be attributed to slowing down of the heart rate, known as bradycardia. Other reasons for a cardiac arrest occurring are respiratory arrest, drowning, electrocution, choking, hypoxia and trauma, and it can occur without any contributing factors.

4. No signs of life. No breathing/abnormal breathing in the form of infrequent noisy gasps. Unconsciousness.

5. Check area for danger/hazards. Assess the patient's response by touching both their shoulders and speaking into both ears. Call for help. Open the airway by performing a head tilt and chin lift. Check the mouth for any debris and if it is easily accessible remove it. Suction may be required. Breathing and circulation is assessed. If none, call the emergency services. If you are alone the patient will have to be left. If help has arrived one of you must phone the emergency services while the other commences cardiopulmonary resuscitation. It is important that the person who makes the call returns to offer assistance and informs that the emergency services are on their way. 30 chest compressions are performed at a depth of 5–6 cm (a third of the chest) over the sternum and at a rate of 100–120 per minute followed by two ventilations. If help arrives request they fetch an automated external defibrillator (AED) if one is available along with a pocket mask and portable oxygen.

6. The child would be assessed in the same way as an adult. If they were not breathing normally five rescue breaths would be administered. If the child was still unresponsive and did not exhibit any sign of life/circulation after 10 seconds then, before calling the emergency services, 1 minute of cardiopulmonary resuscitation is performed by undertaking 15 chest compressions and 2 rescue breaths, using one or two hands for a child elder than the age of 1 to achieve an adequate depth.

7. When the emergency services arrive, have setup and been briefed. If the patient shows signs of regaining consciousness, they move and start to breathe normally, open their eyes or coughs. You become exhausted or in danger.

8. They artificially pump the oxygenated blood around the body.

9. These provide the blood with oxygen to perfuse the vital organs.

10. 30:2.

11. 15:2.

12. The patient might vomit as the stomach is being pressed upon.

13. Ventricles.

14. The pressure provided should be firm, controlled and applied vertically as erratic or violent compressions are dangerous.

15. Between approximately 4 and 6 minutes.

16. Defibrillator.

17. The patient would be managed in the same way except ventilations would not be undertaken, only chest compressions.

Anaphylaxis

1. An extreme, often life-threatening, allergic reaction to an antigen to which the body has become hypersensitive.

2. Latex, foods, medication, administration of a drug, exercise, bee stings, animals, dust and sometimes, unknown causes (idiopathic).

3. Urticaria. Rhinitis. Conjunctivitis. Nausea, vomiting, diarrhoea and abdominal pains.
   Patients might experience a sense of unease and impending doom. Flushing is very common; however, a pale complexion may also occur. Marked upper airway (laryngeal). Oedema of the tongue and upper airway. Bronchospasms may develop, causing strider. Peripheral coldness and cold clammy skin. Rapid/weak impalpable pulse, tachycardia with a rapid drop in blood pressure. Vasodilation leading to a drop in the blood pressure and collapse. Respiratory arrest. Loss of consciousness and cardiac arrest.

4. Remove the cause or stop administration of the drug. Place the patient in the supine position. Maintain the patient's airway and administer 10–15 litres of oxygen per minute. Call the emergency services. The clinician would administer 0.5 ml adrenaline injection 1:1000 intramuscularly (IM) to a semi-conscious patient or one presenting severe bronchospasms and a widespread rash. The dose of adrenaline would be repeated every 5 minutes depending on the patient's vital signs. Continually monitor and reassure the patient. If they lose consciousness, assess for signs of life and breathing and if necessary undertake cardiopulmonary resuscitation, ignoring the occasional gasp. All patients to be transferred to hospital for further assessment, irrespective of their initial recovery. An antihistamine drug, chlorpheniramine maleate (Piriton), and a steroid, hydrocortisone succinate (Solu-Cortef), are useful in the management of an allergic reaction, but they are not first-line drugs and will be administered by the emergency services if necessary.

5. An antihistamine drug, chlorpheniramine maleate (Piriton), and a steroid, hydrocortisone succinate (Solu-Cortef).

6. A few activations of salbutamol would be administered, and if necessary a large-volume spacer device could be used with 4–6 activations of salbutamol being administered every 10 minutes until the emergency services arrive. If the patient showed signs and symptoms that were life threatening, then intramuscular adrenaline would be administered.

7. Adrenaline.

8. Intramuscular.

9. 0.5 ml 1:1000.

10. 0.3 ml 1:1000.

11. It helps to reverse the symptoms of an allergic reaction by improving the blood pressure and accelerating the heart rate.

12. EpiPen or Anapen.

13. It is a vasoconstrictor and therefore, can constrict the vessels to the heart.

14. Biphasic anaphylaxis is the recurrence of symptoms within 1–72 hours with no further exposure to the allergen. This occurs approximately within 6 hours as adrenaline has a short half-life.

15. Within minutes up to hours later.

Adrenal insufficiency

1. This is the condition in which the adrenal glands do not produce sufficient amounts of steroid hormones – cortisol and aldosterone.

2. Pale complexion, abdominal pain, vomiting, nausea, drop in blood pressure, rapid loss of consciousness and low blood glucose levels.

3. Monitor and reassure the patient and lay them flat with their legs higher than their head. Administer oxygen at 10–15 litres per minute. Call the emergency services. Hydrocortisone would be administered.

4. Patients who have been taking corticosteroids for a period of time or have stopped taking them can suffer an adrenal crisis due to physiological stress. This is because insufficient amount of cortisol is being produced by the adrenal glands; therefore, the body might not be able to cope with any kind of major stress, which can be life-threatening.

Angina

1. Angina is pain or pressure localised in the chest that is caused by an insufficient supply of blood (ischaemia) to the heart muscle. It is not a disease but an indication of an underlying heart problem.

2. Angina pectoris.

3. Ischaemia is an insufficient blood supply to an organ, usually due to a blocked artery.

4. Myocardial ischaemia, exercise, stress and hypertension.

5. Pain or tightness in the centre of the chest. Severe retrosternal pain possibly radiating down the left arm and into the neck. Pain can also be experienced within the right arm. Pulse can be regular or irregular. Shortness of breath. Sweating, nausea, light headedness and feeling weak. Women are more prone to experiencing pain in their back, shoulders and abdomen.

6. Reassure and sit the patient up. Glyceryl trinitrate spray to be used and can be repeated three times. Maintain the airway. Oxygen to be administered at 10–15 litres per minute. If the patient is not provided with any relief after 3–5 minutes, the diagnosis would be reconsidered (myocardial infarction). A 300 mg chewable aspirin administered. Emergency services called and patient monitored for deterioration.

7. Laying a patient down would increase their breathlessness and pain.

8. Glycerol trinitrate.

9. Spray or tablets.

10. Sublingual – as the membrane is thin in this area, the medication is absorbed very quickly.

11. As it can result in a headache.

12. Three over a 3–5 minute timeframe.

13. Myocardial infarction.

14. A 300 mg chewable aspirin would be administered and the emergency service called. The patient would be sat up, monitored and reassured.

Asthma

1. A respiratory condition marked by spasms in the bronchi of the lungs, causing difficulty in breathing. It is a chest condition that occurs due to a narrowing of the airways where the lining of the walls swell and become inflamed.

2. Stress, emotion, anxiety, exercise, exposure to an allergen, hay fever colds or chest infections and laughter.

3. Laying a patient down will increase their breathlessness and pain.

4. Salbutamol inhaler.

5. Ventolin.

6. Breathlessness, inability to complete a sentence, wheezing on exhalation with accessory muscles of respiration in action, increased respiratory rate, tachycardia, and anxiety. Life threatening would be bradycardia, a slow pulse rate, decreased respiratory rate, cyanosis of the lips and/or extremities, exhaustion, confusion and a decreased level of consciousness.

7. Reassure and monitor the patient and sit them up. Encourage a few activations from a salbutamol inhaler. If unable to use an inhaler effectively, additional doses should be given through

a large-volume spacer device. Emergency services to be called if the patient does not improve or they deteriorate. Maintain the patient's airway and administer 10–15 litres of oxygen per minute.

8. It works by acting on receptors in the lungs called beta-2 receptors. Stimulating these receptors causes the muscles in the airways to relax. This allows the airways to open and makes it easier to breathe.

9. 100 micrograms per activation.

10. A large-volume spacer device.

11. As it will open the airways shortly before exercising to prevent wheezing.

12. Beclomethasone.

Myocardial infarction

1. Destruction of heart tissue as a result of an obstruction of the blood supply to the heart muscle.

2. Heart attack.

3. Coronary heart diseases lead to blood clot formation. If the clot increases in size, it can cause a narrowing or a complete blockage in the blood pathway to the heart muscle, limiting the oxygen-rich blood, causing a myocardial infarction.

4. Part of the heart muscle becomes damaged and begins to die due to a lack of oxygen.

5. Severe crushing retrosternal chest pain radiating down the left arm and up into the neck. Pain may also be experienced in the right arm. Breathlessness, nausea and vomiting, pale and clammy skin, very distressed patient. Weak, irregular pulse and low blood pressure. Deathly appearance, loss of consciousness and cardiac arrest.

6. Emergency services called. Reassurance provided and the patient sat up. Lay the patient flat if they feel faint. Airway is maintained and oxygen administered at 10–15 litres per minute. If available some clinicians may decide to administer 50% oxygen and 50% nitrous oxide via a relative analgesia machine. A 300 mg chewable aspirin is administered. Glyceryl trinitrate spray can be used. Patient is monitored and watched for signs of a cardiac arrest. Perform cardiopulmonary resuscitation if the patient loses consciousness, stops breathing and/or does not show any signs of life.

7. 300 mg chewable aspirin.

8. It thins the blood.

9. Oxygen or 50% nitrous oxide and 50% oxygen through a dedicated inhalation sedation machine. GTN spray.

Respiratory arrest

1. Respiratory arrest is the cessation of normal respiration due to failure of the lungs to function effectively. A respiratory arrest is different from (but may be caused by) a cardiac arrest.

2. A partial or complete airway obstruction. The most common cause is the tongue obstructing the oropharynx. Causes of an upper airway obstruction could be blood, mucus, vomit, foreign body, spasm or oedema of the vocal cords or trauma. Lower airway obstruction may occur after aspiration of gastric contents, widespread severe bronchospasm or extensive airspace filling processes, that is, pneumonia and pulmonary oedema.

3. The patient collapses and exhibits signs of life, but not breathing.

4. Emergency services called. About 10–12 effective breaths are administered and signs of life rechecked. If breathing is restored, the patient is placed in the recovery position and monitored for any sign of deterioration. In the event of the patient's breathing disappearing, they are placed onto their backs and rescue breathing resumed. If the patient's signs of life disappear, cardiopulmonary resuscitation should be started.

5. Cardiac arrest will quickly follow, because progressive hypoxia will impair cardiac function.

Choking and aspiration

1. It is the inability to breathe due to the trachea being blocked or constricted or swollen shut.

2. A foreign object. The most common causes of choking occur when eating and the food goes down the trachea instead of the oesophagus. This happens if the person inhales before swallowing the food, that is, when they have a sudden urge to cough or swallow too fast without chewing the food enough.

3. Coughing and spluttering, noisy difficult breathing, paradoxical chest or abdominal movements, cyanosis and loss of consciousness.

4. Encourage the patient to cough. If the patient becomes weak, stops coughing or breathing they are left where they are. If possible any obvious foreign objects can be removed carefully. Whether the patient is standing or sitting, the rescuer stands to the side of them, but slightly behind and supports them with one hand. The patient will be leant forward and five sharp slaps between the shoulder blades will be administered using the base of the palm of the hand. These slaps should be fairly forceful and in an upward action. If the object is expelled from the patient's mouth, the slaps must be stopped. If the object is not expelled, then five abdominal thrusts are undertaken by both arms being placed around the upper part of the patient's abdomen, clenching a fist and placing it between the umbilicus and xiphisternum. The fist is grasped with the other hand and pulled sharply inwards and upwards five times. If the object is expelled, the abdominal thrusts must stop. This is repeated. If the patient becomes unconscious, the emergency services are called and cardiopulmonary resuscitation is carried out, adjusting the sequence to suit the age of the patient.

5. Five of each. However, if the item expels before five are administered, they are stopped.

6. Breathing in a foreign object.

7. Coughing and spluttering, noisy difficult breathing, paradoxical chest or abdominal movements, cyanosis and loss of consciousness.

8. Reassure and sit the patient up. Encourage them to cough and ask them to search their clothing. Search the floor to see if the item has fallen. To eliminate the possibility that the item was aspirated into the suction equipment, the practice, if they have the facility (large enough image receptor) could X-ray the suction tubing and pot. The patient should be sent as an emergency for a chest X-ray to establish whether the item has ended up in the stomach or the lungs if it cannot be found. If the patient is wheezing, a few activations of a salbutamol inhaler may be administered.

9. The right lung as the right bronchus is straighter than the left and it is higher up, because the diaphragm is slightly higher on the right than on the left side.

Epilepsy

1. It is a common serious neurological condition in which there is a tendency for seizures to occur that start in the brain. It is usually only diagnosed after a person has had more than one seizure.

2. Stress, tiredness, bright lights, starvation, menstruation, some drugs and alcohol.

3. The patient may have a brief warning or an aura and look and feel detached from their surroundings. They will suddenly lose consciousness, become rigid, fall to the ground and might cry out and in the tonic phase they can become cyanosed. After a few seconds their limbs jerk in thrashing movements and the tongue may be bitten in the clonic phase. They may froth at the mouth and become urinary incontinent.

    The seizure will last for a few minutes and once over the patient may become very floppy and remain unconscious. Recovery will be very slow and can be variable, with some individuals left feeling very dazed and confused.

4. Verbal reassurance is required. Prevent the patient from injury and do not restrain them. Their head can be placed on a pillow or hands can be placed either side of their head to cushion it as it moves from side to side. Whilst they are fitting, an airway is not to be inserted or anything placed between their teeth. When the patient recovers, vital signs are monitored and the patient is placed in the recovery position. Airway to be maintained and oxygen administered at 10–15 litres per minute. Patients are not to be discharged until they are fully fit. If no recovery after 5 minutes or the convulsive movements recur in quick succession, the emergency services must be called. Epistatus can be administered into the buccal sulcus. If the patient remains unconscious, check for breathing (ignoring the occasional gasp) and signs of life, and if necessary start cardiopulmonary resuscitation.

5. When the patient does not recover after 5 minutes or the convulsive movements recur in quick succession.

6. Epistatus.

7. Buccal sulcus.

8. Benzodiazepine.

9. 10 mg/ml.

Hypoglycaemia

1. Diabetes.

2. Low blood glucose levels.

3. If a patient took too much insulin or took the normal amount for that time of day, but ate less than usual or exercised. Not eating or taking their normal dose of insulin or oral hypo-glycaemic agent before attending the dental surgery.

4. The patient could be irritable and aggressive, uncooperative, truculent and have slurred speech. They may be cold, have clammy, sweaty skin, complain of a headache and possi-bly be shaking and trembling. They may appear drowsy, disorientated, find it difficult to concentrate, be vague and confused.

5. If the patient is cooperative, they can be given a glucose drink, milk with some added sugar, dextrose tablets or gel, repeating after 10–15 minutes if necessary. Blood glucose level would be checked.

6. The patient may be fitting and gradually lose consciousness.

7. If the patient's level of consciousness is impaired, they become uncooperative or are unable to swallow, then either buccal glucose gel or intramuscular glucagon is administered. Upon recovery the patient is given some food high in carbohydrates and are not allowed to drive.

8. Glucagon.

9. Intramuscular.

10. 1 mg.

11. 0.5 mg.

12. 4 mmol/l.

Hyperventilation

1. It is an increase in the depth and rate of breathing that is greater than demanded by the body needs.

2. Hyperventilation can be a result of feeling stressed, anxious or a panic attack.

3. When hyperventilating, a person abnormally starts breathing excessively fast (hyperpnoea), resulting in taking in more oxygen than the body normally needs. This causes an imbalance between the body's normal levels of oxygen and carbon dioxide as it retains too much oxygen and causes excessive expulsion of carbon dioxide (hypocapnia).

4. Light headed or faint. Hyperventilation does not normally lead to fainting but can progress to muscle spasms in the face and hands, which is known as tetany.

5. The patient will be reassured and asked to breathe slowly through their nose into a paper bag.

6. The patient will pass out.

7. Re-breathing of carbon dioxide is required to increase the level of carbon dioxide in the blood, thereby restoring to normal.

Airway control and ventilation

Laerdal pocket mask

1. They are clear; therefore, any condensation present as a result of the patient's respiration being restored can be seen. They have 'nose' imprinted on them to aid correct placement and they have a spongy base to allow flexibility and achieve a good seal. A disposable one-way valve is inbuilt, which will prevent the backflow of any expired air to the user, along with an oxygen port to attach tubing.

2. Cardiac and respiratory arrest.

3. 16%.

4. Approximately 6–7 litres per minute.

5. 65–70%.

6. As the oxygen tubing could become detached from the cylinder.

Hudson mask

1. They are made of clear plastic and have exhalation holes, with some having reservoir bags. There is a metal strip over the nose area and an elastic strap, which allows the mask to sit comfortably over the patient's nose and mouth area without the need for it to be held in place.

2. Faint, angina, myocardial infarction, asthma attack, anaphylaxis, epilepsy and hypoglycaemia.

3. Recovering after a general anaesthetic.

4. Flow rate will depend on the clinical diagnosis and condition of the patient, but would be set at approximately 3–6 litres per minute.

Nasal cannulae

1. It is a clear plastic tube with two prongs, which are designed to be placed within a patient's nose, allowing supplementary oxygen to be provided, when a patient is in a stable state.

2. They allow supplementary oxygen to be provided during treatment thereby leaving the mouth free for access.

3. If the patient's oxygen saturation levels drop during treatment, when intravenous sedation is being used or if the patient requires continual long-term oxygen therapy for a medical condition.

4. Approximately 4–5 litres per minute. However, if a patient attended and was on permanent oxygen therapy and the oxygen tubing was disconnected from their supply to the dental practice cylinder or piped system they would advise if the amount of oxygen they are receiving is too little or too much.

Oropharyngeal airway

1. They are curved plastic tubes that are flanged and reinforced at the oral end and used to maintain a patient's airway, especially when or if resuscitation is expected to be prolonged. They are designed to ensure that when inserted the patient's tongue is not displaced backwards and the airway is kept open. They are available in various sizes.

2. Guedel.

3. As there are various sizes available, the correct size is estimated by placing one end on the angle of the patient's mandible with the other at the corner of the patient's mouth.

4. 2, 3 or 4.

5. The patient's mouth must be checked to ensure it is free of foreign bodies. The airway is held in the inverted position and placed into the oral cavity, being rotated 180° as it passes below the palate and into the oropharynx. If the patient retches or coughs, the airway must be removed. Once inserted, the head tilt, chin lift or jaw thrust method must be adopted.

6. Between the tongue and the hard palate.

7. The tongue could be pushed further backwards, possibly into the pharynx causing an airway obstruction.

8. No. If a patient regains consciousness, the airway will be naturally expelled.

9. A head tilt, chin lift or jaw thrust is required in conjunction with an airway adjunct so that they are aligned and functional when in place.

Nasopharyngeal airway

1. They are malleable plastic tubes that are available in various sizes and are bevelled at one end with a flange at the other. They are used to maintain a patient's airway, especially when or if resuscitation is expected to be prolonged.

2. As there are various sizes available, the correct size is selected by measuring the bevelled end against the patient's little finger to establish whether the internal diameter of the airway is approximately the same size.

3. 6–8 mm.

4. The right nostril is checked to ensure it is not blocked. If it is, then the left nostril can be checked and used instead. A safety pin depending on the size of the flange may have to be inserted to prevent the airway being inhaled. The airway is then inserted, bevelled end into the right nostril by using a rotating action to twist it into the airway along the floor of the nose. If any obstructions are felt or difficulties encountered during insertion, the airway must be removed and the left nostril should be used. Once inserted, the head tilt, chin lift or jaw thrust method must be adopted.

5. Patient might vomit or experience a laryngeal spasm.

6. The bevelled end should sit in the pharynx with the flange resting at the nostril.

7. No.

8. A head tilt, chin lift or jaw thrust is required in conjunction with an airway adjunct so that they are aligned and functional when in place.

Oxygen

1. It is administered to patients in order to support life.

2. It is a medical gas.

3. No, it is not flammable but will support combustion.

4. C, D, E, F and G.

5. Approximately 2000 lb per square inch.

6. They are painted black with a white shoulder.

7. The size of the cylinder, batch number, expiry date and its content.

8. It is clear and colourless.

9. No, as it is odourless.

10. When storing cylinders, the full and the empty ones must be separated, with the full stock being kept in date order to avoid expiry going unnoticed.

11. A trolley should be used to avoid any injuries or accidents.

12. When oxygen is under high pressure and grease or oil is present, there is a possibility of explosion/combustion.

13. Approximately every 3–5 years.

Miscellaneous

1. Faint, epilepsy, angina, asthma, myocardial infarction (heart attack), anaphylactic shock, cardiac arrest, respiratory arrest, hypoglycaemia, adrenal insufficiency, panic attack/hyperventilation, choking and aspiration.

2. Faint.

3. Asthma, angina, myocardial infarction, respiratory arrest, choking and aspiration.

4. Epilepsy and hypoglycaemia.

5. Anaphylaxis, adrenal insufficiency, faint and cardiac arrest.

6. All staff to be trained in medical emergency procedures and understanding their role. Undertaking medical emergency simulations. Careful assessment and good patient management. Updating a patient's medical history every time they visit the dental practice. Monitoring a patient's vital signs during and after treatment. Emergency drugs and equipment kept where they are easily accessible. Daily checks undertaken to ensure all drugs are in date and that emergency equipment is functional. Emergency equipment to be serviced at recommended intervals with all documentation being kept. All staff being aware of the contents of the emergency drugs box and know which medication is used for any/each arising condition. Audits of these activities should take place on a regular basis. Recording any incidents in the patient's notes. Scheduling appointments to suit the patient's medical condition. Risk assessments that look at the ergonomics of the practice to establish any difficulties you might encounter should an emergency arise.

7. Surroundings, the condition of the patient and working as a team.

8. By assessing the surroundings to ensure nobody is harmed, assessing the patient, diagnosing their condition and calling for help.

9. Adrenaline (1:1000 1 mg/ml), aspirin, dispersible (300 mg), glucagon (1 mg), glyceryl trinitrate (GTN) spray (400 mcgs/dose), midazolam (5 or 10 mg/ml, buccal or intranasal), oral glucose/tablets/gel/powder, oxygen (D size with a pressure reduction valve and flow meter) and salbutamol (100 mcgs/dose).

10. In a designated place convenient for all who are aware of the location and stored as per the manufacturer's information. Where possible drugs should be drawn into a pre-filled syringe. Daily check sheets should be stored with or close by the drugs box, which contains the name of the drug and its expiry date.

11. Intravenous, intramuscular, inhalation, oral, sublingual, subcutaneous, buccal and nasal.

12. Intramuscular, inhalation, sublingual, buccal and nasal.

13. Different size oxygen face masks with tubing. Portable oxygen cylinder. Pocket mask with an oxygen port. Size 1, 2, 3 and 4 oropharyngeal airways. Self-inflating bag and mask with an oxygen reservoir bag and tubing with different size masks to accommodate both paediatric and adult patients. Portable suction with suction catheters and tubing. A Yankauer sucker.

Different size, single-use sterile syringes and needles. A large-volume spacer device. A blood glucose–monitoring measurement kit. Automated external defibrillator.

14. A sign indicates that a patient is experiencing an emergency, as it would be observed.

15. A symptom is something a patient would experience that would enable them, if it was a regular occurrence, to recognise/realise that the condition was imminent.

16. Hypoglycaemia.

17. A blood glucose–monitoring kit.

18. Epinephrine.

19. Entonox.

20. Status epilepticus.

21. Faint.

22. Asthma.

23. Hypoglycaemia.

24. Cardiac arrest.

25. Epilepsy.

26. Myocardial infarction.

27. Anaphylaxis.

28. Angina.

29. By re-breathing carbon dioxide, the level of carbon dioxide will raise in their blood and therefore they will start to breathe. This is because breathing is dependent on the level of carbon dioxide in blood.

30. Recovery.

31. Lateral.

32. If the patient is not on his or her back, they must be carefully placed in this position with both legs straight. Pockets are emptied and glasses if worn removed. Large rings are turned around so that the bulky area is to the palm side. The airway is opened. The patient's arm that is nearest to the rescuer is placed at right angles to the patient's body with the elbow bent, the palm of their hand being uppermost. The hand that is farthest away is brought across the chest and held in place against their face on the cheek nearest to the rescuer. The leg farthest away, just above the knee, is pulled up so that the foot is as flat as possible on the ground.

The leg is pulled gently so that the patient rolls onto their side. The leg is adjusted so that it is in a right angle position. The patient's airway is adjusted so that it remains open. The hand under the patient's cheek may need adjusting to ensure this. Constant reassurance and monitoring is undertaken throughout.

33. Laerdal pocket mask, bag mask valve, Hudson mask, nasal cannulae, oropharyngeal and nasopharyngeal airways.

34. Hudson mask.

35. Bag mask valve.

36. Nasal cannulae.

37. 15 litres per minute.

38. With a partial obstruction, air movement is reduced and invariably noisy. An upper airway obstruction will cause inspiratory stridor, with any expiratory noise, suggesting that there is an obstruction to the lower airway as it is prone to collapse and obstruct during expiration. A patient might snore if the pharynx is partially blocked by the tongue, whereas a crowing noise will be heard during a laryngeal spasm and if a liquid or a semi-solid foreign body is present, then a gurgling noise would be heard. A patient who has a complete blockage and who is attempting to breathe will exhibit paradoxical chest and abdominal movements, which can often be enhanced by the use of their accessory respiratory muscles.

39. The head must be extended by pushing the forehead backwards and the occiput caudally, whilst placing two fingers under the tip of the mandible to lift the chin, displacing their tongue anteriorly. If it is suspected that the patient has suffered a neck injury, the head can only be tilted if other methods of opening the airway have been unsuccessful.

40. By lifting a patient's head, the neck muscles lift the base of the tongue from the posterior pharyngeal wall and the epiglottis away from the laryngeal inlet. By lifting their chin, it stretches them even further, pulling the mandible and therefore the tongue forward.

41. Any neck injury could worsen. Tetraplegia could occur; however, death through hypoxia is more likely.

42. Thumbs are placed on the chin so that it can be displaced downwards. At the same time, the fingers are positioned behind the angle of the mandible. Pressure is applied in an upward and forward action so that the jaw is lifted forward.

43. Whichever technique is used, it is important to ensure that the airway is patent by the looking, listening and feeling process, because if it is not other possible causes must be explored and managed.

44. Nasopharyngeal.

45. If the patient was suffering from trismus or had trauma to the mouth.

SECTION VIII Answers: Essential anatomy

Heart

1. 72 beats per minute.

2. Pulmonary.

3. Myocardial infarction or fibrillation.

4. Septum.

5. Upper body.

6. Oxygenated.

7. Tricuspid, mitral (bicuspid), semi-lunar and aortic.

8. Prevent the backflow of blood.

9. Systemic.

10. High blood pressure.

11. Low blood pressure.

12. Fast pulse rate.

13. Slow pulse rate.

14. The left atrium.

15. The aorta.

16. Mitral valve (bicuspid).

17. The tricuspid valve.

18. The pulmonary artery.

19. Veins.

20. Two atria and two ventricles.

21. The right ventricle to the right atrium.

22. Oxygenated blood.

23. The pulmonary artery.

Blood

Plasma
1. Straw.

2. 55%.

3. To act as a transport medium.

4. Red blood cells, white blood cells, platelets, hormones, nutrients, proteins, irons, antibodies, clotting substances, gases and waste products.

5. Water.

Red blood cells
1. Oxygen.

2. Red bone marrow.

3. Erythrocytes.

4. Approximately 120 days.

5. Spleen.

6. Haemoglobin.

7. 99%.

8. They carry oxygen from the lungs to the cells and help remove carbon dioxide for transportation to the lungs to be exhaled.

9. Bi-concave (circular with a dip in the middle).

10. Spleen.

White blood cells
1. Leucocytes.

2. Lymphoid tissue.

3. To fight infection.

4. Approximately 13–21 days.

5. Lymph nodes.

6. Lymphatic system.

Platelets

1. 8–10 days.

2. Thrombocytes.

3. Coagulation.

4. Bone marrow.

5. Spleen.

6. Irregular.

7. Spleen.

Diseases/conditions of the blood

1. Anaemia.

2. Leukaemia.

3. Anaemia.

4. Sickle cell anaemia.

5. Half-moon-shaped red cells.

6. Warfarin and aspirin.

7. International Normalised Ratio.

8. Haemophilia, von Willebrand's and Christmas disease.

Miscellaneous

1. Corpuscles.

2. A, B, AB, O.

3. O.

4. White blood cells.

5. Red blood cells.

6. Red blood cells, white blood cells and platelets.

7. 5 litres (8.80 pints.)

8. pH 7.4.

9. White blood cells.

10. White blood cells.

11. Approximately 90%.

12. Platelets.

13. Platelets.

14. Red blood cells.

15. White blood cells.

16. Plasma.

17. Red blood cells.

18. White blood cells.

19. Platelets.

20. White blood cells increase in number when infections are present. They protect the body by engulfing and destroying microorganisms and removing dead or injured tissue.

The respiratory system

The nose and the nasal cavity
1. Cilia.

2. They protect the air passages to prevent any foreign materials from entering the nose.

3. Septum.

4. By sneezing or blowing the nose.

The pharynx
1. Throat.

2. Approximately 5 inches.

3. Nose, mouth and larynx (nasopharynx, oropharynx and laryngopharynx).

4. Oesophagus.

5. Epiglottis.

The larynx

1. Adam's apple.

2. Several cartilages.

3. The vocal cords within the thyroid cartilage.

4. Laryngitis.

5. It initiates the cough reflex and sends any mucous upwards to be swallowed by the pharynx.

6. Cricoid.

7. Cricothyrotomy.

The trachea and the bronchial tree

1. Mucous membrane and cilia.

2. To waft any foreign bodies up into the pharynx to be either swallowed or coughed up.

3. Approximately 12 cm.

4. Incomplete rings of cartilage connected by fibrous tissue.

5. Oesophagus.

6. Primary bronchi.

7. Right.

8. Bronchioles.

9. Alveoli.

10. Alveoli.

The lungs and the pleura

1. Alveoli.

2. The thoracic cavity.

3. Alveoli.

4. Pulmonary artery.

5. Pulmonary vein.

6. 600 million.

7. Right.

8. Left.

9. Right.

10. Three.

11. Two.

12. Superior, middle and inferior.

13. Superior and inferior.

14. Pyramid.

15. Pleural.

16. It allows expansion and contraction and holds the lungs against the chest wall preventing them from collapse.

17. Pneumothorax.

18. During deep breathing.

The diaphragm and the intercostal muscles
1. It moves up and down like a piston to enlarge the chest area.

2. Between the ribs.

Respiration
1. It is the process in which gases in the blood exchange with those present in the tissue cells.

2. It is the process in which the gases in the atmospheric air exchange with the gases in the lungs.

3. 20%.

4. 79% nitrogen, 1.0% trace gases, of which 0.04% is carbon dioxide.

5. Inspiration, expiration and a pause before the next cycle.

6. 16%.

7. Brain.

8. Intercostal muscles and diaphragm.

9. Abdomen, neck and shoulders.

10. Exercise.

11. Alveoli sacs.

12. Diffusion.

13. Oxygen and carbon dioxide.

14. 4%.

15. They will diffuse from a higher to a lower concentration/percentage. They are always in motion and will exert pressure on the container they are held in and if there is a hole they will escape.

16. Hyperventilation.

17. Calm reassurance. Monitor their vital signs. Ask them to breathe in and out of a paper bag. This action will result in them re-breathing their carbon dioxide. This raises the level of carbon dioxide in their blood, resulting in breathing being restored to normal. Under no circumstance should they be given oxygen.

Miscellaneous

1. Larynx.

2. Nose and nasal cavity, pharynx, larynx, trachea, lungs.

3. Inflammation of the pleura and membrane of the lungs.

4. 4%.

5. Cilia.

6. Pulmonary veins.

7. Oxygen and carbon dioxide.

8. The diaphragm.

9. Erythrocyte cells.

10. The trachea.

11. Incomplete rings of cartilage connected by fibrous tissue.

12. Plasma.

13. The pulmonary artery.

14. To trap dirt particles and waft them up to the pharynx for swallowing.

15. Flattened epithelial cells.

16. Numerous capillaries.

17. The diaphragm.

18. Nose, nasal cavity, pharynx and larynx.

19. Trachea, bronchi and lungs.

20. A buildup of carbon dioxide that requires removal as it is a waste gas.

21. To supply the blood with oxygen for transportation to all parts of the body, which takes place through breathing.

22. Energy.

23. Fast breathing.

24. Slow breathing.

The dorsum of the hand and the antecubital fossa

The dorsum of the hand
1. Back of the hand.

2. Dorsal digital network.

3. Cephalic and basilica.

4. If bruising occurs it can be painful.

5. Easy access and more difficult for the patient to bend their hand back.

The antecubital fossa
1. On the inner aspect of the elbow.

2. Cephalic and basilica.

3. Brachial.

4. Depending on the cannula used, the arm may need stabilising to restrict movement, thereby avoiding damage to deeper anatomical structures.

5. Larger veins and if bruising occurs, it can be hidden under clothing.

Miscellaneous

1. Median basilica.

2. Baby finger side of the inner aspect of the arm.

3. Thumb side of the inner aspect of the arm.

4. Use of a tourniquet or the sedation nurse placing both hands around the patient's arm to apply pressure.

CHAPTER 4

Dental implant nursing

Post Registration Qualifications for Dental Care Professionals: Questions and Answers, First Edition.
Nicola Rogers, Rebecca Davies, Wendy Lee, Dominic O'Sullivan and Frances Marriott.
© 2016 John Wiley & Sons, Ltd. Published 2016 by John Wiley & Sons, Ltd.
Companion Website: www.wiley.com/go/rogers/post-registration-dental-care-questions

SECTION I Questions: Indications for dental implant use

LEARNING OUTCOMES

At the end of this section, you should be able to identify any gaps in your knowledge associated with the following:

- How dental implants can be used
- Why dental implants are used

How dental implants can be used

1. What is a prosthesis?

2. What are the examples of fixed prostheses?

3. What is the definition of conventional bridgework?

4. What is a fixed fixed bridge?

5. What is a cantilevered bridge?

6. What are examples of removable prostheses?

7. What is an overdenture?

8. Dental implant-supported prostheses can be used as a method for replacing missing teeth. What are the main reasons for tooth loss?

9. What are the main causes of missing teeth?

10. What is hypodontia?

11. What treatment options should be considered for a patient who has missing teeth?

12. How can dental implants be used to help replace missing teeth?

13. Why do we replace missing teeth?

14. What negative consequences can occur if teeth are not replaced?

15. How can a patient's diet be affected if they have missing teeth?

Why dental implants are used

1. Why are dental implant-supported prostheses often considered as a better treatment option than conventional bridgework for patients with a spaced dentition when they lose a tooth?

2. What advantages do dental implant-supported dentures have over conventional dentures?

3. What differences are seen in how hard a patient can bite if they are moved from conventional denture wearing to implant-supported denture wearing?

4. What differences are seen in how efficiently a patient can chew their food if they are moved from conventional dentures to implant-supported dentures?

5. What differences in patient satisfaction are seen when patients are moved from conventional dentures to implant-supported dentures?

6. What advantages do dental implant-supported bridges have over conventional bridgework?

7. What advantages do a dental implant crown has over the use of a resin retained bridge to replace a missing tooth?

8. What advantages do a dental implant-supported crown has over a conventional bridge to replace a missing tooth?

9. Dental implants are often suggested as a treatment of choice for patients with an unrestored dentition who have a single tooth missing, why is that?

10. Why is it sometimes difficult to use conventional dental prostheses to rehabilitate patients who have had oral cancer?

11. How can dental implants be used in the rehabilitation of patients who have been affected by oral cancer?

12. How can implants be used in the rehabilitation of patients who have been affected by extra-oral cancer of the head and neck?

13. In patients who have hypodontia, what other features may be seen in their remaining teeth which may make conventional bridgework difficult?

SECTION II Questions: Medico-legal aspects of dental implant use

> **LEARNING OUTCOMES**
>
> At the end of this section, you should be able to identify any gaps in your knowledge associated with the following:
>
> • Consent in relation to dental implant treatment
> • The medico-legal considerations of dental implant treatment

Consent

1. How can you assist in helping a patient have informed consent to dental implant treatment?

2. Why is it important that you can understand the treatment plan proposed by the dentist?

3. How can you help to confirm that a patient has given informed consent to treatment?

4. Why is it important to explain to a patient the success rate for dental implants if they are considering dental implant treatment?

5. Why is it important to describe in detail to a patient as part of the consent process the origins of any bone augmentation products that are to be used in a patient's treatment?

6. Why is it important that you do not rely solely on implant company literature to inform patients about the advantages and disadvantages of implant treatment?

7. What are the potential negative aspects of dental implant surgery which patients should be made aware of as part of the consent process?

8. What are the medium and long-term issues that can occur with dental implant prostheses, and which patients should be made aware of as part of the consent process?

Medico-legal considerations

1. What training does a dentist require in the United Kingdom to practise implant dentistry?

2. What are the consequences for a dentist if they undertake implant treatment without appropriate training?

3. Is it essential for a dental nurse assisting in a dental implant treatment to have attended additional dental implant training courses beforehand?

4. Why is it important to record the precise details of the implant components used for each patient including the reference numbers/codes of each component?

5. The majority of patients' complaints regarding dental implant treatment relate to what cause?

6. If a dental implant fails soon after insertion, does this indicate that the surgeon is at fault medico-legally (negligent)?

7. What is medical or clinical negligence?

8. For clinical negligence to be proven against a clinician, what needs to be established?

9. Give some examples of where there may be a failure in the duty of care for a patient?

10. In cases of negligence is the dentist/nurse judged against the best standards of clinical practice that would be expected of a specialist in their field?

11. What is the Bolam test?

12. Very often within implant dentistry, there may be different approaches taken to treat a particular clinical situation with different clinicians taking different points of view. Is it a medico-legal problem if a dentist performs a procedure on a patient which other dentists may not agree is the best option?

13. Why is it important to monitor the failure rate and complication rate of implants in your dental practice?

SECTION III Questions: Role of the dental nurse

> **LEARNING OUTCOMES**
>
> At the end of this section, you should be able to identify any gaps in your knowledge associated with the following:
>
> - Patient assessment and planning for dental implants
> - The surgical phase of dental implant treatment
> - The restorative phase of dental implant treatment
> - The maintenance of dental implants and patient aftercare

Patient assessment and planning

1. What are the main aims of an initial patient assessment for dental implant planning?

2. Why is it important to ask a patient about what their expectations of dental implant treatment are?

3. At the initial examination visit, what basic instrumentation should be laid out for the dentist?

4. When should a medical history be taken?

5. What records/documentation needs to be collected at the initial patient assessment visit?

6. What special tests and diagnostic information may be needed at the initial patient assessment visit?

7. When sending impressions to the dental laboratory how should the impressions be prepared?

8. What information needs to be included on a laboratory prescription?

Surgical

1. It is important for the nurse and surgeon to ensure that drills used to prepare the implant site are suitably irrigated with saline, why is this?

2. It is important to ensure that the drills used for implant surgery are sharp so that they can work efficiently to prepare the site for the dental implant. How often can drills be reused?

3. Does it matter if an instrument or suction tip touches a dental implant before it is placed at the implant site?

4. Sterile drape kits provide the drapes and covers needed for dental implant treatment. What is included in an average drape kit for dental implant surgery?

5. In addition to a sterile drape kit, what other disposable equipment may be needed for implant placement surgery?

6. What personal protection equipment is used to protect the patient during surgery?

7. What personal protection equipment is used to protect the dentist and nurse during implant surgery?

8. When carrying out implant surgery it is important that asepsis is maintained. What does asepsis mean?

9. What does antisepsis mean?

10. Ideally at least two dental nurses should be present prior to and during dental implant surgery. What are their different roles called?

11. An aseptic technique is maintained by each nurse having a clear understanding of their different roles and what areas of the surgery and what equipment they may interact with. What are their different roles in maintaining an aseptic technique?

12. How should the dental surgery be prepared before setting up for the dental implant surgical procedure?

13. Which items and equipment should be gathered for dental implant surgery to be used for setting up and preparing the dental surgery for implant placement?

14. Different surgeons have individual preferences for the instruments that they like to have on an instrument tray; however, what basic instruments should always be on a dental implant surgical tray?

15. What is the general sequence involved in surgical hand scrubbing/cleansing prior to gowning and gloving for surgery?

16. Following hand washing/scrubbing, what should be put on first, the surgical gloves or surgical gown?

17. How is a surgical gown put on?

18. How are surgical gloves put on?

19. What is a bone trap?

20. If a bone trap is used, what precautions need to be taken when aspirating?

21. What is an osteotome?

22. When an implant is placed, what information needs to be recorded about the implant?

23. What post-operative instructions should be given to the patient following implant surgery?

24. Following implant surgery and post-operative instructions, what further arrangements should be made for the patient?

Restorative phase

1. What are the basic prosthodontic stages involved in making an implant-supported crown?

2. What are the basic prosthodontic stages involved in making an implant-supported overdenture?

3. What is a torque wrench?

4. What precautions should be taken when sterilising and storing certain torque wrenches?

5. Are all implant components sterile in their packaging?

6. What is the purpose of an implant-level impression?

7. If the dentist wants to use an open-tray impression technique, how can the special tray be modified?

8. What instruments may be required at the impression stage of implant treatment?

9. What materials may be required at the impression stage of implant treatment?

10. What is a facebow?

11. When might a facebow be used as a part of implant treatment?

12. What is a jaw registration?

13. What materials can be used as part of a jaw registration?

14. What is checked at the try-in stage of an implant prosthesis?

15. What is the difference between laboratory screws and clinical screws in implant prosthodontics?

16. Why is it important to establish whether the laboratory work has been returned with clinical screws ready for fitting in a patient's mouth?

17. When handling small implant instruments and components in the mouth there is a risk of the patient swallowing or inhaling them, how can the nurse help to reduce this risk?

Maintenance and patient aftercare

1. What is usually checked at an implant review appointment?

2. What materials can 'implant-safe' hand scalers be made from?

3. What manual toothbrushes are appropriate and available to be used for cleaning implant abutments and fixed prostheses?

4. How should implant-supported dentures be cleaned?

5. How should implant abutments and single tooth implants be cleaned in the mouth?

6. What oral hygiene aids can be used to clean under an implant-supported bridge pontic?

7. Why is it important to ask a patient to demonstrate their oral hygiene around any new implant prostheses?

8. If a patient reports pain or discomfort from an implant, what advice should you give?

9. If a patient reports bleeding on brushing around an implant, what advice should you give?

10. At the end of each review appointment, what details do you need to confirm with the dentist about the next appointment?

SECTION IV Questions: Implant components and terminology

LEARNING OUTCOMES

At the end of this section, you should be able to identify any gaps in your knowledge associated with the following:

- Implant surgical components
- Implant-supported fixed restorative components
- Implant-supported denture components

Implant surgical components

1. What is an alternative name for a fixture?

2. What does the term endosseous mean?

3. What is the most common metal used for dental implants?

4. Implant surfaces are often roughened to give a 'moderately rough surface', why is this?

5. What is a dental implant abutment?

6. White- or tooth-coloured ceramic materials can be used for dental implants and abutments, what are they made from?

7. What is the name for an implant that lies on top of the bone but under the mucosal tissues?

8. What is the name given to the implant/abutment connection where the connection extends out on the top of the implant platform?

9. What is the name given to the implant/abutment connection where the abutment inserts inside the coronal portion of the implant?

10. What is the name of an implant (blade shaped, cylindrical or root form) surgically placed within bone?

11. What is the general name for an implant that penetrates through the upper and lower borders of the mandible?

12. Some dental implants have a surface that appears to be shiny to the human eye (so-called machined surface implants) but most modern implants have a dull grey surface. What causes the dull grey appearance of these implants?

13. What is a cover screw?

14. What is a healing abutment?

15. How are implant components sterilised by the implant manufacturers?

16. What is internal irrigation?

17. What is external irrigation?

18. What is a zygomatic implant?

Implant-supported fixed restorative components

1. What is the name of the component that connects the implant and the prosthesis?

2. What is a custom-made component?

3. What is an access hole in an implant-supported crown or bridge?

4. What is an implant replica or implant analogue?

5. Some components are known as transmucosal components, what does transmucosal mean?

6. What is the name of the structural component of an implant-supported bridge which connects to the implants or the abutments and which supports all of the artificial teeth?

7. Some dental implant components, crowns and bridges are produced using CADCAM. What does CADCAM mean?

8. What are angled abutments?

9. What are laboratory screws?

10. What are prepable abutments?

11. What are bridge screws or prosthesis screws?

Implant-supported denture components

1. What is an implant overdenture?

2. What methods can be used to retain dentures on implants?

3. What is a Dolder bar?

4. What is an implant ball attachment system?

5. What are Locator™ abutments?

6. What are mini-implants?

SECTION V Questions: Patient assessment for dental implants

> **LEARNING OUTCOMES**
>
> At the end of this section, you should be able to identify any gaps in your knowledge associated with the following:
> - Medical history relevant to dental implant treatment
> - Physical examination for dental implant assessment
> - Relevant imaging for dental implant assessment

Medical history

1. What impact does smoking has on implant success?

2. If a patient has had intravenous bisphosphonate medication, what impact could that have on dental implant treatment?

3. What is osteoporosis?

4. If a patient has osteoporosis, how that may affect implant surgery?

5. Can implants be placed in patients who are diabetic?

6. Are patients with psychological problems suitable for dental implant treatment?

7. If a patient has received radiotherapy to the head and neck, what long-term effects can occur in the tissues?

8. What negative effects can occur if implants are placed in patients who have received radiotherapy at the potential site of the implant placement?

Physical examination

1. What techniques can be used to assess the bone quality available at a potential implant site?

2. Why are study models used as part of implant planning?

3. What is 'ridge mapping'?

4. What impact does periodontal disease has on dental implant treatment?

5. If a patient is diagnosed with uncontrolled periodontal disease at an initial assessment appointment, what steps should be taken prior to them proceeding with dental implant treatment?

6. What is a patient's smile line?

7. Why is a patient's smile line important when replacing teeth towards the front of the mouth?

8. What things should be assessed at a potential implant site during the examination appointment?

9. What is a soft tissue biotype (gingival biotype)?

10. Even though dental implants are not directly affected by dental caries, why is it important to assess the patient's caries risk and carry out any necessary preventive and restorative treatment prior to commencing treatment using dental implants?

11. What are radiographs or 3D CT scans used for at the initial assessment visit?

12. Bone quality is important to assess prior to and during dental implant placement. In general, which jaw tends to have a better bone quality/density?

13. Is it appropriate to consider dental implants for a young patient?

14. Is it appropriate to consider dental implants for very elderly patients?

Relevant imaging

1. What is a radiographic stent or guide?

2. What anatomical structure in the posterior maxilla may reduce the bone height available for dental implant placement?

3. What anatomical structure in the maxillary incisor region provides an upper limit for implant placement?

4. What additional information can be gained for implant planning from a CT scan when compared to a plain radiograph?

5. What nerve must be identified radiographically when implants are planned in the posterior mandible?

6. What is cortical bone?

7. What is trabecular bone?

8. Why is the relative amount of cortical to trabecular bone important when assessing bone at an implant site?

9. What anatomical structures need to be identified on plain radiograph or CT scan prior to placing implants in the maxillary central incisor region?

10. Are all nerves and blood vessels easily identifiable on a CT scan?

11. What is the submandibular fossa, and why is it relevant to dental implant placement in the posterior mandible?

12. What is the usual position of the mental foramen, and how is it relevant to dental implant surgery?

13. What is the most appropriate type of radiograph to use to look for evidence of periapical pathology affecting the teeth adjacent to an implant site?

14. What is the most appropriate type of radiograph to use to assess caries in posterior teeth as part of dental implant planning?

15. What is the most appropriate type of radiograph to use to assess the angulation of tooth roots adjacent to an implant site?

SECTION VI Questions: Implant surgery

LEARNING OUTCOMES

At the end of this section, you should be able to identify any gaps in your knowledge associated with the following:

- Preparation for implant surgery
- Bone grafting and sinus lifts
- Implant placement (first stage) surgery
- Implant uncovering (second stage) surgery
- Surgical complications

Preparation for implant surgery

1. What is tissue conditioning?

2. What is pre-prosthetic surgery?

3. What special care needs to be taken when extracting a tooth which is going to be replaced with a dental implant?

4. What is a periotome?

5. What are socket preservation techniques?

6. What is papilla preservation?

7. What types of techniques can be used for papilla preservation?

8. What are papilla preserving or papilla sparing flaps?

Bone grafting and sinus lifts

1. What is bone resorption?

2. What is a bone graft?

3. What is a simultaneous bone graft?

4. What is a delayed or subsequent bone graft?

5. What is a sinus lift?

6. What different types/approaches of sinus lifts can be used?

7. What is autogenous bone?

8. What is a human allograft?

9. What is an autograft or autogenous graft?

10. What is a xenograft?

11. What is a donor site?

12. What is donor site morbidity?

13. A common donor site for large bone grafts is the iliac crest, where is it?

14. Where are the common places from within the mouth that can be used as donor sites for bone grafting in relation to dental implants?

15. Where are the common places from outside the mouth that can be used as donor sites for bone grafting in relation to dental implants?

Implant placement (first stage) surgery

1. What is periosteum?

2. What is a mucoperiosteal flap?

3. What is a split thickness flap?

4. What can help the surgeon get the exact position of the implant site correct?

5. Does it matter how experienced the surgeon is who is placing the dental implants?

6. A surgical tap is sometimes used when preparing an implant surgical site, what does it do?

7. What does a cover screw do when placed on an implant at the time of surgery?

8. What is an implant osteotomy?

9. What is an osteotome used for in implant surgery?

10. What is a guide drill?

11. What is a piezo-surgery unit?

12. What is a pilot drill?

13. What is bone augmentation?

14. What is an immediate implant?

15. What is guided bone regeneration (GBR)?

16. What is platelet-rich plasma (PRP)?

17. What is implant primary stability?

18. Why is it important that an implant has a good primary stability immediately after it is surgically placed?

19. How can implant primary stability be measured?

20. How can the missing tooth or teeth of a patient be temporarily restored during the healing period following implant surgery?

Implant uncovering (second stage) surgery

1. What is osseointegration?

2. What is second-stage surgery?

3. Is second-stage surgery always needed as a part of dental implant treatment?

4. What is a biopsy punch or mucosal punch?

5. What is the definition of mucosa?

6. What functions does the mucosal layer carry out?

7. What is epithelium?

8. What is connective tissue?

9. What is a connective tissue graft?

10. Why is connective tissue grafting sometimes performed around dental implants?

11. What is a free gingival graft?

12. What is a healing abutment used for at the second-stage surgery?

Surgical complications

1. What advice should be given to a patient if they experience numbness in their lower lip immediately following the placement of an implant in their lower molar region?

2. If a patient experiences numbness of their lower lip following the placement of an implant in their lower left molar region, what nerve may have been damaged?

3. An hour after surgery to have implants placed in their lower jaw a patient telephones the practice to say that they have noticed swelling in the floor of their mouth and bruising under their tongue, which is now making swallowing difficult. What may have happened during surgery?

4. In aforementioned question 3, what advice should be given to the patient?

5. What is osteomyelitis?

6. How can osteomyelitis be treated?

7. How can the risk of infection be reduced for patients having dental implant surgery?

8. What are 'black triangles'?

SECTION VII Questions: Implant restorative procedures

LEARNING OUTCOMES

At the end of this section, you should be able to identify any gaps in your knowledge associated with the following:

- Implant impression techniques
- Implant-supported fixed restorations
- Implant-supported dentures

Impression techniques

1. What is the name of the impression technique where the impression coping projects out of the impression tray into the mouth?

2. What is the name of the impression technique where the impression coping is placed onto the implant but does not protrude through the impression tray when the tray was inserted in the mouth?

3. What is the name of the component that attaches to the implant and is used to register the implant position within an impression?

4. What is the name of the metal component that mimics the shape of the dental implant and is cast into the working model by the laboratory technician?

5. What is a dental articulator?

6. An impression needs to be taken for the construction of a dental implant-supported crown. Which impression materials should be used?

7. What is a pick-up impression?

Implant-supported fixed restorations

1. What is a pontic?

2. What is a bridge abutment?

3. What is a bridge retainer?

4. What is retention in relation to prosthodontics?

5. What is a retentive component?

6. What are the advantages of a cement-retained implant crown or bridge?

7. What are the disadvantages of a cement-retained implant crown or bridge?

8. What is a dental implant abutment for?

9. What two methods can be used to connect a fixed implant prosthesis or bridge to abutments?

10. What is the biggest theoretical advantage of using screws to retain implant components and restorations?

11. In relation to dental implant restorations, what is retrievability?

12. What is the technical name given to the amount of tightening that is applied to screw-shaped components when they are inserted?

13. Why is important to tighten a screw to the correct torque?

14. What is torque?

15. What name is used to describe the procedure whereby a restoration/prosthesis is placed on the implant immediately after surgical placement?

16. What is a superstructure?

17. What is a CADCAM component?

18. What is a prefabricated component?

19. Where can screws be used in a screw-retained prosthesis (in other words, what types of screw-retained prosthesis are there)?

20. What is meant by the term 'loading' in relation to dental implants?

21. What is meant by immediate loading?

22. What is meant by progressive loading?

Implant-supported dentures

1. What materials are used to construct the main parts of an implant-supported overdenture?

2. What is a ball attachment implant overdenture?

3. What is a bar-retained implant overdenture?

4. Although implant dentures are often called implant-supported overdentures, where do they actually get their support from?

5. Why is it important to ask the patient to insert and remove their new implant overdentures in the dental chair at the denture fit appointment?

6. If a patient finds it hard to remove their implant-retained overdentures because the retention is too strong, what can be done to help them?

SECTION VIII Questions: Implant aftercare and maintenance

LEARNING OUTCOMES

At the end of this section, you should be able to identify any gaps in your knowledge associated with the following:

- Oral hygiene in relation to dental implants
- Peri-implant inflammatory disease
- Prosthetic complications of implant-supported crowns, bridges or dentures

Oral hygiene

1. If a patient has generally good oral hygiene prior to an implant being placed, does this mean that they will be likely to have good oral hygiene around the implant when it is restored?

2. What home oral hygiene aids are safe to use around a dental implant?

3. When should Chlorhexidine Gluconate mouthwash use be suggested?

4. Why is it important for patients to maintain an excellent level of oral hygiene around their implants?

5. If you want a patient to improve their oral hygiene, it is often useful to ask them to physically demonstrate their home care routine to you in the surgery, why is that useful rather than simply asking them to describe their routine to you?

Peri-implant inflammatory disease

1. What is the name given to inflammation around a dental implant with bleeding on probing but no bone loss?

2. What is the name given to inflammation around a dental implant with bleeding and/or pus on probing and evidence of bone loss?

3. Bleeding on probing of the mucosa around an implant indicates what?

4. If an implant becomes mobile after being firm for a number of years, what would that mean for the future survival of the implant?

5. During a dental examination, it is noted that a dental implant replacing an upper left central incisor tooth has a 6 mm mesio-buccal pocket with bleeding on probing. A periapical radiograph is taken, and it shows evidence of bone loss around the implant at the bone crest. The most likely provisional diagnosis for the dental implant is?

6. What is the most appropriate imaging technique to use to check the bone levels around a single tooth implant?

Prosthetic complications

1. If a patient is a diagnosed bruxist, what may be the consequences for a fixed implant restoration?

2. If a patient engages in contact sports how this may affect dental implant treatment?

3. If a patient attends the dental practice where you work complaining that their implant-supported crown has become loose, what could be the possible causes?

4. What problems can arise if an abutment or bridge/prosthesis screw fractures during use?

5. If an abutment or bridge/prosthesis screw fractures during use, what can be done to replace the screw?

6. If a patient attends the dental practice where you work complaining that their implant-retained overdentures have become loose after a few years in function. What could be the possible causes?

7. Why is it important for patients who have dental implants to have their occlusion checked periodically at review appointments?

8. Why are dental implant-supported overdentures more prone to wear on their occlusal surfaces when compared to conventional dentures?

9. What is a stripped thread?

SECTION I Answers: Indications for dental implant use

How dental implants can be used

1. It is an artificial device that replaces a missing body part. A dental prosthesis is a fixed or removable artificial device that replaces missing teeth and may also replace missing bone and soft tissue.

2. These include the following:
   - Conventional bridgework
   - Resin retained/adhesive bridgework
   - Implant-supported crown
   - Implant-supported bridgework

3. This is a type of fixed prosthesis designed to replace a missing tooth or teeth. In a conventional bridge, the tooth or teeth next to the space are prepared for a crown preparation by the reduction of the tooth in width and height. A bridge is made of metal, metal/ceramic or all-ceramic, which then fits over the prepared teeth with missing teeth replaced with pontics on the bridge attached to the crown retainers.

4. This is a bridge design where the bridge is attached to, and supported by, teeth or implants at both ends of the bridge. Fixed–fixed bridges can be conventional, resin retained or implant supported.

5. This is a bridge design where the bridge is attached to, and supported by, a tooth or implant at only one end of the bridge. Cantilever bridges can be conventional, resin retained or implant supported.

6. These include the following:
   - Complete dentures
   - Partial dentures
   - Overdentures
   - Implant-supported overdentures

7. It is a denture that sits on top of mucosa and also over remaining tooth roots and/or dental implants. The tooth roots/implants provide support and sometimes retention for the denture.

8. Reasons for tooth loss include the following:
   - Periodontal disease
   - Dental caries
   - Endodontic failure
   - Trauma

9. Reasons for missing teeth can include teeth lost due to the reasons in 8:
   - Periodontal disease
   - Dental caries
   - Endodontic failure
   - Trauma
   In addition, teeth may not develop and erupt correctly due to hypodontia.

10. Hypodontia is characterized by congenitally missing teeth. About 5% of the population have at least one tooth missing; however, only about 0.3% of the population are affected with severe hypodontia where six or more permanent teeth are absent. In addition to missing teeth, people with hypodontia may have small or very conical teeth. Sometimes the jaw bone in the missing tooth spaces does not develop as much as when teeth are present, which can make dental implant planning difficult, and any permanent teeth that are present may erupt late. Where permanent teeth are missing, the overlying deciduous teeth may be kept for many years into adulthood.

11. Several options can be considered including the following:
    - No replacement of the missing teeth
    - Orthodontic treatment to close spaces
    - Removable partial dentures
    - Complete dentures
    - Conventional or adhesive bridgework
    - Implant-supported crowns, bridges or dentures
    - Transplantation of another tooth into the missing tooth/teeth spaces

12. They can be used to support a crown, bridge or overdenture. They can be used to provide both support and retention for the prostheses.

13. Many patients have individual reasons for having their teeth replaced. The common reasons for wishing to replace teeth are to improve appearance, to improve function (mastication, speech) and to maintain oral health (e.g. to prevent the unwanted movement of other teeth). It is not always appropriate to replace missing teeth, and both the patient and dentist must feel that it is appropriate to consider tooth replacement.

14. If missing teeth are not replaced, there may be no negative consequences. In some cases though negative consequences can occur including the following:
    - Tilting or drifting of teeth adjacent to the missing tooth site
    - Overeruption of teeth opposing the space
    - Functional issues affecting mastication and speaking
    - Aesthetic issues due to the appearance of anterior tooth spaces

15. Teeth are not essential to maintain life; however, they do play a role in effective mastication of food. If patients have a reduced number of effective tooth contacts, their masticatory efficiency is affected; this can affect the types of food that they choose to eat and how well they are chewed. Patients may avoid eating in social situations and may report a reduced enjoyment of eating food. Patients often adapt their diets as they lose multiple teeth. This can have an impact on older patients in particular who also often reduce the volume of food consumed as they get older and may struggle to maintain effective calorific and nutritional intake.

Why dental implants are used

1. In a patient with a spaced dentition, it is difficult to construct fixed conventional bridgework. The connectors between the bridge abutments and the pontics would be visible in the spaces

between the teeth. The use of dental implants allows a prosthesis to be constructed that does not need to be attached to adjacent teeth.

2. Implant-supported dentures have greatly improved retention when compared to conventional dentures, this leads to less movement of the dentures when eating and talking and reduces the risk of social embarrassment experienced by patients with loose conventional dentures. They also allow the patient to masticate food with much greater efficiency than conventional dentures. The improved chewing ability that comes with implant-supported dentures allows patients to eat a broader range of foods than patients with conventional dentures in most cases. In addition, there is some evidence that the implants help to maintain alveolar bone in the region of the dental implants. Because implant-supported dentures are less reliant upon mucosal coverage for retention, it is possible to make dentures that are smaller and cover less soft tissue surface in the mouth. This can be helpful in patients with a severe gag reflex.

3. Biting force increases when a patient moves from conventional denture wearing to implant-supported denture wearing. Activity in the patient's muscles of mastication also increases, and in some patients this can lead to an increase in muscle tone and masseter muscle thickness.

4. Chewing efficiency improves when a patient moves from conventional denture wearing to implant-supported denture wearing. Food can be chewed more effectively, and patients often report that they can eat tougher, more challenging foods with implant-supported dentures.

5. In general, patients report much higher levels of satisfaction with implant-supported dentures when compared to conventional dentures.

6. The main advantage of using dental implants to support bridgework is that an implant-supported bridge does not rely upon using teeth adjacent to the edentulous space for support. Conventional bridgework requires the tooth or teeth adjacent to the edentulous space to be prepared as bridge abutments. This involves removing tooth tissue and/or restorative material from the tooth/teeth and usually reduces the strength in the crown of the tooth/teeth and also requires that there is sufficient sound tooth tissue after tooth preparation to support the additional occlusal load of a bridge. The replacement of teeth with an implant-supported bridge can add occlusal support to a patient's dentition and improve function for the patient without compromising additional teeth.

7. A resin-retained bridge is a minimal intervention bridge; however in some cases, it still requires some minor preparation of the abutment tooth or teeth. An implant-supported crown allows a tooth to be replaced without the need to involve the teeth on either side of the missing tooth. This can be particularly useful in patients with a spaced dentition where bridge connectors may show between the teeth. Although a single tooth implant crown requires careful oral hygiene, it is often easier for patients to clean a single implant-supported crown than to clean under the pontic of a resin-retained bridge and particularly the region of the bridge where the pontic attaches to the abutment tooth or teeth. Although the longevity of resin-retained bridges has improved greatly, they do still tend to debond earlier than a dental implant crown would debond or require replacement.

8. The main advantage of using a dental implant-supported crown is that it does not rely upon using teeth adjacent to the edentulous space for support. Conventional bridgework requires the tooth or teeth adjacent to the edentulous space to be prepared as bridge abutments. This involves removing tooth tissue and/or restorative material from the tooth/teeth and usually reduces the strength in the crown of the tooth/teeth. It also requires that there is sufficient sound tooth tissue after tooth preparation to support the additional occlusal load of a bridge. Although a single tooth implant crown requires careful oral hygiene, it is often easier for patients to clean a single implant-supported crown than to clean under the pontic of a bridge and particularly the region of the bridge where the pontic attaches to the abutment tooth or teeth. The replacement of a missing tooth with an implant-supported crown can add occlusal support to a patient's dentition and improve function for the patient without compromising additional teeth.

9. In patients with an unrestored dentition, a single tooth dental implant has the advantage that a tooth can be replaced with a fixed prosthesis without attaching a prosthesis to adjacent teeth or covering the hard and soft tissues of the mouth with a denture. Any restoration or preparation of teeth can lead to unwanted complications for the patient and is usually avoided where possible. The use of a removable denture is often unpopular with patients only wishing to replace a single tooth, and if poorly maintained can lead to problems related to poor oral and denture hygiene as well as potential long-term traumatic damage to the mouth. Dental implants obviously carry their own risks and complications, and the assumptions above assume that the other potential complications of dental implant treatment have been explained to the patient, and that the single tooth implant is placed carefully with appropriate planning. Patients should have the advantages and disadvantages of each treatment option explained to them to allow them to make an informed decision.

10. Treatment for oral cancer can often involve radiotherapy, chemotherapy and/or surgical excision of teeth as well as hard and soft tissues of the mouth. Preparation for radiotherapy can involve extraction of any teeth that may have an uncertain prognosis, and patients can therefore suffer the loss of a number of teeth quite suddenly. There can be insufficient teeth left to support fixed prostheses, and the loss of tissue within the mouth may make it difficult to stabilise and retain a removable prosthesis adequately. Radiotherapy can make the soft tissues of the mouth thin and vulnerable to trauma, as well as leading to a reduced saliva flow in patients, which can also make denture wearing difficult.

11. Patients who have had surgery as part of the treatment for oral cancer often suffer the loss of teeth and significant amount of hard and soft tissues within the oral cavity. This can make the process very difficult to prepare satisfactory prostheses for these patients as part of their rehabilitation. There is also often inadequate or less than ideal distributions of remaining teeth and hard and soft tissues to support conventional dentures, obturators or fixed prostheses. In addition, the soft tissues of the mouth can be atrophic and vulnerable to trauma and discomfort from the movement of removable prostheses during function. Dental implants can provide fixed attachment points to support these prostheses with subsequent improvements in comfort and function.

12. Bone-anchored implants can be used to attach prostheses to replace missing hard and soft tissues lost following surgery for extra-oral cancer of the head and neck. These can be used to anchor and support prostheses. Common types of prostheses are ear, eye and nose prostheses,

but they can be used to replace a wider range of missing facial tissues with flexible prostheses that can be attached to the implants using magnets or clip attachment systems.

13. Hypodontia patients may have conical or small teeth in addition to the teeth that fail to develop. These teeth are often not ideal as bridge abutments due to their size and lack of coronal tooth tissue. They also often retain teeth from the primary dentition, which are again unsuitable as bridge abutments in most cases.

SECTION II Answers: Medico-legal aspects of dental implant use

Consent

1. You may speak to patients to give them general information regarding dental implants and to reassure them about aspects of treatment. You may organise and provide relevant literature and patient information leaflets to support the dentist during patient assessment and treatment planning visits.

2. It is important that you can understand the explanation and treatment plan described to a patient including its advantages, disadvantages and alternative options. If you cannot understand the suggested plan, then it is likely that the patient may not understand the treatment plan either and this may lead to a lack of informed consent to treatment. It is also important that you understand the treatment plan so that you can provide the correct information when the patient asks you questions regarding the plan at a later date. It will also facilitate treatment and ensure that the whole team is aware of the proposed treatment plan.

3. It is important that the consent process is witnessed wherever this is practical by a third party. This can help to ensure that the dentist's explanation of the proposed treatment plan is clear to the patient and that risks of the treatment have been explained fully. It is important that a consent form is signed as a written record of the consent process. You should ensure that a copy of the consent form is stored correctly for future reference if needed and that the patient also receives a copy or printout of the form.

4. Some patients may not realise that dental implant treatment can be associated with complications and failure rates. Advertising material that is available to patients including Internet resources often only project a very positive view of dental implant treatment. It is important that patients are fully informed of the likelihood of a particular treatment option being successful. It is also important that they are made aware of the consequences of treatment failure as well as the benefits that may come with successful treatment.

5. The origins of bone augmentation products vary, but some are animal- or human-derived products. The patient may have religious or ethical concerns about the use of animal or human products in general or about the use of animal products from certain species of animal on religious grounds. Some patients may also have concerns about the potential of disease being transmitted from the products. Although steps are taken to reduce the potential of disease transmission, it is important to fully disclose information about all implanted materials so that the patient can make a fully informed decision.

6. Implant company literature is largely sales literature that can place too much emphasis on the advantages of dental implant treatment and usually do not go into details about the advantages and disadvantages of alternative treatment options or of the risks and consequences of implant treatment. It is important that this type of literature is supplemented by discussion with the patient as well as other more detailed literature or practice-specific information for patients.

7. Surgical aspects that patients should be aware of include normal consequences of oral surgery including the following:
    - Pain and/or discomfort following surgery
    - Post-operative swelling
    - Post-operative bruising
    - Bleeding from the surgical site
    - Risk of post-operative infection.
      In addition, patients should be warned about the following:
    - Potential risks of damage to any nerves close to the implant site (e.g. lower lip paraesthesia due to inferior alveolar nerve damage)
    - Potential involvement in the maxillary antrum if implant placement is in the posterior maxilla
    - Potential implant loss.

8. Medium and long-term problems/issues that patients should be made aware of include the following:
    - Aesthetic issues (e.g. soft tissue recession, loss of interdental papillae, need to place prosthesis in relation to the available bone/implant position)
    - Oral hygiene difficulties that may be associated with different prostheses
    - Need for prosthesis maintenance, repair and replacement
    - Need for meticulous oral hygiene
    - Peri-implant inflammatory disease

Medico-legal considerations

1. Although there is no legal requirement in the United Kingdom for a dentist to have specific training in implant dentistry, there are minimum suggested training standards available. The General Dental Council supports the Training Standards in Implant Dentistry, published by the Faculty of General Dental Practice (UK). The council expects education providers and dentists who wish to practise implant dentistry to refer to these standards as the authoritative source of training standards for implant dentistry for dentists in the United Kingdom. This includes the recommendation that dentists should follow a reputable training course in conjunction with mentoring from an experienced implant clinician.

2. Dental implant treatment requires experience and detailed knowledge in order to achieve predictable and high-quality outcomes for patients. The most immediate consequence of inadequate training is that the dentist may carry out treatment that is inappropriate for a patient and may not achieve the best outcome or potentially may even cause a patient to be harmed. If a complaint is made about the dentist, then they would be vulnerable to criticism, professional regulation or even prosecution. The General Dental Council refers to the Training Standards in Implant Dentistry, published by the Faculty of General Dental Practice (UK) in cases where complaints are raised by patients involving dental implant treatment and may

consider that the dentist is practising beyond the limits of their competency if they have not been adequately trained.

3. No, it is not essential that dental nurses need to attend specific dental implant training in order to assist in dental implant procedures. It is advisable though to try to undertake additional training if possible and particularly if you are nursing for implant surgery and is considered to be best practice.

4. As a medical device, it is important to record the precise details of any components used in the event of a future problem. Implant companies will require details of the exact components used in the event of a component mechanical failure. They will use these details to look at their own quality assurance processes and to determine whether other patients may be affected. It is also important to record clearly that each component was used within its allotted shelf-life, which is displayed on the component packaging when appropriate.

5. The majority of complaints relate to poor communication between the dentist and patient. This often relates to dentists not giving enough information about alternative treatment options and also the relative advantages and disadvantages of dental implant treatment. Patients often may have read misleading, overly positive information in the media or in the Internet, and it is the task of the dentist and nurse to explain the correct information regarding the likely advantages and disadvantages of treatment. Any potential problems in the treatment as well as any risks of surgery should be clearly described.

6. No, a small failure rate can occur in dental implant treatment. Failure can occur for several reasons, and it does not always indicate a failure on the part of the surgeon. It is important that as part of the consent process, the patient is fully informed about the risks and consequences of implant failure.

7. Clinical negligence, also known as 'medical negligence', is a legal definition referring to the process of claiming financial compensation for physical and mental injuries and other conditions suffered as the result of a medical or dental professional's negligence.

8. In order for negligence to be proven, a claimant (usually the patient themselves) must show the following:
   - The clinician owed a duty of care to them.
   - The clinician was negligent in their management.
   - The patient suffered harm as a result.
   The claimant has to succeed on both liability and causation to obtain compensation:
   - *Liability* to show that the clinician must have been found to have acted in a manner that no other similar professional would have done.
   - *Causation* that harm has resulted which would not otherwise have occurred (on the balance of probability, that is, the action of the clinican was more than 50% likely to have caused the harm).

9. There are a number of situations that may be classified as a breach of duty of care, they include, but are not limited to:
   - failure to give due warning of risks involved in treatment administered;
   - failure to obtain consent to perform a procedure;
   - taking insufficient care in performing a procedure;

- performing a procedure without appropriate training;
- delayed referral to specialists;
- failed or delayed diagnosis of medical/dental problems
- prescribing incorrect medication.

10. No, cases are judged against the standard of care, which would be expected to be provided by a similar, reasonable practitioner. The standard of care is not judged against the standard of the best specialist in the field. This, however, does not excuse practitioners from working outside their level of competency.

11. The Bolam test takes its name from a legal case (Bolam vs. Friern Hospital Management Committee). It outlines key principles that are still important when clinical negligence claims are assessed. A doctor/dentist/nurse is not guilty of negligence if they have acted in accordance with a practice accepted as proper and reasonable by a responsible body of fellow professionals. The implication of this when working in primary care is that the standard against which you would be judged is that of your own peers – not that of the wisest and most experienced doctor/dentist/nurse who exists.

12. Many treatments in implant dentistry fall into this category, where different clinicians may recommend different treatment options or approaches. If a difference of opinion exists about a preferred treatment approach in the dental profession, this should be explained to a patient as part of the consent process, including the relative advantages and disadvantages of the various choices. It is defensible medico-legally to carry out such a procedure as long as it would be considered the treatment of choice of a representative group of reasonable practitioners (the Bolam test). This should be evidence based where possible and always in the best interests of the patient. It is important that the rationale behind the treatment is logical and would stand up to independent scrutiny. In other words, just because a group of clinicians feels a treatment is appropriate, this is not enough of a justification in itself to carry it out if the treatment is not logical. Their decision should be supported by evidence and a logical rationale, not just based on an eccentric belief (the Bolitho test).

13. Failure rates for dental implant treatment have been well established in many studies. It is important that any dental practice where implant treatment is taking place monitors their failure and complication rates and compares them against published failure rates in the research literature. The use of audit can confirm that the treatment of patients within the practice complies with established best practice seen in other centres. Patients are entitled to ask about the success and failure rates of implant treatment provided by the practice and also for the dentist carrying out their treatment. Failure rates and complication rates should always be monitored regularly because an increase in the failure or complication rate may indicate a problem with training, personnel, equipment, treatment protocols or materials and should be investigated.

SECTION III Answers: Role of the dental nurse

Patient assessment and planning

1. The aims of this visit are to identify what the patient's problems, requests and concerns are and their expectations of treatment and to explore their medical and dental history as well as

relevant aspects of their social history. This should be followed by a physical extra-oral and intra-oral examination to assess the current status of the patient's mouth and peri-oral tissues as well as to identify any active disease or dental problems. Further special tests and investigations can then be undertaken to refine the initial diagnoses and assess the patient's suitability for dental implant treatment. The information gathered from this visit helps to develop an initial list of potential treatment options and then refine this, following further consultation with the patient, into a definitive treatment plan.

2. It is important to ask about a patient's expectations from dental implant treatment for several reasons. It is important that any treatment plan attempts to address the concerns of the patient and is not driven purely by what the dentist thinks are the patient's needs. It is also important to make sure that the patient's expectations are realistic and achievable. Because of the relative cost of dental implant treatment compared to other treatment options, sometimes patients may have unrealistic expectations of what can be achieved. It is the task of the dental team to help manage the patient's expectations and provide them with realistic advice.

3. Mouth mirror, straight probe No. 6, periodontal probe (Basic Periodontal Examination (BPE) or periodontal pocket measuring probe), college tweezers, Gauze and cotton wool rolls, cold spray and electric pulp tester, PPE (personal protection equipment) for the patient, clinician and dental nurse, for example, safety glasses, bib, mouthwash.

4. It is essential that a full medical history is taken for all patients being assessed for dental implant treatment. This can take the form of a questionnaire that the patient fills out, but this should always be supplemented and checked by speaking to the patient. This information should be updated at each visit to ensure that the patient's medical history has not changed since the last visit. It is both the clinician's and dental nurse's responsibilities to ensure this happens.

5. It is important to record an up-to-date medical history, dental charting, BPE scoring and if indicated a full periodontal charting.

6. Radiographs and/or if indicated a cone beam CT scan (CBCT), study models and photographs may be necessary. The vitality/sensibility of teeth may be necessary to exclude periapical endodontic problems.

7. The impressions should be disinfected and sealed in a transparent plastic bag with a label indicating the disinfection process used. The impressions should be placed carefully in a location where they will not be damaged and ready for transfer to the dental laboratory. The impressions should be accompanied by a laboratory prescription, which should clearly indicate the required information to allow the laboratory work to be completed.

8. The prescription should include the following information:
   - Dental practice address and contact telephone number.
   - The prescribing dentist.
   - The patient's name/identification number.
   - A description of the required laboratory work in writing and if necessary in diagrams.
   - Where appropriate a tooth shade and details of any specific requirements (e.g. tooth shape, material choices).
   - The implant system used and the implant/component names and diameters used (if appropriate).

- A next appointment date for the work to be returned by.
- An indication of the disinfection process used for the impressions (this may also be directly on the bag holding the impressions/clinical records).
- Often an indication whether the work is private or National Health Service (NHS).

Surgical

1. It is important that the drills are kept cool to prevent the bone overheating at the implant site. If the bone temperature rises to 47 °C or above for one minute, the bone cells can die and lead to bone necrosis and cell death at the implant site. This may cause the implant to fail to heal successfully.

2. Some implant manufacturers produce reusable drills. The manufacturer has a recommended number of times that each drill can be reused. You should have a system to record how often a drill is reused to ensure that drills do not become blunt. Most manufacturers now offer single-use drills. These have the advantage of guaranteed sharpness and efficiency, but they also have the advantage of improved cross-infection control. It is important to determine whether drills are reusable or single use.

3. Yes, it does. For an implant to successfully integrate, it is important that the implant surface does not become contaminated with any foreign material. If another material contacts the dental implant, then contamination can occur and foreign material can be deposited on the dental implant surface that may interfere with osseointegration.

4. Sterile gowns (×2 or ×3), theatre caps (×2 or ×3), sterile face masks, patient drape to cover the whole body, sterile bench or bracket table covers, sterile bag and/or sleeve for the drill equipment, gauze, aspiration tubing cover and light handle covers. Some kits will also include sterile aspiration tubing and tip, and sterile shoe covers.

5. Sterile gloves, face mask/visor, sterile surgical blades usually No. 11/12/15, sutures, sterile saline bag (commonly 500 ml IV bag), topical anaesthetic, local anaesthetic cartridge, handle and needle, chlorhexidine scrub, chlorhexidine mouthwash. Some surgeons may also want additional disposable surgical equipment such as bone trap or disposable drills.

6. Safety glasses, bib, drapes, theatre cap (sometimes used), chlorhexidine mouthwash.

7. Safety glasses/visor, theatre gown, theatre cap, surgical gloves, face mask.

8. Asepsis means the absence of living organisms. Aseptic technique is a set of specific practices and procedures performed under carefully controlled conditions with the goal of minimizing contamination by pathogens.

9. Antisepsis is the prevention of infection by inhibiting or arresting the growth and multiplication of microorganisms (infectious agents) usually by washing and/or chemical intervention. Antisepsis implies that all areas in close proximity to the surgical area are scrupulously clean and free of all living microorganisms. Skin microorganisms should be removed and reduced via careful hand washing as far as possible.

10. One nurse is the circulatory or non-sterile nurse, the other nurse is the sterile or scrub nurse.

11. The circulatory or non-sterile nurse is generally able to move around the surgery freely; however, they must not enter or reach over the sterile area. They should stay at least 30 cm away from all sterile areas and should not touch sterile equipment or materials, which are due to be used in the surgical procedure. The sterile or scrub nurse can touch sterile equipment and materials to be used in the surgical procedure, and they can reach over and touch objects within the sterile area. They must not touch anything that is not sterile or anything that may be of doubtful sterility. All objects within the sterile area must be sterilised or covered with a sterile protective barrier.

12. All unnecessary items should be removed from the room. The floor should be cleaned, and routine cleaning of the room should have been carried out in line with normal practice. Only fixed items or equipment and materials to be used in the procedure should remain in the room. All horizontal surfaces should be wiped down with a suitable hard surface disinfectant.

13. Surgical instrument kit, local anaesthetic items (local anaesthetic syringe and needle, re-sheathing device if a safety syringe is not used, cartridges of local anaesthetic, topical anaesthetic), dental examination tray (dental mirror, straight probe, periodontal probe, college tweezers), chlorhexidine mouthwash, saline, sterile drape pack, suture, scalpel blades, implant drill unit and hand piece, implant components (drills, implants, cover screw(s), healing abutment(s) and so on as required), suction tubing, radiographic viewer (if traditional radiographic films need to be displayed), bone augmentation/graft materials and surgical stent (soaked in chlorhexidine for a minimum of 1 hour prior to surgery). A checklist is ideally used to ensure that all equipment and materials are available.

14. Mirror, straight dental probe, college tweezers, periodontal measuring probe, scalpel handle, periosteal elevator, tissue forceps, suture holder, scissors, tissue retractor(s), syringe, artery forceps and curette.

15. Remove all hand jewellery from hands and wrists. Wet hands and forearms under running water. Clean carefully under each fingernail with a stick or brush. Holding arms up above elbow level, apply the antiseptic scrub agent. Using a circular motion, beginning at the fingertips, thoroughly lather and scrub the whole area of one hand with the other. Then swap hands and repeat the process of lathering and cleansing of the other hand. Each hand and arms should then be rinsed under running water, starting at the fingertips, holding the hands above elbow level. Using a sterile towel, the arms and hands should be dried starting at the fingertips and using a different towel for each arm. Following hand washing/scrubbing, the hands should be kept above waist height with the hands above the elbows, making sure not to touch anything before putting on sterile gloves.

16. The surgical gown should be put on first.

17. The scrub nurse should take the gown (which is folded with the inside folded outwards), they should put their hands through the gown sleeves and slip the gown up the arms and over the shoulders assisted by the circulating dental nurse. The circulating dental nurse should take hold of the inside of the gown and pull the gown up into the correct position. The circulating nurse then ties the gown from behind. After the scrub nurse has put on the surgical gloves, they may wrap the tie around their waist and tie it with the assistance of the circulating

nurse. The scrub nurse hands the card tag attached to one tie to the circulating nurse, the scrub nurse then rotates on the spot and pulls away from the circulating nurse until the circulating nurse has access to both ties and can tie the gown around the waist.

18. The circulating nurse opens the surgical glove packaging containing the gloves. The sterile scrub nurse takes the inner sterile pack of gloves and opens it. The fingers of one hand are placed into the appropriate glove, and the folded cuff of the glove is grasped with the other hand. The glove can be pulled onto the fingers of the hand. The fingers of either hand should only touch the inside surface of the glove. Once this has been completed, the fingers of the gloved hand are inserted into the fold of the other glove and the glove is pulled onto the other hand. The outside of the gloves should never be touched by the fingers of either hand. Once the glove is on the hand, the folded cuffs can be folded down onto the elasticated cuff of the gown.

19. It is a small disposable filter that is attached to the aspiration system at the time of implant site preparation. It collects bone particles during the implant site preparation. The device can then be used to compress the bony particles into a paste, which can be applied as a bone augmentation material around the dental implant.

20. It is important to try to reduce the number of microorganisms and other debris in the collected bone particles. The bone trap must only be attached to an aspiration tip, which is collecting bone debris and irrigation saline from the implant site. A separate aspiration tip and tubing should ideally be used to collect any other saliva, blood and debris from the mouth. Alternatively, the bone trap and aspiration tip should be removed from the system when it is being used away from the implant site for functions other than to collect bone.

21. It is a cylindrical or tapered cylindrical surgical instrument, which can sometimes be used to expand and develop the shape of the hole at an implant site. It is inserted carefully and firmly into the hole and pushed or tapped apically in order to expand the implant site and condense the bone around the instrument.

22. The position, length, diameter and type of implant must be recorded in the patient's notes. Each implant package will have information regarding the manufacturing date, reference number and batch code as well as the use by date. This information must also be recorded so that if there were to be problems with the implant at a later date, the manufacturer can identify the implant and look into possible manufacturing errors. Most implant packages now hold this information on easy-peel labels, which can be stored in written records for future reference. This information should be recorded in the patient's notes and also in a separate implant log.

23. Instructions should include the following:
    - Warn the patient that they may experience swelling and possibly bruising.
    - They may be advised to use an ice pack or cool pack to reduce swelling.
    - An analgesic may have been prescribed or the patient may be advised to use over-the-counter analgesics for pain relief.
    - If the patient has been prescribed antibiotics, then they should complete the course.
    - Sterile gauze should be provided, and the patient told to apply pressure to the tissues if bleeding occurs.
    - Oral hygiene advice should be given.

- Saline or chlorhexidine mouth rinsing should be advised.
- If surgery involved the maxillary sinus/antrum, then patients may be advised to avoid blowing their nose during the healing period and they may be prescribed nasal drops in some cases.

24. A follow-up appointment should be made to check wound healing and remove any sutures still present. The patient should also be given a phone number to call in an emergency. Patients who have received sedation should be transported and escorted home. For all patients, it is important to ensure that they feel able to return home and if necessary that they have transportation and an escort.

Restorative phase

1. The basic stages involved are as follows:
   - Removal of healing abutment
   - Abutment connection (radiograph taken to confirm the fit of the components)
   - Abutment torqued to final tightness
   - Impression taken, jaw registration and shade taken
   - Temporisation
   - Try-in and cementation or screw connection of crown onto implant abutment.
     These stages can be changed or omitted depending on the technique used. Sometimes an abutment may not be connected before an impression is taken. Then the impression of the implant is taken, and this is used to fabricate either an abutment and crown or a combined crown and abutment that can be attached directly to the implant.

2. The basic stages involved are as follows:
   - Removal of healing abutments
   - Abutment connection
   - Primary impressions
   - Secondary impressions
   - Jaw/bite registration
   - Try-in appointment
   - Fit appointment
   - Review appointment
     These stages can be changed or omitted depending on the technique used.

3. It is a device that can be used to tighten screw joint components together to an accurate predetermined tightness.

4. Torque wrenches vary in complexity and design. Some torque wrenches have multiple parts and may have central spring components, which need to be handled carefully during sterilisation and later storage. It is important to follow the manufacturer's instructions regarding cleaning, disinfection and storage to avoid corrosion and damage to the torque wrench. If poorly maintained, then the accuracy of the torque wrench may be affected.

5. No, implant surgical components are always sterile within the packaging; however, some of the restorative components of some implant systems are not sterile and may require sterilising

before they are fitted for a patient. It is always important to read the manufacturer's instructions before use to ensure that the correct advice has been followed.

6. The purpose is to locate the relative positions of the implant(s), adjacent teeth and soft tissues for planning and prosthesis construction.

7. The special tray must have an opening above the implant(s) to allow the pick-up impression copings to stick out above the top of the tray. The dentist may have to use an acrylic trimming bur and straight handpiece to modify this opening.

8. Mirror, probe, periodontal probe (or abutment height-measuring probe), college tweezers, local anaesthetic syringe, sterile scalpel handle and blade, handheld implant screwdrivers for the implant cover screw and/or healing abutment and impression coping, bone mill (if required to remove bone overgrowth onto the implant head), impression copings, impression tray, scissors, handpiece with acrylic trimming bur, spatula and mixing pad (if cementing temporary crown(s)), shade guide and facebow.

9. Local anaesthetic, tray adhesive, alginate, silicone impression material or polyether impression material, pink modelling wax (to cover open-tray holes in the impression tray), temporary crowns (if required), temporary crown cement (if required), temporary crown resin (e.g. integrity or trim) and jaw registration paste.

10. It is a device that is used to record the relation of the maxilla/maxillary teeth to the hinge axis of the temporomandibular joints. This measurement can then be transferred to a dental articulator onto which casts of the patient's teeth and soft tissues are mounted in the same relation. This allows a more accurate simulation of the positions of the jaws, teeth and temporomandibular joints to be reproduced when treatment planning or constructing prostheses.

11. A facebow may be used as part of the treatment planning process or during the construction of fixed or removable prostheses.

12. It is a record of the relationship between the mandible and maxilla of a patient. Jaw registration records can be taken with the patient biting in different positions depending on the intention of the jaw registration.

13. Jaw registration (bite registration) can involve the use of a number of different materials. For a simple jaw registration, the patient may be asked to bite into a softened wax sheet shaped to their dental arch. Alternatively, jaw registration pastes may be used. These are usually dispensed in the form of an automixing paste/gun system. The dentist syringes the paste onto the surfaces of the mandibular teeth and asks the patient to bite together and hold the position while the paste sets. The set wax/paste can then be removed from the mouth and sent to the dental laboratory. If a patient is edentulous or partially edentulous to a degree where a paste/wax sheet record would not be stable, then wax occlusal rims may be needed. These are trimmed and adjusted so that they fit comfortably in the mouth and allow the patient to bite together in the correct position. The occlusal surfaces of the rims should touch lightly together in the desired position once they are trimmed. The rims are then fixed together to record the jaw position using either wax or a paste registration material between the rims.

In addition, more specialised methods are also available for the recording of jaw positions; however, these are not commonly used in practice.

14. The shape of the final restoration, the fit of the prosthesis to the implant abutments/implants, the patient's thoughts on the prosthesis (appearance, contours, tooth arrangement) and the occlusion, if any adjustments are required.

15. Laboratory screws and clinical screws are essentially the same shape and size in most implant systems and are made from similar materials. The laboratory screws are used by the laboratory technicians when they are making the prosthesis in the laboratory. Clinical screws are the screws that are used in the clinic to try in and attach the prosthesis in the patient's mouth.

16. Laboratory screws are often used repeatedly and they become weakened over time. They should not be used to attach a prosthesis in a patient's mouth as they may not have sufficient strength to withstand the forces that a prosthesis is subjected to during function. New clinical screws should always be used to fit a prosthesis. To help identify lab screws, some implant systems colour code their laboratory and clinical screws in different colours or they use a slightly different shape for the two screw types so that it is difficult or impossible to fit a lab screw by accident in a patient's mouth.

17. Small screwdrivers should have dental floss tied to the handles of the instruments to help to retrieve them if dropped. The use of a small gauze pack placed in the patient's mouth can also help to catch any small components that are dropped (e.g. bridge screws). The nurse should watch the procedure closely so that the exact location of any dropped component is identified quickly and if requested by the dentist, aspirated (although this will obviously mean that component cannot be reused).

Maintenance and patient aftercare

1. A typical implant review appointment would involve the following:
   - Asking the patient about any concerns they have.
   - An update of the patient's medical history
   - An update of the patient's dental history if their general dental care is provided elsewhere.
   - A clinical examination that should include the following:
     - Oral hygiene assessment
     - Prosthesis hygiene assessment
     - Soft tissue examination of the mouth
     - Peri-implant probing to measure peri-implant probing depths as well as to look for the presence of bleeding and/or suppuration on probing
     - Occlusal assessment of the implant prosthesis
     - Quality assessment of the prosthesis to look for evidence of wear or fractures
     - Check of the retention of removable prostheses
     - Radiographic assessment of the implant and peri-implant bone levels

2. It is important that hand scalers are made from material, which will not damage the implant surface. *Implant safe* scalers are made from plastic, carbon–fibre, gold or titanium tipped.

3. Conventional manual toothbrushes are appropriate for cleaning around implant prostheses and abutments. In addition the use of interdental and single-tuft interspace brushes can be useful particularly for cleaning around fixed bridgework and under implant-supported bars. There are also a number of specialist implant brushes available which have been designed to help clean around dental implants. They often have smaller heads to aid access to small gaps and spaces and they also often have additional bends in the head of the brushes to allow the brushes to access lingual and palatal to prostheses, bars and abutments.

4. Implant-supported dentures should be cleaned in the same way that conventional dentures are cleaned. They should be cleaned after every meal when possible and left out at night. When cleaning a denture, the denture should be held over a bowl of water and gently cleaned with a soft toothbrush or denture brush using a plain soap. A smaller headed brush is sometimes useful when cleaning around intricate denture clips to help to dislodge any food debris that may collect around them. For patients with impaired vision, it is important to ensure that they can see adequately to clean the dentures effectively (e.g. make sure they are wearing glasses if they need them and that they are working in a well-lit area). The dentures should then be rinsed in clean water and either returned to the mouth or stored in water when they are not being worn.

5. They should be cleaned with a manual or electric toothbrush using a conventional low abrasion toothpaste. Patients should also be encouraged to use interproximal cleaning aids such as floss and interdental brushes to clean around the implants and slightly under the gum line. Specialist implant toothbrushes can also be useful.

6. In addition to using a manual or electric toothbrush, patients should be encouraged to clean under a bridge pontic using other oral hygiene aids. Conventional dental floss or tape can be used; however, often patients may find that thicker crown and bridge floss is more effective under the pontic area. Interdental brushes are also effective as well as some of the specialist implant toothbrushes designed to clean under implant superstructures. Some patients prefer the use of a Waterpik™/waterjet device; however, in general these are less effective for cleaning under implant-supported bridgework than brushes/floss.

7. Patients need reasonable manual dexterity to clean effectively under bridgework and around implant-supported superstructures and this should be assessed at the chairside in the dental practice to ensure that patients can understand, as well as physically see and carry out the required oral hygiene measures.

8. Pain and discomfort related to dental implants is extremely unusual. Patients should be advised to arrange an appointment as soon as possible for the implant(s) and prostheses to be examined.

9. Simple oral hygiene measures should be advised and the patient should be encouraged to arrange an appointment for the implant and the peri-implant tissues to be examined for evidence of peri-implant inflammatory disease as soon as possible.

10. The key information you need to ask for is the following:
    - The time interval before the next appointment
    - Who the next appointment should be with
    - What the next appointment is for
    - The length of the next appointment.

SECTION IV Answers: Implant components and terminology

Implant surgical components

1. A dental implant.

2. Within bone.

3. Titanium or an alloy of titanium (such as titanium–aluminium–vanadium alloy).

4. To enhance osseointegration/growth of bone onto the implant's surface.

5. It is a mass manufactured or custom-made component that connects to the top of the implant. They can be used to shape the soft tissues above the implant during healing, and different designs can also be used to connect to the final prosthesis. They can be made from a variety of materials, in a variety of shapes and have a number of functions.

6. Zirconia or zirconium oxide, some older implants used hydroxyapatite.

7. Subperiosteal implant.

8. External connection.

9. Internal connection.

10. Endosseous implant.

11. Transosseous implant.

12. Machined surface implants are so-called because their surface is the result of the machining process used to manufacture them in a milling machine. Some implants are then treated to roughen and change the implant surface to speed up bone growth on the implants' surface and improve osseointegration. These surface treatments can include acid etching, blasting the surface, anodisation or coating the surface, and these treatments lead to a change in the surface colour from a shiny metallic surface to a dull grey appearance.

13. It is a small component which can be screwed into the implant and which covers the coronal connection area of the implant and the internal connection and screw threads. By covering the connector surface of the implant, the cover screw can prevent bone and soft tissue growing over the implant connector surface and down into the internal threads of the implant. They are often placed on implants when a two-stage surgical technique is used. The soft tissues can be closed over the top of the cover screw to allow healing to take place. At the second-stage surgery to uncover the implant, the cover screw can be removed and the coronal connector surface and internal threads of the implants are available for use having been protected during the healing period.

14. It is a prosthetic component that may be cylindrical in cross section but widens in diameter towards the coronal aspect. The shape of the healing abutment is designed to guide the soft tissues to form a suitably shaped peri-implant sulcus.

15. Gamma irradiation.

16. It is irrigation during the implant site preparation that is delivered through the contra-angle handpiece and the through the drill itself. This is not widely used as it requires drills with hollow internal spaces that are difficult to sterilise, and external irrigation is more commonly used.

17. This is the most common type of irrigation used for surgical procedures and implant surgery. In this technique, the irrigation saline is delivered via an external irrigation tube that is attached to the contra-angle handpiece.

18. It is a long endosseous implant that is placed using a complex surgical procedure into the zygoma as an alternative to bone grafting for patients who have a severely atrophic maxilla. It is a long screw-shaped implant that is placed with its apex in the zygoma on the affected side and then it runs down the lateral wall of the antrum to exit with the coronal portion of the implant in the patient's palate. These are usually placed in a specialist or hospital environment.

Implant-supported fixed restorative components

1. The abutment, transmucosal abutment or TMA (transmucosal abutment) screw.

2. It is a component that is specifically manufactured for an individual patient. Custom-made components are usually specifically made for an individual location in the mouth (e.g. a custom-made abutment will usually be made to connect to the implant in a specific position with the coronal portion of the abutment ideally shaped to connect to the prosthesis).

3. It is a hole through a replacement tooth's occlusal or lingual/palatal surface that provides access to the abutment or prosthesis screw for insertion or removal.

4. It is an implant component that has one surface, which exactly duplicates the connection surface of a dental implant. The component is typically cast into the master/working laboratory cast so that the dental technician can have an accurate model in which copies of the dental implants are placed in the correct positions.

5. It means 'across the mucosa'. These components such as transmucosal abutments attach to a dental implant beneath the mucosa at one end and to a prosthesis or superstructure at the other.

6. The implant superstructure.

7. Computer-aided design and computer-aided manufacture.

8. These are abutments that attach to the implant at one end, but there is then a change in angulation of the abutment body so that the long axis of the coronal part of the abutment is at a different angulation than the angulation of the implant. They are used when the angulations of the implants would not be ideal for the creation of a satisfactory prosthesis. The angled abutments allow correction for implant angulation problems.

9. They are abutment or bridge/prosthesis screws that are used by the dental laboratory technician when producing the implant-supported crown or bridgework in the laboratory. When implant-supported laboratory work is constructed, components have to be screwed and unscrewed many times and the screws can become worn, weakened or damaged. It is important that different screws are used in the laboratory than those that are used to attach the final components and prosthesis in the mouth.

10. These are abutments that can be adjusted and prepped to alter their shape. The coronal portion of the abutment may be shaped in a form similar to a basic crown preparation that would be prepared on a tooth, and they are available in different diameters and heights. Their basic shape can be adjusted by the use of dental burs and abrasives to give the ideal preparation.

11. They are small-diameter screws that connect through the access holes in the occlusal or lingual/palatal surfaces of the prosthesis and when correctly tightened into position hold the prosthesis in place on the implants or abutments.

Implant-supported denture components

1. A complete or partial removable prosthesis that covers and is supported by dental implants, which usually gains support from the implants and the mucosa on which it rests.

2. Broadly the types of retention mechanisms that can be used to retain implant-supported dentures can be grouped into the following categories:
   • Bar clip, with a bar attached to the implants and retentive clips in the denture.
   • Stud clip, with abutments attached to the implants that have an undercut element into which clips in the denture can engage for retention.
   • Ball end-clip, with ball-shaped abutments attached to the implants and retentive clips in the denture.
   • Magnets, abutments attach to the implants with magnets housed within the denture for retention when the denture is inserted.
   • Tapered crown technique, tapered abutments on the implants fit into matching tapered inserts in the denture. The friction fit of the abutments into the inserts keeps the denture in place.

3. A prefabricated bar that connects implant abutments together (and can also be used on retained tooth roots) to provide support and retention to an implant-supported overdenture. The retentive clip is a single sleeve which is processed into the fit surface of the denture and which clips on to the Dolder bar when the denture is inserted.

4. It is an attachment system to help support and retain implant-supported overdentures. An abutment is connected to a dental implant and has a ball at the coronal end of the abutment that sits just above the mucosa. A matching component which clips onto the ball attachment is processed into the denture base. When the denture is inserted, the denture components clip onto the ball abutments and act as a source of retention and support for the denture.

5. They are abutments that attach at one end to the implant and emerge through the mucosa as a gold-coloured cylinder. The top of the cylinder has a lip and the retentive clip in the denture clips over this retentive lip when the denture is inserted. The strength of the retention can be

altered by changing the plastic insert inside the denture clip. Different retention strengths are denoted by a different colour of the plastic inserts.

6. Mini-implants are poorly defined, but in general it is the name given to implants that have a small diameter (<3 mm) and a threaded implant at one end, which is inserted into bone, and a ball-shaped abutment attached to the implant as a single component at the other end. The implants are inserted into bone surgically until the ball end is at the correct height above the mucosa. The retentive element is often a simple O-ring clip, which is processed into the denture. They can be used for denture retention sometimes as a temporary measure while wider diameter implants are healing or they can be used for longer term retention of a denture.

SECTION V Answers: Patient assessment for dental implants

Medical history

1. It increases the chances of problems with post-operative healing and also increases the risk of peri-implant disease and implant loss.

2. They are at higher risk of osseous necrosis. This is a condition where normal bony healing fails to take place, it can be very difficult to control and can cause excessive tissue destruction.

3. It is a generalised bone disorder characterised by a low bone mineral density and a change in the microarchitecture of the bone with thinning of the cortical bone and reduction in the number and size of the trabeculae in trabecular bone.

4. Osteoporosis does not affect implant success and is not a contraindication to having dental implants; however, they may be on medication, such as bisphosphonates, which does have an impact on implant surgery.

5. Yes, implants can be successful in patients who are diabetic. It is important though that patients with uncontrolled diabetes are stabilised before being considered for dental implant surgery.

6. Patients with psychological problems can be successfully provided with dental implants (depending on their individual status). It is very important that patients with psychological problems are assessed very carefully before committing to dental implant treatment.

7. Radiotherapy causes vascular changes at the site of radiation exposure with a reduction in the blood flow to the tissues. The tissues have a reduced vascularity, reduced cellularity and a reduced oxygen perfusion. This has a potentially negative effect on wound healing and the success rate of dental implants. In general, the effect of radiotherapy varies depending on the amount of radiation administered, the exact path of radiation and the amount of radiation that the bone at the implant site received.

8. The area may fail to heal following implant placement; osseointegration may be affected; and there is a higher risk of implant failure and loss. In some cases, there may be necrosis of the bone with subsequent ischaemic necrosis of the mucosa and exposure of the necrotic bone in the mouth. This is known as osteoradionecrosis. This can be very difficult to manage clinically and resolve.

Physical examination

1. Clinical examination, plain film radiographs, bone ridge mapping, CT scanning, Cone Beam Computed Tomography (CBCT) scanning and rarely MRI scanning can all be used.

2. They can be used to carry out a diagnostic wax up of the proposed prosthesis, to show the patient, to plan implant placement, to produce a radiographic guide and to produce a surgical guide for implant placement.

3. It is a technique where direct measurements are taken through anaesthetised mucosa at a proposed implant site, these depths can be transferred to a study model sectioned at the same site so that the thickness of the soft tissue and the bone contour can be drawn onto the cast. It was more commonly carried out before 3D scanning was available but is still sometimes useful.

4. Implants placed in patients with a history of periodontal disease are at greater risk of developing peri-implant inflammatory diseases (peri-implant mucositis and peri-implantitis).

5. The diagnosis and the effect of periodontal disease on dental implant treatment should be explained to the patient. An active course of periodontal treatment should be prescribed by the dentist. The patient should be reviewed and their periodontal condition monitored. Their periodontal condition should be improved and stabilised prior to the placement of dental implants.

6. It is the relationship of the upper and lower lips to the gingival margins of the anterior teeth. In other words, how much tooth and gum does the patient show when they talk and smile.

7. It is important to look at how much of the patient's teeth and gums are shown when the patient talks and smiles. Some patients do not show the gingival margins of their front teeth at all, even when smiling broadly; however, some patients show large amounts of their front teeth and gums. If dental implants are to be planned, the dentist has to plan carefully to ensure that the appearance of the final prosthesis will look good and that the patient has the greatest aesthetic result that can be achieved.

8. The following conditions should be considered at a potential implant site during the examination appointment: the space available between the teeth next to the proposed implant site; the space between the mucosa at the implant site and the teeth of the opposite arch; the thickness and shape of the ridge at the implant site; the condition, type, shape and thickness of the mucosa and bone at the implant site.

9. It is a categorisation of the thickness of the soft tissues around teeth and/or implants. It can give an indication of the likelihood of soft tissue changes following periodontal or implant surgery. Generally, soft tissues are classified as thick, thin or sometimes thin-scalloped. A thick biotype is characterised by a thick and wide area of keratinised tissue at the buccal/labial aspect of the tissues. These patients are more resistant to recession following surgery. A thin biotype is characterised by thin periodontal/peri-implant tissues, this tissue type can be prone to gingival/mucosal recession particularly after surgery. A thin-scalloped biotype is characterised by a disparity between the height of the gingival margin on the buccal/lingual

surfaces of the teeth/implants and that found interproximally. The buccal/labial tissues in these patients are again prone to recession.

10. Caries can lead to the loss of teeth ultimately if untreated. Extensive caries can severely weaken the structure of affected teeth, even when the teeth are restored, and it is important to identify teeth that may be lost and also teeth that may be compromised. These teeth need to be considered as part of an overall treatment plan.

11. They are used to assess the patient's bone quantity and quality at the proposed implant site(s). In addition, it is important to identify important anatomical structures in the region where implants may be placed. Any pathology should be identified (e.g. periapical pathology, periodontal defects) and treatment provided where appropriate.

12. Although variable between patients, in general the bone of the mandible tends to have the denser/higher quality bone.

13. Implant placement is not recommended in young patients who are still growing. Dental implants when osseointegrated will not move with the developing bone, teeth, mucosa and gingivae. This can lead to the appearance of the implants submerging in the tissues (infraoccluding). It is generally accepted that it is better to wait until the patient is at least 18 years old. Completion of growth is usually earlier in females than in males.

14. There is no upper age limit for dental implants. Wound healing can be delayed in older patients, and they may also have an increased risk of other health-related issues that may impact on dental treatment. If the patient is fit and well and is suitable to undergo surgery, then their age does not have a direct impact on implant success.

Relevant imaging

1. It is an acrylic resin guide constructed with markers that are radiopaque placed in the positions of a patient's missing teeth. The patient can wear the stent or guide when having either plain radiographs or CT scans taken. It allows identification of the proposed site for implant placement on the radiographic image so that a more accurate assessment can be made of the bone quality and quantity at the implant site(s).

2. The maxillary sinus or antrum.

3. The nasal floor or floor of the nose.

4. Three-dimensional (3D) details and relationships as well as being able to take exact measurements more reliably.

5. Inferior alveolar nerve or inferior dental nerve.

6. As its name suggests, cortical bone forms the outer shell or cortex of most bones. It is much denser, harder and stronger than the other type of bone found in the body (cancellous bone). The primary functional and anatomical unit of cortical bone is the osteon.

7. Trabecular or cancellous bone is a light, porous bone enclosing numerous large spaces that give a honeycombed or spongy appearance. The bone matrix, or framework, is organized into a 3D latticework of bony processes, called trabeculae, arranged along lines of stress. The spaces in between are often filled with marrow. It is less dense and less strong when compared to cortical bone.

8. The quality of bone at an implant site is an important indicator of implant success. A higher ratio of cortical bone at an implant site is indicative of a higher bone density and quality. Implants placed into high-quality bone have a higher success rate when compared to implants placed into bone of poor quality.

9. The structures in the upper central incisor region relevant to dental implant placement that can be identified on a plain radiograph include the following:
   - The floor of the nose
   - The apices and root angulations of the adjacent teeth
   - The incisive foramen
   - The bone ridge crest (to assess bone height)

   Additionally, on a CT scan, 3D information regarding these structures can be seen, as well as an assessment of the bone width and contour in the area.

10. No, although, in general, the 3D nature of a CT scan makes it easier to identify and map anatomical structures, there can still be a degree of uncertainty about the exact extent of certain smaller structures such as nerves and blood vessels in some cases. This can be due to the structures being very small and ill-defined. It may also be difficult to identify structures if the scan is affected by significant scatter from adjacent metallic implants/restorations/prostheses.

11. The submandibular fossa (or fovea) is a depression on the medial surface of the mandible below the mylohyoid line. The submandibular salivary gland sits within the fossa. It is important to identify its size and position when placing implants in the posterior mandible as it limits the amount of bone height and width available for implant placement in the region.

12. The mental foramen is most commonly located in the line of the long axis of the lower second premolar tooth in the mandible. It contains the mental nerve and vessels as they exit the mandible to supply the lower lip on each side of the lower jaw. If the nerve is cut or compressed during implant treatment, the patient may suffer nerve damage with resultant paraesthesia to the lower lip on the affected side.

13. A long cone periapical radiograph (LCPA or PA). In some circumstances, it may also be appropriate to consider the use of a 3D imaging technique such as a cone beam CT (CBCT) image if the 3D extent of a periapical lesion needs to be assessed more fully.

14. Left- and right-bitewing radiographs to diagnose the extent of any carious lesions in the posterior teeth.

15. A long cone periapical radiograph (LCPA or PA) is the most suitable for a small region, a dental pantomogram (DPT) may be used if the assessment needs to involve a number of edentulous spaces, evaluate other anatomical structures or look for the presence of retained roots. In some circumstances, it may also be appropriate to consider the use of a 3D imaging technique such as a CBCT image if the 3D relationship of the tooth roots to other anatomical structures needs to be assessed.

SECTION VI Answers: Implant surgery

Preparation for implant surgery

1. It is the process of restoring health to the denture-bearing soft tissues of the mouth. A firm elastomeric material (tissue conditioner) is usually used and applied to the fit surface of a removable prosthesis to more evenly distribute the occlusal load to the damaged tissues. The tissue conditioner may have to be reapplied, and interim prostheses have to be modified to allow the soft tissues to recover. Tissue conditioning may be necessary in patients where they have been wearing ill-fitting dentures and the soft tissues have become hyperplastic and damaged.

2. It is a surgery that is aimed to make the construction of a prosthesis easier and more successful for a patient in the longer term. Examples of pre-prosthetic surgery include the removal of bony undercuts, removal of prominent bony lumps and tori and reducing and smoothing sharp bony edentulous ridges.

3. It is important to maintain bone at the implant site. When a tooth is extracted with the aim of replacing it with a dental implant, it is important to extract the tooth carefully, preserving the maximum amount of bone possible at the extraction site. Different techniques can be used to remove the tooth atraumatically. Bone removal should be avoided if at all possible.

4. It is a surgical instrument consisting of a fine blade that can be inserted into the periodontal ligament of a tooth to aid its removal atraumatically, attempting to preserve bone at the extraction site.

5. They are techniques used after the extraction of a tooth in order to try to reduce the amount of bone loss at the extraction site after the tooth is taken out.

6. It is a measure or series of measures taken to maintain and preserve the interdental papilla following tooth extraction.

7. A number of measures can be used including the use of atraumatic tooth extraction techniques, the use of special surgical flap designs, the augmentation of bone and/or soft tissues, the careful placement of implants in the correct position to favour papilla growth and the correct shaping of temporary and final fixed prostheses to maintain the correct space for papillae to be preserved.

8. They are surgical flap designs where the incision does not include the interdental papilla. This preserves the blood supply to the papilla tissues and avoids post-surgical scarring and loss of the papillae.

Bone grafting and sinus lifts

1. It is an essential physiological process within the body. Osteoclast cells demineralise the bone around them and also secrete enzymes that break down the organic components of the bone. It is a process which is an essential part of bone healing as well as part of physiologic bone remodelling. Problems can occur if bone resorption is excessive.

2. It is a procedure where bone is taken from a donor site of the same patient or from another source and placed into an area of bone deficiency. Following a healing period, it can integrate with the bone at the recipient site, rebuilding the area of bone deficiency. It is usually used to augment an area of poor bone quantity.

3. It is when a bone graft is placed at the same time as dental implants are placed.

4. It is when a bone graft is placed and allowed to heal and integrate initially. Following a suitable healing period, dental implants are then placed into the healed bone site as a separate procedure.

5. It is procedure where the inferior lining of the maxillary antrum (sinus) is raised in order to encourage new bone formation in the antral floor, increasing the amount of available bone for dental implant placement.

6. In general, a sinus lift can be performed via the lateral wall of the antrum or via the crest of the maxillary ridge. In the lateral window technique, a modified Caldwell–Luc operation is used to gain access to the sinus cavity. A bony window is created in the lateral maxillary wall; the Schneiderian membrane is elevated; and bone grafting material is placed under the membrane. In the crestal technique (one variant of which is the summers lift), access is usually made via a small hole in the maxillary ridge prior to implant placement. The Schneiderian membrane is elevated, and bone grafting material is placed via this approach. Different instruments can be used to help access the antrum depending on the technique used.

7. It is bone taken from the patient and used to build up areas of deficiency at an implant site, it can be used as a block graft or ground down into a granular form or taken as shavings.

8. It is a graft of tissue from one human to another. Most commonly, this is in the form of graft material taken from donated human cadavers.

9. It is a tissue graft taken from one area of a patient's body and transplanted to another part of their body such as a gingival graft or a bone graft.

10. It is a graft taken from an individual of another species.

11. It is the site from which tissue is taken in a grafting procedure.

12. It refers to the pain, swelling, limitation of movement, changes in sensation, discharge or other complications, which may arise at the donor site in a grafting procedure. It is important to warn patients of these potential issues as part of the consent procedure. It is also important that clinicians, practices and hospitals monitor morbidity rates for all relevant procedures.

13. The iliac crest or ilium is the largest and uppermost portion of the hip bone. The hip bone is the broadest bone in the skeleton and is located in the sidewall and anterior wall of the pelvis. The size of the bone allows relatively large bone grafts to be taken and used as intraoral bone grafts.

14. Bone is most commonly taken from the ramus and the chin. Additional sites that can be used include the maxillary tuberosity, anterior nasal spine, zygomatic buttress and coronoid process.

15. If significant volumes of bone are needed, then they can be commonly taken from the iliac crest, cranium, fibula or tibia.

Implant placement (first stage) surgery

1. It is a thin outer layer of connective tissue covering the mineralised outer surface of any bone (except the articulating surface of joints). Periosteum is divided into an outer fibrous layer and an inner deep layer. The dense fibrous layer contains fibroblasts and blood vessels, while the inner layer contains more loosely arranged collagenous fibres and thin elastic fibres. Periosteum is attached to bone by strong collagenous fibres called Sharpey's fibres. It also provides an attachment for muscles and tendons. Blood vessels passing through it provide an important blood supply to the bone tissue beneath.

2. It is the most common type of surgical flap used in oral surgery procedures. It involves making an incision through the mucosa and periosteum. The full thickness of the mucosa and periosteum can be then raised together and lifted away from the bone to expose the surgical site.

3. It is a surgical flap that includes the epithelium and part of the subepithelial connective tissue but does not include the periosteum.

4. A surgical guide should always be made and used to help guide the surgeon during the implant surgery. Some standardised guides are also made by different implant manufacturers; however, a customised guide should ideally be used for each patient.

5. Yes, it does, it has been shown that inexperienced surgeons have higher implant failure rates and complication rates. It is very important that anyone placing dental implants has undergone suitable training and that they have been mentored by a suitably experienced clinician.

6. It cuts a threaded channel in the bone ready to receive an implant.

7. It prevents hard and soft tissue growth into the implant and prevents the build up of infective material within the implant.

8. The surgical implant site.

9. An osteotome in implant dentistry is a cylindrical or gently conical instrument used to widen an implant site with apical and lateral pressures, it can be used by hand or with a surgical mallet.

10. It is usually a small round bur used to create the initial entry point for the implant surgical site. The terminology for this does vary between different implant systems.

11. A piezo-surgical unit uses ultrasonic frequency vibrations of the unit handpiece to surgically cut hard tissues.

12. It is a drill with a smaller diameter non-cutting tip and a wider diameter upper cutting section. It is used to widen a smaller diameter hole to a wider diameter. In some implant systems, it

refers to a small diameter drill used after the guide drill to create the initial path for subsequent implant drills to follow.

13. It is when a deficiency in the bone is built up with a bone-substituted material such as autogenous bone, synthetic mineral-based materials or animal-derived xenograft material. It is a form of grafting technique designed to increase the volume of tissues. In dental implantology, it usually relates to bone augmentation designed to increase the volume of bone around a dental implant for support and/or for aesthetic reasons.

14. It is an implant placed immediately following the extraction of a tooth, usually into the tooth socket.

15. It is a form of bone augmentation. Barrier materials (or membranes) can be placed over bone defects to exclude fast growing cell types such as epithelium and connective tissue, which then allows slower growing bone tissue to form in the defect area. Many different Guided Bone Regeneration (GBR) membrane materials have been used and are either nonresorbable materials which have to be removed after the new bone tissue has formed or resorbable membranes which do not have to be removed.

16. Platelet-rich plasma (PRP) is a preparation obtained from a patient's own blood, which is centrifuged to produce a limited volume of plasma enriched with platelets. The platelets contain a number of growth factors, which are known to play a role in hard and soft tissue healing. PRP has been used in a number of regenerative periodontal and implant procedures including sinus lift and soft tissue augmentation procedures.

17. It is the ability of an implant to resist movement immediately after placement in the bone. In effect, it is a measure of how firmly the implant is held within the bone.

18. It is important that an implant is able to resist microscopic movements during the early healing period immediately after surgery in order that osseointegration can take place. If the implant has a low primary stability, it is less likely to be able to resist micromovement during the healing phase, and there may be an increased likelihood of the implant failing to osseointegrate. A number of factors can affect how stable the implant is after placement. The surgical technique used, the implant design and the bone quality are the main factors. It is much harder to gain a high primary implant stability in bone of very poor quality.

19. A number of techniques have been suggested to measure implant primary stability. The most commonly used is the feel of the implant during placement. An experienced implant surgeon is able to feel whether an implant is very stable following placement because of how much force was needed to insert the implant into the bone (in other words, how firm did it feel). As an extension of this technique, some clinicians and implant manufacturers recommend the use of insertion torque as an indirect measure of primary stability, again this measures how much force was needed to screw the implant into position. Another widely used technique is to use a vibration test called resonance frequency analysis to assess how firmly the implant is held in bone. The instrument (Ostell™) uses a probe that is connected to the implant and a measuring device that gives a numerical reading to indicate the implant stability. The higher the number, the better the implant stability. Other techniques that have been tried have involved tapping the implant either by hand or using an electronic device (Periotest); however, this is less commonly used.

20. The space(s) can be temporarily restored with the following:
   - Temporary denture
   - Temporary bridge (conventional or adhesive/resin-retained)

   The space may also be left unrestored if that is acceptable to the patient.

Implant uncovering (second stage) surgery

1. It is a direct, structural and functional connection between an implant and living bone.

2. It is the surgical uncovering of an integrated dental implant. Sometimes it simply involves the use of a round 'biopsy punch' to remove a disc of mucosa over the head of the implant so that the implant cover screw can be removed and a healing abutment be placed. In other cases, it may be necessary for a wider surgical flap to be raised to gain access to the implant, particularly if further surgery is needed to improve the soft tissue contour around the implant.

3. It is not always needed. If it is intended to bury the implant during the healing period, then a two-stage surgical procedure is needed to uncover the implant after the healing period. In some cases, though a single-stage approach is used whereby a long healing abutment is attached to the implant during the healing period. This healing abutment protrudes through the mucosa during the healing period. Following implant integration, this healing abutment can simply be unscrewed to access the implant, removing the need for a second surgical procedure to uncover the implant.

4. It is a cylindrical surgical instrument that can be used to remove a disc of soft tissue from above a dental implant. One end of the instrument has either a short fingergrip or longer handle, the other working end of the instrument is usually a typical metal cylinder of 4 or 5 mm in diameter and with a cutting edge, which is used to cut the soft tissue using gentle pressure and a slight rotating movement over the implant.

5. It is a membrane tissue rich in mucous glands. It is the mucous lining of body passages and cavities including the lining of the mouth and nose. It consists of epithelium, basement membrane, lamina propria and lamina muscularis mucosae.

6. It is involved in a number of functions and processes including protection, support, nutrient absorption and the secretion of enzymes, salts and lubricant mucus.

7. It is the soft tissue covering of the internal and external surfaces of the body. It consists of cells joined together to form a tissue layer. It is classified on the basis of the shape of the surface cells and the number of layers deep.

8. It is soft tissue consisting of various cells (e.g. fibroblasts and macrophages), interlacing protein fibres (e.g. collagen) embedded in a chiefly carbohydrate ground substance that supports and bonds the other tissues together. It has a strong regenerative capacity. In the mouth, it is found beneath the epithelium surface and can be harvested for surgical use.

9. It is a soft tissue augmentation procedure adopted from periodontal surgery using connective tissue usually harvested from a patient's palatal donor site.

10. It is often difficult to rebuild the soft tissues around a dental implant. Connective tissue grafting is just one surgical procedure, which can be used to enhance and augment the tissues around a dental implant in order to try to improve the soft tissue appearance. This can be performed as a part of the first-stage surgical procedure, second-stage surgical procedure or as a separate procedure at a later time.

11. It is a soft tissue grafting procedure where a small layer of tissue is removed from the palate of the patient's mouth and then relocated to the site of gingival/mucosal recession. The graft is sutured into place and allowed to heal and repair the soft tissue defect. This procedure can be used to increase the height and thickness of gingival and peri-implant tissue.

12. It is connected to the implant and screwed into place. The soft tissues are closed around the healing abutment and, if necessary, sutured into place. The soft tissues heal around the healing abutment, and the shape of the abutment controls the shape of the soft tissues above the implant and generates an emergence profile for the future abutment and implant crown.

Surgical complications

1. They should contact the practice immediately and return to be examined by the dentist who may withdraw the implant slightly or completely in order to attempt to decompress the inferior alveolar nerve.

2. The inferior alveolar or inferior dental nerve.

3. During implant surgery, a blood vessel may have been damaged either within the mandible or more likely within the sublingual tissues adjacent to the implant site. This vessel may have led to bleeding within the sublingual tissues with consequent swelling. As the swelling progresses, the tongue becomes raised and swallowing and eventually breathing may be obstructed. Bleeding into these tissues may not be apparent immediately after surgery, and there have been reported cases of bleeding not being apparent for several hours after the surgery.

4. This is potentially a medical emergency as the sublingual bleeding may obstruct the airway. The patient should be told to get to the nearest hospital accident and emergency department immediately. Ideally, the surgeon who placed the implants should attempt to attend the hospital to help provide support and help the patient and medical team if possible. Patients have unfortunately died from this complication following dental implant surgery, and so it must be taken seriously if seen or reported by a patient and action taken swiftly.

5. It is an infection of the bone. In the mouth, it most often affects the mandible and may develop as a result of periapical pathology, dental extractions, oral surgery or bone fractures. It is caused by oral bacteria especially anaerobes.

6. In the early stages, treatment may be aimed at removing any sources of infection and the administration of antibiotics. In the later stages of more severe cases, surgical treatment may be considered to remove necrotic bone tissue and improve wound healing.

7. The use of an aseptic surgical technique and the use of pre-sterilised surgical components are the most important measures to reduce post-operative infection. In addition, the use of a

pre-operative Chlorhexidine Gluconate mouthwash to reduce the level of viable microorganisms can be useful. The use of antibiotics, either at the time of surgery or in the post-surgical period, is a matter of some debate with conflicting opinions and research evidence regarding how effective they are. Some surgeons will however suggest the use of antibiotics to reduce post-operative surgical infection risk, and this is still commonly used worldwide. Post-operative instructions regarding wound care, rinsing with a Chlorhexidine Gluconate mouthwash and effective oral hygiene should also be emphasised to patients.

8. They are the visible dark spaces seen interproximally when an interdental papilla is absent. Interdental papilla are often damaged, lost or reduced in size adjacent to dental implants. Multiple techniques are available to help maintain or rebuild interdental papillae in order to reduce black triangles adjacent to dental implants and improve the aesthetic result.

SECTION VII Answers: Implant restorative procedures

Impression techniques

1. Open-tray impression technique.

2. Closed-tray impression technique.

3. An impression coping.

4. The implant replica or analogue.

5. It is an apparatus designed to mechanically position the elements of the masticatory system (maxilla, mandible, teeth, temporomandibular joints) in the correct position to one another in order to simulate their respective positions in a patient's mouth. They can be used during the planning stage of complex dental implant work and during the fabrication of the implant-supported prostheses.

6. Addition cured polyvinylsiloxane (silicone impression material) or a polyether impression material should be used. These materials are accurate, stable and flexible enough to be used for dental implant working impressions.

7. It is an impression where a component or superstructure that was seated securely in the mouth is 'picked up' within the impression and removed from the mouth within the body of the impression. It allows the technician to fabricate a cast where the contours and position of the component/superstructure as well as the adjacent soft tissues can be captured accurately.

Implant-supported fixed restorations

1. It is an artificial tooth replacement that is part of a fixed or removable partial prosthesis. It is usually placed in the position of the crown(s) of the tooth or teeth being replaced.

2. It is a tooth, tooth root or implant component that acts as a supporting and/or retentive element for a dental prosthesis.

3. In general, it is a device or structure that is used to retain and stabilise a prosthesis. In fixed prostheses, it refers to the crown, inlay or coping that attaches to the abutment teeth or implants to provide retention and support for the prosthesis.

4. It is the ability of a prosthesis or restoration to maintain its intended position during function. For a removable prosthesis, it is the resistance to displacement along the path of insertion of the denture.

5. It is a component or element that aids retention of a prosthesis.

6. Sometimes, these prostheses may have a better appearance (aesthetically more pleasing) because there is no need to have a screw hole in the crown or bridge. The prosthesis also does not have to fit as precisely as a screw-retained crown as the cement can fill in minor inaccuracies between the abutment and the crown or bridge. Because the stages of cementation of the crown is similar to conventional crown and bridgework, dentists and nurses may feel more familiar with the techniques involved that may also be seen as an advantage.

7. It can be difficult to remove the crown or bridge at a later date if required. In general, screw-retained prostheses are 'retrievable' and can be removed relatively easily if required. It can be difficult to remove excess cement from beneath the soft tissues. Excess cement in the soft tissues can lead to tissue irritation and possible infection and bone loss.

8. They can have a number of functions:
   - They bridge the soft tissue space between the implant and the prosthesis.
   - They can bridge and help to alter any difference between the implant angulation and the angulation required by the prosthesis.
   - They are used for the retention of the final prosthesis whether a fixed or removable prosthesis and have specific design features to aid retention.

9. Screw or cement retained.

10. It allows the components or prosthesis to be removed relatively easily.

11. It is the ability to remove a prosthesis or implant component easily, this tends to be used in connection with screw-retained restorations.

12. Torque.

13. The correct torque is needed to ensure that the components are firmly held together, too little torque and the components may come apart, too much torque and the screw may break.

14. It is a force acting around a rotation, it is a measure of how tight a screw joint is secured when a screw is tightened. In implant dentistry, it is quoted in Ncm (Newton centimetres).

15. Immediate loading.

16. It is the structural support component for the implant prosthesis. It usually connects to the implant or abutment and supports the prosthetic materials and/or components.

17. It is a Computer-Aided Design and Computer-Aided Manufactured component.

18. It is a component that is manufactured in a standardised form, it is not custom made for a specific patient.

19. Screws can be used in different ways to retain a prosthesis:
- A screw can be used to attach the prosthesis directly to the internal screw thread in the implant.
- A screw can be used to attach the prosthesis to an abutment or abutments, which in turn attach to the implant(s).
- A lateral screw can be used to attach the prosthesis to a custom-made abutment, these are usually used to hide the screw hole by placing it on the lingual or palatal surface of the prosthesis.

20. It is the name given to the application of a load or force to an object. In relation to dental implants, it relates to an implant having a load applied to it by connecting the prosthesis to the implant.

21. This relates the connection of a temporary or permanent prosthesis to an implant immediately after implant placement or at least within the early healing period immediately after the implant is placed (<48 hours after implant placement).

22. As the name implies, this relates to the gradual increase in the amount of functional load that is applied to an implant. This is done by changing the design of the prosthesis in stages, allowing the implant to be progressively loaded more and more in function as time goes on. It is based on the assumption that the bone will strengthen and adapt as time goes on, improving the quality of the bone around the implant and avoiding overloading the implant in the early stages.

Implant-supported dentures

1. Implant-supported dentures are generally constructed from acrylic resin and/or metal alloy in a similar way to conventional dentures. Implant overdentures are subjected to high forces in the mouth and so dentures with acrylic bases (particularly lower dentures) are often strengthened with a metal strengthener.

2. A mucosa-supported denture constructed in a similar way to a conventional denture but which sits over and clips onto ball-shaped abutments that are in turn connected to the dental implants. The clips give the denture an added retention and also some support.

3. A mucosa-supported denture constructed in a similar way to a conventional denture but which sits over and clips onto a bar. The bar is attached to dental implants in the mouth. The clips give the denture retention and also some support.

4. In reality, most dentures gain support from the soft tissues on which they rest and also from the implants.

5. The retention that can be achieved with an implant overdenture can be considerable. Some patients may have difficulty with manual dexterity and also in their hand strength, and they may struggle to insert and remove new implant-retained overdentures. It is important to check that a patient can easily insert and remove their implant overdentures before they leave the surgery.

6. Most retention systems are adjustable. It should be possible to reduce the level of retention in the implant clips and therefore make it easier for the patient to remove their dentures. Some systems have interchangeable inserts with different degrees of retention that can be changed easily at the chairside, other systems can be adjusted within the denture by the use of specific tools that increase or decrease the level of retentive force in the denture clips.

SECTION VIII Answers: Implant aftercare and maintenance

Oral hygiene

1. Although a patient with a good general level of oral hygiene prior to implant placement is likely to have a similar standard of oral hygiene around their implant, it is not necessarily the case. The shape of the implant and prosthesis, as well as the soft tissue shape around the implant can make it more difficult to carry out oral hygiene measures around an implant when compared to a natural tooth. Oral hygiene around a new implant should always be checked for each patient.

2. All conventional home oral hygiene aids are safe to use around an implant. This includes manual and electric toothbrushes, floss/tape, interdental and interproximal brushes as well as more specialist implant brushes. The use of abrasive products and aids that could scratch the titanium implant and abutment surfaces should be avoided.

3. Chlorhexidine mouthwash can be useful during the immediate post-surgical wound healing phase. It can also be useful for periods when the soft tissues around the implant may show evidence of acute inflammation. It should not be advised as part of a long-term regular home care regime.

4. There is a link between the level of oral hygiene around an implant and the likelihood of that implant developing peri-implant inflammatory disease. It is important for patients to have a good level of oral hygiene in order to maintain the healthy status of the hard and soft tissues around their implants.

5. A number of patients do not use oral hygiene aids correctly or effectively. Although they may be able to describe the use of tooth brushes and floss in reality, they may have difficulty using the oral hygiene aids effectively, particularly if they have reduced manual dexterity. It is often useful to ask patients to demonstrate their home care routines in the dental surgery so that they can be observed and any errors in technique corrected.

Peri-implant inflammatory disease

1. Peri-implant mucositis.

2. Peri-implantitis.

3. The presence of inflammation in the peri-implant tissues.

4. A successfully osseointegrated dental implant should not move within the tissues of the mouth. If an implant becomes mobile, then it is not sufficiently osseointegrated to function correctly and should be removed. Clinical and radiographic assessment of the implant should be carried out to confirm the cause of the mobility.

5. Peri-implantitis

6. A long cone periapical radiograph.

Prosthetic complications

1. There may be a high load placed on the restoration by the bruxist activity. This can lead to the fracture of components and/or the materials that the prosthesis was constructed from.

2. If dental implants are placed especially at the front of the mouth, they may be vulnerable to damage when subjected to trauma during contact sports. It should always be advised that patients involved in contact sports consider having a sports mouthguard made to protect their natural teeth and implants from trauma when playing sports.

3. The implant and crown need to be carefully assessed clinically and radiographically to confirm the reason for the loose crown. A loose implant crown can have several causes:
   - If the crown is cement retained, then it may have simply become decemented.
   - If the crown is screw retained, then the crown may have become unscrewed or the screw retaining the crown may have fractured.
   - The abutment under the crown may have become unscrewed, or the abutment screw or the abutment itself may have fractured.
   - The implant may have fractured.
   - The implant may have become mobile due to peri-implant bone loss.

4. If an abutment or bridge/prosthesis screw fractures during use, the prosthesis may become loose or may move during function which the patient may be able to detect. If the prosthesis is no longer securely held in place due to the fractured screw, then additional load may be placed on other screws or components putting them at higher risk of damage unless the problem is identified and dealt with appropriately. The fractured portion of the screw in the abutment or implant is often fractured within the body of the implant or abutment making removal difficult.

5. It can be difficult to replace a fractured implant screw, as often a portion of the screw is fractured within the implant or abutment. It may be possible to unwind the fractured portion of the screw with the use of a dental probe. Alternatively if this is not possible, then most implant companies have specialised components or kits to remove fractured screw remnants. A replacement screw can then be placed, restoring the patient to normal function.

6. Conventional checks of the denture should be made to make sure that the denture is still stable and well-fitting in the mouth. If the dentures had previously been retentive and are still well-fitting, then the most likely change would be that the retentive clasps within the denture have become worn, damaged or lost. These can be replaced or in some cases the clasps may have interchangeable inserts, which can be changed to return the clasps back to full retention. It would also be important to make sure that there is no damage or loss from the implant abutments or implant bar if present in the mouth. In very rare situations, it may be that the implant(s) themselves have become loose and this would indicate a catastrophic loss of integration.

7. Changes in a patient's occlusion can have a serious impact on the load that is applied to their dental implants. If their remaining natural teeth wear down, change shape because of being restored or are removed, then the force that is applied to the dental implant prosthesis may change. An increase in the load can be damaging to the implant components, the implant-supported prosthesis or the opposing teeth/prosthesis and should be identified early in order to correct it.

8. Patients can bite with much higher forces with dental implant-supported overdentures when compared to conventional dentures. This can lead to increased wear of the denture materials. In addition, it is common for patients to adapt their diets and many patients with implant-supported overdentures may have a more varied and challenging diet, which may be more abrasive and lead to increased denture wear.

9. It is when a screw-shaped component loses its thread shape because the screw was inserted and tightened incorrectly or because the screw was pulled out forcibly without unscrewing it correctly.

CHAPTER 5

Dental radiography

Post Registration Qualifications for Dental Care Professionals: Questions and Answers, First Edition.
Nicola Rogers, Rebecca Davies, Wendy Lee, Dominic O'Sullivan and Frances Marriott.
© 2016 John Wiley & Sons, Ltd. Published 2016 by John Wiley & Sons, Ltd.
Companion Website: www.wiley.com/go/rogers/post-registration-dental-care-questions

SECTION I Questions: Radiation physics

LEARNING OUTCOMES

At the end of this section, you should be able to identify any gaps in your personal knowledge associated with the following:
- A basic understanding of atomic structure
- Properties of X-rays
- The components of the X-ray tubehead
- Production of X-rays
- Interactions of X-rays with matter

Atomic structure

1. Define an **atom** and name its constituent parts.

2. What are the charges of the atomic particles?

3. Name the two innermost shells orbiting the nucleus of an atom.

4. What is the maximum number of electrons that can exist on these two innermost shells?

5. Define **atomic number**.

6. Define **atomic mass number**.

7. What are **isotopes**?

8. What is a **radioisotope**?

9. What are the similarities between a **neutron** and a **proton**?

10. In what ways do electrons differ from protons?

11. What is a **neutral atom**?

12. Define an **ion**.

13. Name the process whereby an electron is removed from an atom resulting in a positive ion.

14. Name the process whereby the atom remains neutral but an electron is displaced from an inner shell to an outer shell.

15. What is **electron binding energy**?

Properties of X-rays

1. Name the German physicist who discovered X-rays by chance.

2. Why were they named X-rays?

3. Which German dentist took the first dental radiograph?

4. What is an **X-ray**?

5. X-rays are part of which spectrum?

6. Name the other types of radiation in this spectrum?

7. What is the difference between **ionising** and **non-ionising** radiation?

8. List the main properties of X-rays.

9. Can human senses detect X-rays?

10. What are the two main uses of X-rays in medicine?

11. Name two types of industries that utilise ionising radiation?

12. X-rays obey the **inverse square law**, what does this mean and what is its significance?

Dental X-ray generating equipment

X-ray tubehead

1. What are the three main components of dental X-ray generating equipment?

2. List five components of the X-ray tubehead.

3. What is the function of the **step-up transformer**?

4. What is the function of the **step-down transformer**?

5. What is the function of the outer **lead casing**?

6. If a crack is noted in the outer casing of the X-ray tubehead prior to a radiographic examination, should the procedure be postponed?

7. Which component in the X-ray tubehead has a similar function to the copper? What is the function?

8. What is the function of the **aluminium filter**?

9. What is the optimal shape of the collimator in the tubehead?

10. Does the collimator affect the mean energy of the X-ray beam?

11. What is the legal **focus to skin distance** (FSD) for dental X-ray sets operating above 60 kV?

X-ray tube

1. Draw a simple diagram of a **glass X-ray tube** labelling the main components.

2. What material forms the **cathode filament**?

3. What material houses the tungsten target at the anode? What is its function?

4. Detail the properties of tungsten that ensures it is a good material in dental X-ray equipment.

5. Is tungsten a more efficient thermo conductor than copper?

6. What is the purpose of the **leaded glass housing**?

7. What is the function of the **cathode**?

8. What is the purpose of the **focusing cup**?

9. What is the function of the **anode**?

10. Name the electrical potential that is applied to the X-ray tube between the cathode and anode.

11. What effect does this electrical potential have on the electrons?

12. Name the electrical current that flows through the X-ray tube.

Production of X-rays

1. What are the three principal electrical quantities that control X-ray production?

2. How are electrons produced at the cathode?

3. What accelerates the electrons across the vacuum towards the anode?

4. What helps to aim the electrons towards the focal spot on the anode target?

5. When high-speed electrons bombard the target, there are two main types of collisions with the tungsten target, of which one is X-ray producing collisions. Name the other.

6. In a 70 kV dental X-ray set, what is the approximate percentage of each type of collision during a radiation exposure?

7. What X-ray producing collision is linked to the **continuous spectrum** of radiation? Briefly describe this interaction at the atomic level.

8. Do low-energy or high-energy X-ray photons predominate in this interaction?

9. In the continuous X-ray spectrum on what is the maximum photon energy dependent?

10. What X-ray producing collision is linked to the **characteristic/line spectrum** of radiation? Describe this interaction at the atomic level.

11. What is the energy requirement of the bombarding electron to displace a K shell tungsten electron in order to produce a K line on the characteristic spectrum?

12. Can characteristic K line photons be produced in an 85 kV dental X-ray set?

13. Can characteristic K line photons be produced in a 65 kV dental X-ray set?

14. Which spectrum predominates in the intensity of the diagnostic X-ray beam?

15. Define the **combined spectrum**.

16. Define the term **quality** of the X-ray beam.

17. What principally determines the quality of the X-ray beam?

18. Define the term **intensity** of the X-ray beam.

19. What effect does increasing kV have on the contrast of the image?

20. What effect does increasing kV have on patient dose?

21. What effect does increasing mA have on the image?

22. What effect does increasing mA have on patient dose?

23. What effect does increasing exposure time have on the image?

24. What effect does increasing exposure time have on patient dose?

25. How many volts supply a dental X-ray machine?

26. What happens to this voltage to enable X-ray production?

27. The mains voltage is an alternating current. Is the positive or negative half of the cycle required for X-ray production?

28. When considering alternating current (**AC**) or direct current (**DC**) dental X-ray sets, which are more efficient at X-ray production and why?

The control panel and circuitry

1. List the main components of the control panel of dental X-ray equipment.

2. Which setting on the dental X-ray control panel is commonly set and cannot be adjusted?

3. State one type of exposure time selection on a control panel.

4. Can a non-trained employee set the exposure parameters and conduct a medical exposure?

5. Can a non-trained employee press the exposure button once a trained operator has prepared the patient and set the exposure parameters for a dental exposure?

6. If a medical X-ray exposure fails to terminate, what actions need to be taken?

Interactions of X-rays with matter

1. Name the four possible interactions that X-ray photons may have when they enter a patient's tissues.

2. Define **attenuation** with respect to X-ray interactions.

3. Define **scatter** with respect to X-ray interactions.

4. Define **absorption** with respect to X-ray interactions.

5. Name the two X-ray interactions with matter, at the atomic level, which are relevant to dental radiography.

6. Which interaction predominates with low-energy X-ray photons?

7. Which interaction predominates with high-energy X-ray photons?

8. Which interaction is a process of absorption and scatter?

9. Which interaction is a process of pure absorption?

10. In which interaction does the incoming photon interact with a bound inner shell electron?

11. In which interaction does the incoming photon interact with a loosely bound or free outer shell electron?

12. Which interaction is not dependent on the atomic number so that it will occur in all tissues equally?

13. Is the probability of the photoelectric effect proportional to the Z^3?

14. Why is lead used in radiation protection?

15. Which of the interactions results in ionisation of the tissues?

16. Which interaction allows intensifying screens, in extra-oral cassettes, to emit their excess energy as light in order to create a radiographic image?

SECTION II Questions: Radiation dose and the biological risks associated with X-rays

---

LEARNING OUTCOMES

At the end of this section, you should be able to identify any gaps in your personal knowledge associated with the following:
- The definitions in radiation dosimetry
- Sources of radiation
- The classification of the biological effects of ionising radiation
- How X-rays cause damage and the magnitude of risk in dental radiography
- Annual dose limits and dose monitoring

Dosimetry

1. Define the term **radiation-absorbed dose (D)**.

2. What is the special name of the unit of measurement for the radiation-absorbed dose?

3. Define the term **equivalent dose (H_T)**.

4. What is the special name of the unit of measurement for the equivalent dose?

5. Define the term **effective dose (E)**.

6. What is the special name of the unit of measurement for the effective dose?

7. Define the term **collective dose**.

8. Let us assume that a periapical radiograph dose is 0.001 mSv. Does this describe the absorbed, equivalent, effective or collective dose?

Sources of radiation

1. What is **radiation**?

2. Define **background radiation**.

3. List the sources of natural background radiation.

4. List the sources of artificial radiation.

5. What is the estimated annual dose of background radiation that a person in the United Kingdom receives?

6. The Radiation Protection Division of the Health Protection Agency estimates the average annual doses to the UK population from various sources of ionising radiation. What approximate percentage is made up from natural background radiation versus artificial radiation?

7. What is the dominant source of artificial radiation that contributes to the average annual UK dose?

Biological effects of ionising radiation

1. Define **tissue reactions** (deterministic effects).

2. Why does the International Commission on Radiation Protection (ICRP) now use the term **tissue reactions** rather than **deterministic effects**?

3. Define the **stochastic** effect.

4. The stochastic effects can be subdivided, the heritable (genetic) effect is one, name the other.

5. Define the **heritable (genetic)** effect.

6. Which of these effects is of primary concern in dental radiography and why?

7. Name some of the tissue reactions that are expected following radiotherapy (for cancer treatment) to the head and neck.

8. With routine dental radiography would you expect to see a tissue reaction (deterministic effect)?

9. Can a dose as low as a bitewing radiograph produce a stochastic effect?

X-ray damage and risk in dental radiography

1. Name the two proposed mechanisms of X-ray damage at the cellular level.

2. Describe the basic method of cell damage for each mechanism.

3. Name factors that may determine what happens to the cells following damage from ionising radiation.

4. Is the risk of biological damage from ionising radiation age dependent?

5. What is the estimated risk of fatal radiation-induced malignancy from a dental panoramic radiograph?

6. What is the estimated risk of fatal radiation-induced malignancy from a bitewing or periapical radiograph using 70 kV, rectangular collimation and F speed film?

7. Consider two periapical radiographic exposures, the first using 70 kV, circular collimation and D speed film and the second using 70 kV, rectangular collimation and F speed film. Which of the two examinations has a higher estimated risk of inducing a radiation-induced malignancy?

8. What is the estimated background radiation equivalent (in days in the United Kingdom) to that of a dental panoramic radiograph?

9. Is comparing equivalent background radiation dose to the effective dose of an exposure a good way of explaining dose and risk?

Annual dose limits and dose monitoring

1. What are **dose limits**?

2. Why are dose limits in place?

3. Are radiation workers allowed to exceed a dose limit?

4. Under which legislation were the dose limits revised in 1999?

5. Are there different dose limits for individuals?

6. What is the annual dose limit for patients?

7. What is the annual dose limit for the general public?

8. Radiation workers have been separated into two categories, what are they?

9. What is the maximum annual dose limit for each classification of radiation worker?

10. Which organisation sets the annual dose limits for radiation workers?

11. A dentist or radiation trained nurse in dental practice would generally work under which of the two categories?

12. Do both groups of workers require compulsory dose monitoring and annual health checks?

13. What types of personal radiation dose monitoring devices do you know?

14. Which is most commonly used in dental radiography?

15. Should a female employee working with ionising radiation inform their employer if they are pregnant?

16. You inform the employer that a person undergoing a medical examination was exposed to a lot more radiation than intended (×20 times) due to a defect in the X-ray equipment. Which regulatory agency should be notified of this event?

SECTION III Questions: Radiation protection

LEARNING OUTCOMES

At the end of this section, you should be able to identify any gaps in your personal knowledge associated with the following:
- An understanding of current UK legislation and guidelines
- Methods of dose reduction in dental radiography

Legislation

Ionising radiation regulations 1999

1. What are the principal considerations of the Ionising Radiation Regulations 1999 (IRR 99)?

2. Who must be notified of the routine use of dental X-ray equipment in a dental practice or of any modifications or repositioning of X-ray equipment?

3. What does **RPA** stand for?

4. Define an RPA?

5. Does a dental practice using ionising radiation require an RPA?

6. Can a dental nurse with a certificate in dental radiography be an RPA?

7. What does the RPA advise on?

8. What does **RPS** stand for?

9. Is an RPS mandatory?

10. Are local rules relating to radiation protection mandatory?

11. Who is responsible for implementation of the local rules?

12. What information must be included in the local rules?

IR(ME)R 2000

1. What does **IR(ME)R 2000** stand for?

2. What is the principal concern of IR(ME)R 2000?

3. New positions of responsibility are defined in the IR(ME)R regulations. Name and briefly describe the duties of each recognised position.

4. In dental practice, can a dentist perform all of the defined roles?

5. In dental practice, can a dental nurse perform all of the defined roles?

6. What IR(ME)R position defines your role?

7. Define **justification** with respect to a medical exposure.

8. Who is responsible for justifying a medical exposure?

9. In dental practice, is there justification to take X-rays of a patient prior to a clinical examination?

10. If a radiographic image is poor and deemed non-diagnostic (grade 3), should the operator repeat the exposure?

11. As a practising IR(ME)R operator who regularly takes radiographs, is continued education required?

12. As a practising IR(ME)R operator who only processes radiographs, is continued education required?

Dose reduction in dental radiography

1. What is meant by the term **dose optimisation**?

2. What should be the principal consideration when deciding whether a radiographic examination is required?

3. What do you understand by the term **dose constraints** as suggested by the Ionising Radiation Regulations 1999?

4. What is a **DRL**?

5. Who measures DRLs in a dental practice?

6. How often are National DRLs revised by the Health Protection Agency?

Radiation protection of radiation workers and the general public

1. Define **general public** with respect to radiation protection.

2. What radiation protection measures must be in place to protect the general public from ionising radiation?

3. How may radiation workers inadvertently receive a radiation dose?

4. How can an operator limit their risk of radiation exposure?

5. Who is responsible for a risk assessment prior to commencement of ionising radiation within a dental practice?

6. With respect to ionising radiation, what is the minimum number of employees in a dental practice that warrants a mandatory risk assessment to be performed?

7. Risk assessments should be subject to review. What is the recommended interval between reviews?

8. Does a film-monitoring badge provide a retrospective or prospective assessment of radiation exposure?

9. Do X-ray monitoring devices protect against radiation exposure?

10. Is there a limit on the number of dental radiographs a single operator can perform?

11. What is the **controlled area**?

12. Where should the operator position himself or herself with respect to the controlled area during an X-ray exposure?

13. Who is allowed in the controlled area during an X-ray exposure?

14. Why must the mains switch to the X-ray generating equipment be sited outside of the controlled area?

15. Who advises on all aspects of the controlled area?

16. Do IR(ME)R operators in dental practice routinely wear lead protection?

17. Can an employee continue to take radiographs while pregnant?

18. Must a pregnant employee, who acts as an operator in dental radiography, wear a lead apron during working hours?

19. Should an operator wear a thyroid collar?

20. If an employee or member of the general public is required to be in the controlled area during a radiation exposure, for example, as a comforter/carer, do they require lead protection?

X-ray equipment and dose reduction to the patient

1. Why are direct current (constant potential) **DC** X-ray generating units favoured over alternating current **AC** units?

2. Why is filtration within the X-ray tubehead a method of dose reduction?

3. What material is used in the filtration process?

4. For X-ray tube voltages up to and including 70 kV, what thickness of filtration material is required?

5. For X-ray tube voltages above 70 kV, what thickness of filtration material is required?

6. What is the minimum required focus to skin distance (fsd) for a dental X-ray set operating above 60 kV?

7. What effect would a short focus to skin distance (fsd) have on the image?

8. What is the typical kV range for an intra-oral dental X-ray set?

9. What is the typical kV range for a panoramic X-ray set?

10. Which dental X-ray set would produce higher patient dose, a set operating at 50 kV or 70 kV?

11. Is film-based image contrast better in a set operating at 50 kV or 70 kV?

12. Which collimator shape, in combination with optimal operator technique, is dose saving, rectangular or circular?

13. You are asked to perform a periapical radiograph of the upper left canine tooth on an adult patient. You have two films available E speed and F speed. Which would you choose for dose optimisation and why?

14. You are asked to perform a periapical radiograph of the upper left canine tooth on an adult patient. You have two image receptors to choose from conventional **F speed film** and a **solid-state digital sensor**. Which method is generally considered the lower dose technique?

15. Name the two periapical radiographic techniques that an operator may use.

16. Which periapical radiographic technique is optimal for reproducibility and diagnostic quality?

17. What are the benefits of using image receptor holders?

18. In an extra-oral cassette for film-based imaging, intensifying screens are used as a dose reduction method. How do they work and what types of screens do you know?

19. Which screen type is the fastest and most efficient?

20. Is resolution of the image improved with intensifying screens?

21. What is the first line of dose reduction?

22. What evidence-based guidelines are in place to aid dentists in the justification process?

23. You have been asked by the dentist to perform a periapical radiograph of a lower left first molar tooth on a female patient prior to extraction of the tooth. You find a periapical radiograph of this tooth in the notes that was taken 5 months ago during endodontic treatment. What should you do?

24. The dentist asks you to take a dental panoramic radiograph of a 12-year-old boy for the purposes of orthodontic assessment. While positioning the patient for the examination he starts hiccupping, what should you do?

25. The dentist asks you to take left and right lateral oblique radiographs on a 5-year-old girl for caries assessment. She was unable to tolerate bitewing radiographs and was getting distressed. You have not used this technique for over 10 years and you are not confident in the procedure, what should you do?

26. Should patients be given a lead apron during a dental radiographic procedure?

27. Can pregnant patients have dental radiographs?

28. Is it a legal requirement to provide a pregnant patient with a lead apron during dental radiographs?

29. What is the minimum thickness of lead in protective aprons that should be provided for any adult who acts as a comforter/carer in the controlled area?

30. How should lead aprons be stored?

31. Is it a legal requirement to provide a thyroid collar to a patient having dental radiographs?

SECTION IV Questions: Image receptors and processing

LEARNING OUTCOMES

At the end of this section, you should be able to identify any gaps in your personal knowledge associated with the following:
- the components and action of direct and indirect radiographic film;
- the components and action of digital sensors;
- image processing to include chemical and computer digital processing.

Direct action film

1. Are direct action films primarily sensitive to light or X-ray photons?

2. Why are direct action films given their name?

3. List common dental radiographic examinations that use direct X-ray film.

4. Other than the X-ray film, name the contents of the direct action intra-oral film packet and discuss the purpose of each component.

5. What feature of the film packet helps the operator to orientate the film?

6. What distinguishing feature on the radiographic image would inform the operator that they had placed the film the wrong way round in the patient's mouth?

7. What are the components of the radiographic film? Discuss the action of each part.

8. Define the **latent image** with respect to direct action film.

9. What is the most common silver halide crystal used in direct action film?

10. How do the silver halide crystals affect film speed?

11. What effect does faster film speed have on the image?

12. What effect does faster film speed have on patient dose?

13. How can you visually distinguish an 'E speed' film from an 'F speed' film?

14. What film speed should be used as standard in dental radiography?

15. What is the approximate dose reduction of F speed film compared to E speed film?

16. What is the approximate resolution (in line pairs per millimetre) of direct action film?

17. What cross-infection control measure can be an additional component of the intra-oral direct action film?

Indirect action film

1. Are indirect action films primarily sensitive to light or X-ray photons?

2. Why are indirect action films given their name?

3. List dental radiographic examinations that use indirect X-ray film in dental practice.

4. What are the three components of an indirect action dental image receptor?

5. How are indirect action films commonly orientated?

6. What is an **intensifying screen**?

7. What are the components of an intensifying screen?

8. Name the two main types of phosphor materials that have been used in intensifying screens?

9. Which type of phosphor is used in modern intensifying screens and why?

10. How do intensifying screens work?

11. Do intensifying screens work by the photoelectric or the Compton effect?

12. Does having an intensifying screen in a cassette increase or decrease radiation dose to the patient?

13. Do intensifying screens in a cassette increase or decrease resolution?

14. What is the approximate resolution (in line pairs per millimetre) of indirect action film?

15. Which has better resolution, direct or indirect action film?

16. How does the silver halide emulsion differ in its action between direct and indirect film?

17. Why is it important to use a specific film and intensifying screen combination?

18. What will be the result of poor film/screen contact in a cassette?

19. Define **screen speed**.

20. What affects the speed of intensifying screens?

21. What affect does high screen speed have on patient dose?

22. What affect does high screen speed have on image detail?

23. If it is noted on inspection that a screen is damaged, should it be used?

24. You notice damage to the hinge on a film cassette, what should you do?

Digital image receptors

1. What is the difference between direct and indirect digital image acquisition?

2. What type of digital image receptor is termed a 'solid-state' sensor?

3. Why are the solid-state sensors termed 'real-time' systems?

4. What are the main basic components of a solid-state sensor?

5. Describe basically how a solid-state sensor produces a radiographic image.

6. What are the basic components of a phosphor plate sensor?

7. What is the typical phosphor used in phosphor plate sensors?

8. Do phosphor plates provide 'real-time' imaging?

9. Describe simply how a phosphor plate produces a radiographic image.

10. Once the phosphor plate has been read, what has to be done before the plate can be re-used?

11. Which types of digital image receptors can be used for both intra-oral and extra-oral dental radiographies?

12. Which type of digital receptor is almost identical in size and shape to conventional intra-oral film?

13. Which type of digital receptor is generally used for occlusal radiography?

14. Do solid-state sensors generally have a larger or smaller surface area than phosphor plates?

15. Which type of digital image receptor is generally connected to the computer by a cable/cord?

16. What component of the solid-state sensor converts X-ray photons into light?

17. Name a disadvantage of the connecting cable or cord present on solid-state sensors.

18. Which of the digital sensors can commonly be used with standard conventional film holders?

19. Are solid-state sensors thicker than phosphor plates?

20. Which are more expensive solid-state sensors or phosphor plates?

21. Which type of digital sensor would you least like to drop and break?

22. Which sensors do patients tend to tolerate better in their mouths.

23. Are solid-state sensors autoclavable?

24. Are phosphor plate's autoclavable?

25. Why are intra-oral digital detectors barrier wrapped?

26. Do extra-oral digital detectors require barrier wrapping?

Conventional versus digital imaging

1. Which is considered lower dose, conventional or solid-state intra-oral digital radiography?

2. Why is extra-oral digital radiography reportedly less dose saving compared to conventional film than intra-oral digital radiography?

3. Do the principal radiographic techniques differ between conventional and digital dental radiography?

4. What is the main similarity of the radiographic images with both conventional and digital techniques?

5. Should different X-ray generating equipment be used for conventional and digital intra-oral radiographies?

6. Can film holders be used in both conventional and digital intra-oral imagings?

7. As digital imaging does not require chemical processing solutions, is a quality assurance programme required?

8. List some advantages of digital over film-based imaging.

9. List some disadvantages of digital over film-based imaging.

Image processing

Chemical processing

1. Define **image processing**.

2. What is the **latent image**?

3. Is the latent image visible?

4. What are the two main methods of chemical film processing available in dental practice?

5. Can you think of a third method of practical chemical processing of film?

6. How many processing stages are there in converting film emulsion into the visible radiographic image during manual processing?

7. How many processing chemicals are required?

8. What is the processing stage whereby the unsensitised silver halide crystals in the emulsion are removed to reveal the transparent or white areas of the image?

9. At what processing stage is the emulsion hardened?

10. What is the processing stage whereby the sensitised silver halide crystals in the emulsion are converted to black metallic silver to produce the grey to black areas on the image?

11. How many washing stages are there?

12. What is the purpose of the washing stages?

13. Which of the washing cycles is the longest in manual film processing?

14. If films are processed manually in a darkroom, why should the room be light tight?

15. What is present on an automatic processor that eliminates the need for a darkroom?

16. Why should a darkroom be well ventilated?

17. What are the safelight requirements in a darkroom?

18. What does the **coin test** measure?

19. Can the coin test be carried out in automatic processors as well as darkrooms?

20. In manual processing, what is the recommended time that the film should be left in the developer solution?

21. In manual processing, what is the recommended temperature of the developer?

22. In manual processing, what is the recommended time that the film should be left in the fixer solution?

23. Films should be fixed for double the clearing time. What is the clearing time?

24. Name the developer agents in the developing solution.

25. Name the constituent of the fixer solution that removes the unsensitised silver halide crystals.

26. Name the preservative used in both the developer and fixer solutions.

27. Is developer acidic or alkaline?

28. Is fixer acidic or alkaline?

29. How often should the developing solutions be replaced?

30. Why does developer need to be replaced?

31. What will be the effect on the radiographic image if the film is over developed?

32. What will be the effect on the radiographic image if the film is under developed?

33. What will be the effect on the radiographic image if the developer solution is too hot?

34. What will be the effect on the radiographic image if the developer solution is too cool?

35. What can happen to the film if the developer solution is contaminated with fixer?

36. What should you do if the developing solution has been contaminated?

37. What advice should you follow with respect to chemical processing concentrations?

38. What will happen to a film if it has been inadequately fixed?

39. What are the advantages of automatic processing over manual processing?

40. What are the disadvantages of automatic processing over manual processing?

41. Describe a self-developing film.

42. What are the advantages of self-developing film compared to other methods of chemical processing?

43. What are the disadvantages of self-developing film compared to other methods of chemical processing?

44. In what situations may a self-developing film be the optimal choice?

45. There are occasions when a second radiograph or copy of the original is required. Is there a means of producing two identical radiographic images for a patient in one conventional radiographic exposure?

46. Can chemical processing influence the quality rating of a radiograph?

Digital processing

1. Define a **pixel**.

2. What does a pixel measure?

3. Each pixel has an *x*- and *y*-coordinate and is allocated a number. What is the typical range of numbers allocated?

4. What colour relates to a pixel assigned number 0? Explain your answer.

5. What colour relates to a pixel assigned number 255? Explain your answer.

6. What is the total number of shades of grey that the computer can typically allocate to a pixel?

7. What is the general size range of a pixel in dental digital imaging?

8. What effect does pixel size have on the radiographic image?

9. What is the approximate resolution (in line pairs per millimetre) of digital sensors?

10. Which type of digital sensor inputs the pixel information directly to the computer's analogue-to-digital converter?

11. Which type of digital sensor is not directly linked to the computer and requires an additional processing stage?

12. Digital images can be manipulated to enhance the image. List the types of enhancement techniques that you know?

13. Which two image enhancement techniques are most often used?

14. What happens to the image if brightness is increased?

15. How is increasing brightness achieved in digital processing?

16. What would the resultant image look like if each pixel were assigned the number 255?

17. What happens to the image if contrast is increased?

18. How is increasing contrast achieved in digital processing?

19. What would the resultant image look like if each pixel were either assigned the highest number (255) or the lowest number (0)?

20. What is **blooming**?

21. Which type of sensor does blooming affect?

22. Can blooming be reduced by software manipulation?

23. If a solid-state sensor is positioned the wrong way round in the patient's mouth, what internal components of the sensor become visible on the digital image?

24. Depending on the brand of phosphor plate, what circular shadow may be cast on the resultant digital image if the plate is positioned the wrong way round in the patient's mouth?

25. If a phosphor plate is scratched, what will be seen on the digital image?

26. If a phosphor plate is dirty and there is debris on the plate, what will be seen on the digital image?

27. What will happen to an image if an irradiated phosphor plate is exposed to light prior to being placed into the reader?

28. What is the disadvantage of obtaining hard copy digital images using thermal, ink jet or laser printers?

29. Name a 3D digital imaging modality used in dental implant planning.

SECTION V Questions: Image quality and quality assurance

LEARNING OUTCOMES

At the end of this section, you should be able to identify any gaps in your personal knowledge associated with the following:
- The basic concepts of the radiographic image
- General radiographic image faults
- Quality assurance programme relevant to dental radiography

The radiographic image

1. What are the main limitations of viewing the 2D radiographic image of a 3D object?

2. What do the **radiopaque**, white shadows on a radiographic image represent?

3. What do the **radiolucent**, black shadows on a radiographic image represent?

4. Give two examples of dense structures in a patient that form radiopaque shadows on the image.

5. Give two examples of structures in a patient that form radiolucent shadows on the image.

6. Name three factors that affect the image density of an object.

7. What is **contrast** with respect to the radiographic image?

8. Does an increase in kV increase or decrease contrast?

9. For optimal imaging technique (e.g. a periapical radiograph) how should the object, image receptor and X-ray beam be positioned relative to one another?

10. What effect does increased patient size have on subject contrast?

11. Define **image sharpness**.

12. How can definition on a radiograph be lost?

13. Define **image resolution**?

14. How is image resolution measured?

15. What can affect resolution?

16. Overall, what practical factors have an impact on the radiographic image quality?

17. What are the features of an **ideal** radiographic image?

Film-based radiographic faults

1. List the possible causes of a pale film.

2. List the possible causes of a dark film.

3. List the possible causes of a marked film.

4. List the possible causes of low contrast.

5. List the possible causes of a blurred or unsharp image.

6. What is **coning off**?

7. Does film fogging show as a white or dark area on the film?

8. What can cause geometric distortion of an image?

9. Can geometric distortion be seen in both film-captured and digital dental radiographs?

10. What is cervical burnout?

11. Describe the faults you can see on this film-captured bitewing radiograph. How could the operator attempt to prevent the problems when retaking the radiograph? (Figure 5.1)

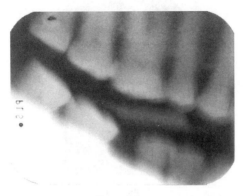

Figure 5.1

12. Describe the faults you can see on this film-captured bitewing radiograph. How can the operator prevent these faults when repeating the radiograph? (Figure 5.2)

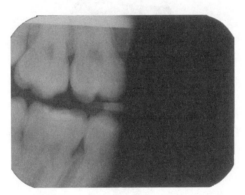

Figure 5.2

13. Describe the main fault demonstrated in this film-captured radiograph? How has this occurred? (Figure 5.3)

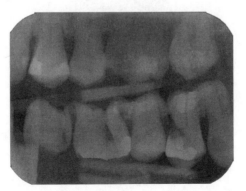

Figure 5.3

14. Describe any faults you can see on this film-captured vertical bitewing radiograph. (Figure 5.4)

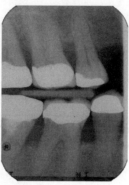

Figure 5.4

15. Describe the main fault that you can see on this film-captured periapical radiograph. How may this problem be rectified? (Figure 5.5)

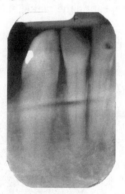

Figure 5.5

16. Describe the main fault of this film-captured periapical radiograph. How may this problem be rectified on the repeat radiograph? (Figure 5.6)

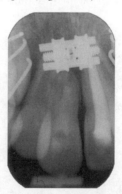

Figure 5.6

17. Describe the main fault in this film-captured periapical radiograph. How may this problem be rectified on the repeat radiograph? (Figure 5.7)

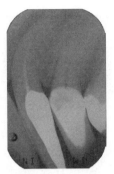

Figure 5.7

18. Describe the faults on this image-captured panoramic radiograph. (Figure 5.8)

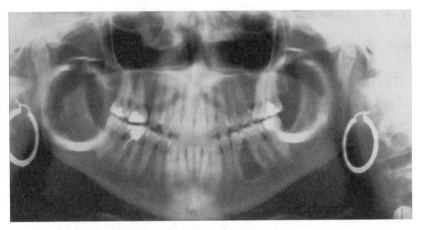

Figure 5.8

19. Describe the film faults on this film-captured bitewing radiograph. What may have caused these faults? (Figure 5.9)

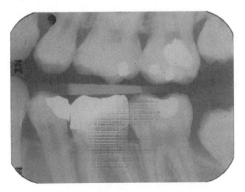

Figure 5.9

20. Describe the film fault on this film-captured bitewing radiograph. What may have caused this film fault? (Figure 5.10)

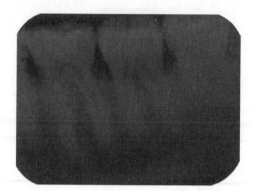

Figure 5.10

Quality assurance

1. In radiography, what is meant by the term **quality control**?

2. In radiography, what is meant by the term **quality assurance**?

3. According to the World Health Organisation definition, what are the aims of a **quality assurance programme** in dental radiography?

4. Is a quality assurance programme mandatory in a dental practice using digital radiography?

5. Is a quality assurance programme mandatory in a dental practice using film-based radiography?

6. Who is responsible for a quality assurance programme in dental practice?

7. Should a quality assurance programme be documented?

8. List the five essential quality control procedures within a programme suited to dental radiography.

9. What additional procedures should be considered with digital radiography?

10. Name the guidance notes that provide a basis for a recommended quality assurance programme for film-based radiographs.

11. Define a Grade 1 film-captured image.

12. Define a Grade 2 film-captured image.

13. Define a Grade 3 film-captured image.

14. Should a Grade 1 film be retaken?

15. Should a Grade 2 film be retaken?

16. Should a Grade 3 film be retaken?

17. Can digitally captured images be quality rated?

18. When quality rating an image what fact is important to consider?

19. According to the 2001 Guidance Notes, what are the minimum long-term targets in a practice for the percentage of Grade 1 films taken?

20. According to the 2001 Guidance Notes, what are the minimum long-term targets in a practice for the percentage of Grade 2 films taken?

21. According to the 2001 Guidance Notes, what are the minimum long-term targets in a practice for the percentage of Grade 3 films taken?

22. According to the 2001 Guidance Notes, after how many years of introducing a quality assurance programme should a dental practice aim to achieve the image rating targets?

23. What method of assessment is commonly used in dental practice to assess standards of image quality and to confirm that any implemented changes lead to improvement?

24. What is the aim of a reject logbook and what would you expect to see recorded?

25. Name four reasons for film rejection.

26. How can image quality be simply assessed on a daily basis?

27. Part of a quality assurance programme is to keep dose ALARP, what does **ALARP** mean?

28. With respect to quality assurance equipment measures, what is a **critical examination**?

29. Who should undertake the critical examination?

30. What is an **acceptance test**?

31. Who is responsible for ensuring that an acceptance test is performed?

32. How often should the X-ray equipment be routinely tested as part of the quality assurance programme?

33. When is a re-examination report required?

34. Should the documentation of any critical, acceptance, re-examination and routine tests be retained?

35. What daily equipment checks can be carried out as part of the quality assurance programme?

36. An up-to-date inventory of each piece of X-ray equipment should be available in the practice. What information should be included in this document?

37. Darkroom processing is now less common, but what safety considerations within a quality assurance programme should be given to this technique of processing?

38. What effect does light have on an unprocessed film?

39. Name a quality control test that may be used in manual and automatic film processing to assess for film fogging.

40. How can light tightness of an extra-oral film cassette be checked?

41. How can film/screen contact of an extra-oral cassette be checked?

42. What information should be included in the written instructions on chemical processing solutions?

43. How often should chemical solutions be changed?

44. How often should a cleaning film be run through the automatic processor?

45. How often should an automatic processor transport mechanism and tank be cleaned?

46. What is shown in the diagram below and what is its use in quality control? (Figure 5.11)

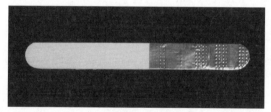

Figure 5.11

47. How often should processing equipment be tested?

48. What are the ideal storage conditions for X-ray film?

49. What are the ideal storage conditions for digital sensors?

50. What care should be given to intensifying screens and why?

51. A quality assurance programme should hold a register of all staff involved with any aspect of radiography. What information is required in this document?

52. Is training of IR(ME)R practitioners and operators a legal or a desirable requirement?

53. How often is it recommended that practitioners and operators attend a continuing education course in radiography?

54. Should dental nurses who are qualified to act as operators have continued education and training in dental radiography?

55. Define clinical audit?

56. As an IR(ME)R operator in dental practice what audits relevant to dental radiography could you implement?

57. In a quality assurance programme, what is included in the working procedures documentation?

SECTION VI Questions: Patient care

LEARNING OUTCOMES

At the end of this section, you should be able to identify any gaps in your personal knowledge associated with the following:
- General patient considerations in dental radiography
- Control of infection and waste disposal

Patient care during dental radiography

1. What aspects of dental radiography do you think may concern or scare patients?

2. What type of patient in particular may need more support than others during a radiographic procedure?

3. As the operator, how can you help to make the experience as easy for the patient as possible?

4. What instructions do you need to give a patient before a dental radiographic procedure?

5. Why should the operator observe a patient during a medical radiation exposure?

6. Why should the exposure variables on the control panel be set prior to positioning the image receptor and tubehead?

7. What should be removed from a patient prior to a dental radiographic procedure?

8. Why should a necklace be removed during a dental panoramic radiograph?

9. How may the selection of intra-oral image receptors vary between adults and children?

10. List some anatomical difficulties that a dental operator may encounter when radiographing a patient.

11. Discuss some of the difficulties that an operator may encounter when radiographing children.

12. Discuss some of the disabilities that a patient may have that make dental radiography difficult.

13. You are asked by the dentist to obtain a dental panoramic radiograph on a 6-year-old boy who requires multiple extractions. You are concerned that the patient will not stay still during the procedure. What are your options?

14. You are asked by the dentist to obtain bitewing radiographs on a 10-year-old girl with mild learning difficulties. Her mother informs you that having her hair stroked calms her down. How may you manage this situation?

15. You are asked by the dentist to obtain a periapical radiograph of the upper left first premolar tooth on a 35-year-old man for the purposes of endodontic treatment. The patient informs you that he has a severe gag reflex. How could you manage this situation?

Control of infection

1. Which 1974 UK Act states that 'every person working in hospitals or general practice has a legal duty to take all the necessary steps required to prevent cross infection in order to protect themselves, their colleagues and patients'?

2. Is dental radiography primarily considered an invasive or non-invasive prone procedure?

3. What is the main cross-infection contamination risk in dental radiography?

4. Why is it important to carry out cross-infection control measures when taking a radiograph?

5. Which form of hepatitis should all clinical staff be vaccinated against?

6. What extra precautions should be given for a patient with a known infection risk?

7. What cross-infection control measures would be carried out prior to taking a radiograph?

8. When taking a radiograph what cross-infection control measures does the operator perform?

9. What cross-infection control measures would be carried out after a radiograph has been taken?

10. How often should X-ray image receptor holders be sterilised?

11. How often should the X-ray generating equipment controls be disinfected?

12. What is the benefit of using barrier-wrapped image receptors?

13. Can digital image receptors be sterilised in an autoclave?

Waste disposal

1. In which waste bin should the outer packaging of a non-barrier wrapped X-ray film packet be placed?

2. In which waste bin should the inner black paper of an X-ray film packet be placed?

3. Where should the lead foil from inside the X-ray film packet be disposed?

4. How should you dispose of spent processing solutions?

5. What classification of waste is spent processing solutions?

6. Are radiography chemical processing solutions considered under the COSHH regulations?

7. What does **COSHH** stand for?

8. In which bin would the barrier wrap from an X-ray film packet be placed after use?

9. In which bin would the barrier wrap from a solid-state sensor be placed following use?

10. In which bin would the protective barrier envelope from a phosphor plate be placed following use?

11. In which bin would the phosphor plate be placed after use?

12. In which bin should the personal protective equipment be disposed after undertaking cross-infection measures?

SECTION VII Questions: Dental radiography

LEARNING OUTCOMES

At the end of this section, you should be able to identify any gaps in your personal knowledge associated with the following:
- The uses and technique of intra-oral radiography
- The uses and technique of extra-oral radiography
- Advantages, disadvantages and limitations of the different radiographic procedures

Bitewing radiography

1. Is a bitewing radiograph an intra-oral or extra-oral radiographic technique?

2. What anatomy should a bitewing radiograph demonstrate?

3. What is the main clinical indication for a bitewing radiograph?

4. Can bitewing radiographs assess periodontal status?

5. Horizontal or vertical bitewing techniques can be employed. Which is the most common technique used?

6. What is the difference in the horizontal and vertical bitewing image receptor positioning?

7. Why might the vertical bitewing technique be used rather than horizontal bitewings?

8. Which teeth should be demonstrated on a bitewing radiograph in a fully dentate adult?

9. Is the entire root morphology demonstrated on a bitewing radiograph?

10. What methods are used to support the image receptor in the patient's mouth and which technique is optimal?

11. What are the three main components of custom-made bitewing image receptor holders?

12. When positioning the image receptor in the patient's mouth, what is its ideal relation to the teeth?

13. Which age group is most likely not to tolerate bitewing holders well?

14. How should you position the patient for a bitewing radiograph?

15. Should the image receptor be positioned perpendicular or parallel to the long axis of the teeth?

16. In the horizontal bitewing technique, where should the anterior edge of the image receptor be positioned with respect to the teeth in a fully dentate patient?

17. In the horizontal bitewing technique, where does the posterior edge of the image receptor generally extend with respect to the teeth in a fully dentate patient?

18. At what angle should the X-ray beam meet the teeth and image receptor?

19. What image faults may result from incorrect tubehead positioning in the horizontal plane?

20. What image faults may result from incorrect tubehead positioning in the vertical plane?

21. Why is it important that the X-ray beam passes between the contact points of the teeth?

22. As the operator, what technical considerations should you give to performing horizontal bitewing radiographs on a young child?

23. List three advantages of the bitewing image receptor holder technique compared to the tab technique.

24. List three disadvantages of the bitewing image receptor holder technique compared to the tab technique.

25. In bitewing caries assessment, why is good contrast essential?

26. For primary periodontal assessment purposes, why should under exposure of the image receptor be achieved?

27. Are carious lesions generally perceived as smaller or larger radiologically than clinically?

28. Give a quality rating to this film-captured bitewing radiograph, which was justified for caries assessment. Explain your answer. (Figure 5.12)

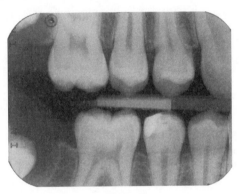

Figure 5.12

29. Give a quality rating to this film-captured bitewing radiograph, which was justified for caries assessment of the molar teeth. Explain your answer. (Figure 5.13)

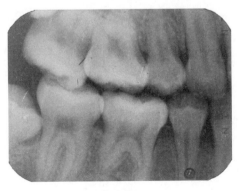

Figure 5.13

Periapical radiography

1. Is a periapical radiograph an intra-oral or extra-oral radiographic technique?

2. What anatomy should a periapical radiograph demonstrate?

3. What are the main clinical indications for a periapical radiograph?

4. Can periapical radiographs assess caries status?

5. Which teeth do periapical radiographs image that bitewing radiographs do not?

6. When positioning the image receptor in the patient's mouth, what is the ideal relation of the image receptor to the teeth?

7. Should the image receptor be positioned perpendicular or parallel to the long axis of the teeth?

8. How should the image receptor be positioned with respect to its long axis for the incisor and canine teeth?

9. How should the image receptor be positioned with respect to its long axis for the premolar and molar teeth?

10. At what angle should the X-ray beam meet the teeth and image receptor?

11. There are two periapical techniques, the **paralleling** and **bisecting angle technique**. Which one is considered more reproducible?

12. Which of the periapical techniques utilises image receptor holders?

13. Which of the periapical techniques is considered best practice and should be used whenever possible?

14. Describe the **bisecting angle technique**.

15. With respect to the bisected angle technique, what is the vertical angulation of the X-ray tubehead?

16. What happens to the image if the vertical angulation is incorrect?

17. What happens to the image if the horizontal angulation is incorrect?

18. Describe the **paralleling technique**.

19. With respect to the paralleling technique, what determines the vertical and horizontal angulations of the X-ray tubehead?

20. What are the three main components of custom-made periapical image receptor holders?

21. With respect to both techniques, how should you position the patient for a periapical radiograph?

22. Of the two images shown in Figures 5.14 and 5.15, which one demonstrates the paralleling periapical technique in use?

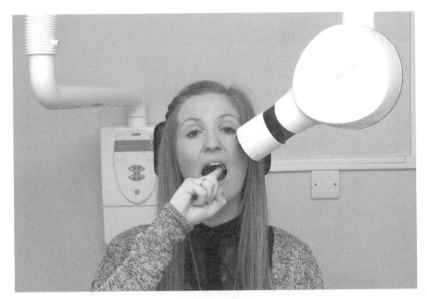

Figure 5.14

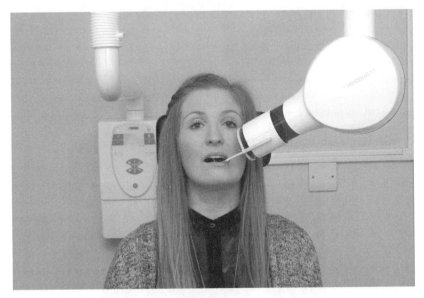

Figure 5.15

23. Which periapical technique does not allow the image receptor and teeth to be in close contact?

24. What is the effect on the image when the image receptor and tooth are not closely approximated? How is this effect overcome?

25. List the main advantages of the paralleling technique.

26. List the main disadvantages of the paralleling technique.

27. List the main advantages of the bisecting angle technique.

28. List the main disadvantages of the bisecting angle technique.

29. In periapical radiography, how many image receptors (22 × 35 mm) are generally required to image the maxillary incisor and canine teeth?

30. In periapical radiography, how many image receptors (22 × 35 mm) are generally required to image the mandibular incisor and canine teeth?

31. In periapical radiography, how many image receptors (31 × 41 mm) are generally required to image the maxillary premolar and molar teeth in one quadrant?

32. In periapical radiography, how many image receptors (31 × 41 mm) are generally required to image the mandibular premolar and molar teeth in one quadrant?

33. How many periapical radiographs generally make a full-mouth survey in a fully dentate adult patient.

34. When positioning radiographic film for a periapical radiograph, where should the orientation dot be positioned and why?

35. Can radiographic film be placed in holders?

36. Can phosphor plates be placed in holders?

37. Can solid-state sensors be placed in holders?

38. Which teeth would you image with the image receptor holder set up as shown in Figures 5.16 and 5.17?

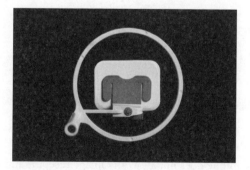

Figure 5.16

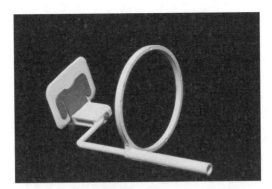

Figure 5.17

39. Which teeth would you image with the image receptor holder set up as shown in Figures 5.18 and 5.19?

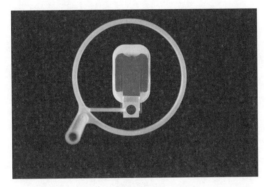

Figure 5.18

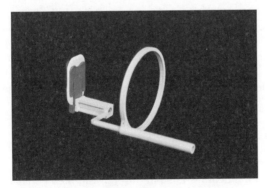

Figure 5.19

40. Which teeth could you image with the image receptor holder set up as shown in Figures 5.20 and 5.21?

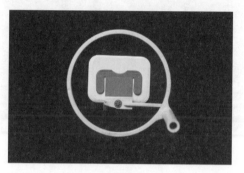

Figure 5.20

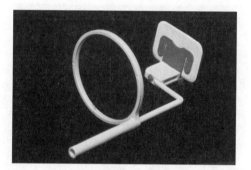

Figure 5.21

41. What are the challenges that the operator faces when taking a periapical radiograph of a tooth that has endodontic instruments *in situ* for working length assessment?

42. Can a holder be used to radiograph a tooth that has a pre-set endodontic file *in situ*?

43. What are the challenges that the operator faces when taking a periapical radiograph of an edentulous ridge?

44. What positioning faults are demonstrated in this periapical film-captured image? (Figure 5.22)

45. What positioning fault is demonstrated in this film-captured periapical image? (Figure 5.23)

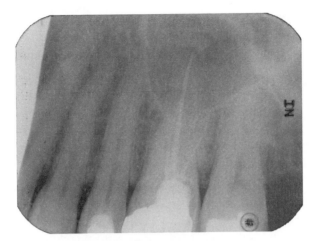

Figure 5.22

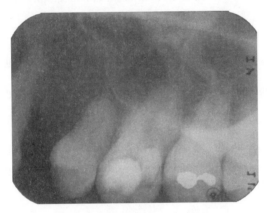

Figure 5.23

46. What positioning fault is demonstrated in this digitally captured periapical image? (Figure 5.24)

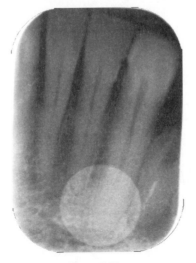

Figure 5.24

Occlusal radiography

1. Is an occlusal radiograph an intra-oral or extra-oral radiographic technique?

2. Are image receptor holders required for occlusal radiography?

3. Which one of the following occlusal projections is no longer routinely used in dental radiography?
   - Upper standard occlusal
   - Upper oblique occlusal
   - Vertex occlusal
   - Lower 90° occlusal
   - Lower 45° occlusal
   - Lower oblique occlusal

4. What is the receptor size generally used for occlusal radiography in adult patients?

5. What anatomy should the upper standard occlusal radiograph demonstrate?

6. What are the main clinical indications for an upper standard occlusal radiograph?

7. How should you prepare and position the patient for an upper occlusal radiograph?

8. In an upper occlusal radiograph, which side of radiographic film is placed facing uppermost in the patients mouth?

9. You are taking an occlusal radiograph in an adult patient. How should you normally position the long axis of the image receptor in the mouth?

10. You are taking an occlusal radiograph in a child patient. How should you normally position the long axis of the image receptor in the mouth?

11. How is the image receptor held in position?

12. In an upper occlusal radiograph where is the X-ray tubehead positioned with respect to the patient?

13. What is the required angle between the X-ray tubehead and the image receptor?

14. What are the main clinical indications for an upper oblique occlusal radiograph?

15. How should you prepare and position the patient for an upper oblique occlusal radiograph?

16. What are the differences in the image receptor positioning between an upper standard occlusal and an upper oblique occlusal radiograph?

17. In an upper oblique occlusal radiograph, where is the X-ray tubehead positioned with respect to the patient?

18. What is the required angle between the X-ray tubehead and the image receptor?

19. Should the patient wear a thyroid collar during an upper occlusal radiographic procedure?

20. Should the patient wear a thyroid collar during a lower occlusal radiographic procedure?

21. What is another name for the lower 90° occlusal radiograph?

22. What anatomy does the lower 90° occlusal radiograph demonstrate?

23. What are the main clinical indications for a lower 90° occlusal radiograph?

24. In a lower 90° occlusal radiograph, which side of the radiographic film is placed facing uppermost in the patient's mouth?

25. How should you position the patient's head for a lower 90° occlusal radiograph?

26. In a lower 90° occlusal radiograph where is the X-ray tubehead positioned with respect to the patient?

27. What is the required angle between the X-ray tubehead and the image receptor?

28. Can a lower 90° occlusal radiograph be performed on one side of the mandible only?

29. What is another name for the lower 45° occlusal radiograph?

30. What anatomy does the lower 45° occlusal radiograph demonstrate?

31. What are the main clinical indications for a lower 45° occlusal radiograph?

32. In a lower 45° occlusal radiograph, which side of the radiographic film is placed facing uppermost in the patient's mouth?

33. How should you position the patient's head for a lower 45° occlusal radiograph?

34. In a lower 45° occlusal radiograph, where is the X-ray tubehead positioned with respect to the patient?

35. What is the required angle between the X-ray tubehead and the image receptor?

36. What anatomy does the lower oblique occlusal radiograph demonstrate?

37. What are the main clinical indications for a lower oblique occlusal radiograph?

38. In a lower oblique occlusal radiograph, which side of the radiographic film is placed facing uppermost in the patient's mouth?

39. You are taking an oblique occlusal radiograph in an adult patient. How would you normally position the long axis of the image receptor in the mouth?

40. How should you position the patient's head for a lower oblique occlusal radiograph?

41. In a lower oblique occlusal radiograph, where is the X-ray tubehead positioned with respect to the patient?

42. What is the required angle between the X-ray tubehead and the image receptor?

43. Which of the occlusal radiographic techniques may not be achievable in a patient with poor mobility of the neck?

44. Which occlusal technique is being performed in the image? (Figure 5.25)

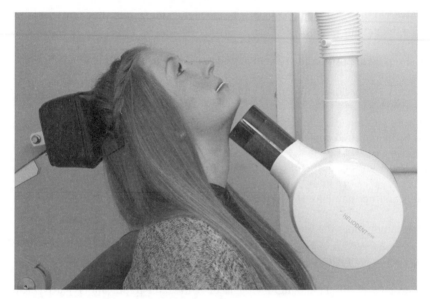

Figure 5.25

45. Which film-captured occlusal radiograph is shown in Figure 5.26?

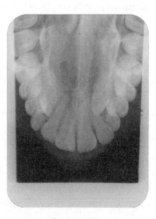

Figure 5.26

Panoramic radiography (PR)

1. Is a dental panoramic radiograph an intra-oral or extra-oral radiographic technique?

2. What aspect of the dentition is shown on a panoramic radiograph?

3. According to the UK Dental radiography Selection Criteria Guidelines (2013), what are the main clinical indications for a dental panoramic radiograph?

4. Should a panoramic radiograph be used as a 'screening' tool for new patients?

5. The panoramic radiograph is also known under several other names and abbreviated terms. How many can you name?

6. Define **tomography**.

7. Define **tomograph**.

8. Define **tomogram**.

9. Which type of tomography is used to create the dental panoramic radiograph?

10. Define **focal trough** with respect to dental panoramic radiography.

11. What are the anatomical features to consider with respect to the focal trough in dental panoramic tomography? How is the tomographic equipment designed to produce a satisfactory representation of the patient's jaws?

12. What determines the vertical height of the focal trough?

13. If a panoramic exposure is terminated halfway through, will the entire image receptor have been exposed to X-rays?

14. Is X-ray production, in modern equipment, continuous or intermittent in an uninterrupted dental panoramic cycle?

15. Name the main components of a dental panoramic unit.

16. What features can an operator adjust on a dental panoramic control panel?

17. Does the X-ray beam of a dental panoramic unit angle upwards or downwards?

18. What angle is the X-ray beam with respect to the horizontal?

19. What is the approximate exposure time of a panoramic radiograph for an adult patient?

20. What is the approximate exposure time of a panoramic radiograph for a child patient?

21. What is the normal range of tube potential for panoramic radiography equipment?

22. What types of image receptor can be used in modern dental panoramic equipment?

23. What should the patient be asked to remove prior to a dental panoramic radiograph?

24. Do rings and bracelets need to be removed?

25. What information should the operator give to the patient prior to a panoramic radiographic exposure?

26. How should the operator position the patient for a dental panoramic radiograph?

27. Why is it so important to position the patient's head accurately in the dental panoramic unit?

28. What advice should the patient be given with respect to their tongue position and why?

29. Should the patient's lips be open or closed during a panoramic radiographic exposure?

30. Should every patient wear a lead apron during a panoramic radiographic exposure?

31. Should every patient wear a thyroid collar during a dental panoramic exposure?

32. What do you understand by the term **ghost shadow** with respect to dental panoramic tomography?

33. If a ghost shadow is cast from a left earring that has not been removed, which side of the image will the ghost shadow be seen?

34. Is a ghost shadow magnified or minified with respect to the real object?

35. Is a ghost shadow positioned higher or lower with respect to the real object?

36. Is the ghost shadow more defined or blurred than the real object?

37. Name some anatomical bony structures that cause ghost shadows on a panoramic radiograph?

38. List some limitations of a dental panoramic image.

39. By what method is the panoramic image anatomically orientated?

40. Which is higher resolution, dental panoramic radiographs or intra-oral radiographs?

41. What is the most common fault seen on a dental panoramic radiograph?

42. It is the operator's responsibility to position a patient correctly in the panoramic unit during the radiographic exposure. What failings may lead to poor image quality?

43. At what stage should the operator watch the patient during the X-ray exposure?

44. Describe the panoramic X-ray fault if the patient is positioned too close to the image receptor?

45. Describe the panoramic X-ray fault if the patient is positioned too far from the image receptor?

46. What will be the effect on the panoramic image if the patient is asymmetrically positioned with the head turned to either the left or right?

47. What will be the effect on the panoramic image if the patient's chin is positioned too low?

48. What will be the effect on the panoramic image if the patient's chin is positioned too high?

49. Describe the positioning error shown in Figure 5.27. What effect will this error have on the resultant image?

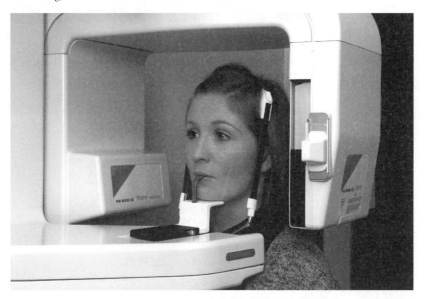

Figure 5.27

50. Describe the positioning error shown in Figure 5.28. What effect will this error have on the resultant image?

51. List the faults demonstrated on this film-captured panoramic radiograph? (Figure 5.29)

52. List the positioning fault demonstrated on this film-captured panoramic radiograph? (Figure 5.30)

53. List the fault demonstrated on this digitally captured panoramic radiograph. (Figure 5.31)

54. You have been asked by the dentist to perform a panoramic radiograph on a young adult patient for left and right wisdom tooth assessment. The lower wisdom teeth are in a position that means periapical radiographs are inappropriate. What can you do to optimise the dose without compromising the diagnostic quality that the clinician requires?

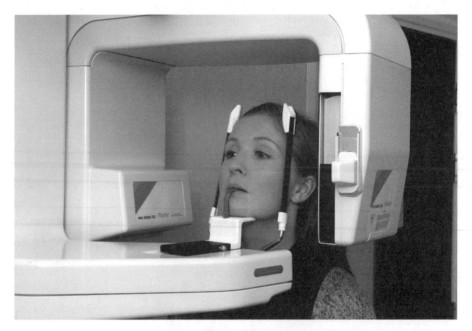

Figure 5.28

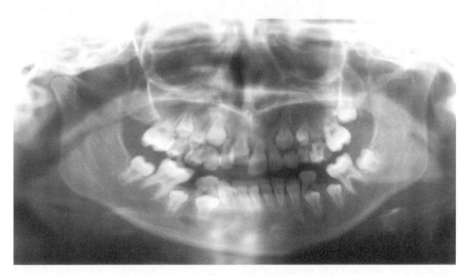

Figure 5.29

55. You have been asked by the dentist to perform a panoramic radiograph on an elderly male patient who suffers with involuntary muscle movements of the head and neck. The indication is for review of an apicectomy of the upper left central incisor tooth. Should you perform this procedure?

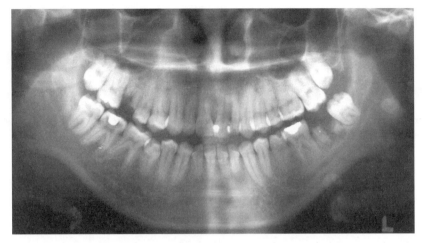

Figure 5.30

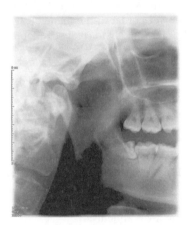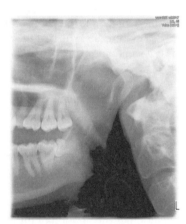

Figure 5.31

Oblique lateral radiography

1. Is an oblique lateral radiograph an intra-oral or extra-oral radiographic technique?

2. What aspect of the dentition is shown on an oblique lateral radiograph?

3. What are the main clinical indications for an oblique lateral radiograph?

4. Which has a faster exposure time, an oblique lateral radiograph or a dental panoramic radiograph?

5. In a true lateral radiograph, is the image receptor and sagittal plane of the patient's head parallel or perpendicular to one another?

6. In a true lateral radiograph, is the image receptor and X-ray beam parallel or perpendicular to one another?

7. How does an oblique lateral radiograph differ from a true lateral radiograph?

8. What equipment is needed to perform an oblique lateral radiograph?

9. There are various oblique lateral projections of the jaws. Describe how the cassette is generally positioned with respect to the patient.

10. Describe how the patient is positioned during an oblique lateral radiograph.

11. What is the **radiographic keyhole**?

12. Is the X-ray tubehead positioned on the same or opposite side of the patient's head to the cassette?

13. During an oblique lateral radiographic procedure, the X-ray beam can be either passed through the radiographic keyhole or beneath the lower border of the mandible, depending on the area of interest. Which of the two methods is most likely to create overlapping of the dental contact points?

14. Which of the two methods described in question 13 will create some distortion of the teeth in the vertical plane? Explain your answer.

15. Which of the two methods described in question 13 will create the shadow of the mandibular body on the maxillary teeth?

16. Which of the two methods described in question 13 is designed to assess the posterior maxillary and mandibular teeth?

17. What determines the position of the cassette and the X-ray tubehead?

18. What information should the operator know prior to performing an appropriate oblique lateral radiograph?

19. How can you, as the operator, stabilise a young patient in the chair for an oblique lateral radiograph?

20. What is the suggested area of interest in this oblique lateral technique? (Figure 5.32)

Cephalometric radiography

1. Is a lateral cephalometric radiograph an intra-oral or extra-oral radiographic technique?

2. What anatomy is shown on a lateral cephalometric radiograph?

3. Which dental specialist commonly requests a cephalometric radiograph?

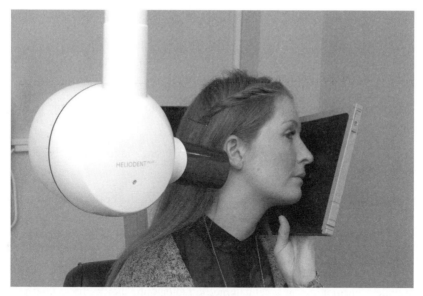

Figure 5.32

4. What are the main clinical indications for a lateral cephalometric radiograph?

5. Which selection criteria guidelines assist the clinician in the justification process for lateral cephalometric radiography?

6. What is the important difference between a lateral cephalometric radiograph and a lateral skull radiograph?

7. What equipment is required to produce a cephalometric radiograph in a film/intensifying screen-based system?

8. Can film/intensifying screens be replaced with photostimulable phosphor plates?

9. Is the equipment used to obtain the cephalometric radiograph considered a stand-alone unit?

10. Which apparatus stabilises the patient's head during a cephalometric radiographic procedure?

11. What is the function of an anti-scatter grid?

12. What is the function of an aluminium wedge filter?

13. What shape is the X-ray beam ideally collimated to in order to image the areas of interest but avoid irradiating the skull vault and cervical spine?

14. Cephalometric equipment that uses solid-state sensors does not commonly use aluminium wedge filters. How is the soft tissue profile viewed?

15. At what general distance is the X-ray-generating equipment placed from the cephalostat and image receptor?

16. In a lateral cephalometric projection, is the image receptor and sagittal plane of the patient's head parallel or perpendicular to one another?

17. In a lateral cephalometric projection, is the X-ray beam and sagittal plane of the patient's head parallel or perpendicular to one another?

18. In a lateral cephalometric projection, are the X-ray beam and the image receptor parallel or perpendicular to one another?

19. In the patient positioning for a cephalometric radiograph, the **Frankfort plane** needs to be considered. What anatomical boundaries define the Frankfort plane?

20. In the patient positioning for a cephalometric radiograph, should the Frankfort plane be parallel or perpendicular to the floor?

21. In the patient positioning for a cephalometric radiograph, should the sagittal plane of the patient's head be parallel or perpendicular to the floor?

22. In the patient positioning for a cephalometric radiograph, where exactly are the ear rods placed?

23. If the patient has been correctly positioned, through which point should the X-ray beam be centred?

24. How can accurate measurements of the patient's skeletal pattern, incisor inclinations and relationships of the jaws to the cranial base be made?

25. Which transverse plane through the skull represents the line joining orbitale and porion?

26. In cephalometric radiography, what should be the position of the teeth relative to one another?

SECTION VIII Questions: Radiological interpretation

LEARNING OUTCOMES

At the end of this section, you should be able to identify any gaps in your personal knowledge associated with the following:
- Optimal viewing conditions of radiographs
- Basic radiographic anatomy of the dentition and supporting structures
- Basic introduction into radiographic interpretation to include dental caries, periapical and periodontal disease
- Localisation of teeth by understanding the principle of parallax

Dental terminology

1. Define **radiology**.

2. Define **dental radiology**.

3. Define **dental radiography**.

Image interpretation

1. Why are dental radiographs taken?

2. Should every radiograph taken be viewed?

3. Does a radiographic image require a written radiographic report?

4. Why is it essential to review the entire radiographic image rather than just the area of interest?

5. Who is responsible for the radiographic report?

6. What role does a dental nurse acting as radiographic operator have in assessing the radio-graphic image?

7. What are the essential requirements for interpretation of dental radiographs?

8. You critically assess an image you have taken and are unsure as to whether it provides enough information for the dentist. What should you do?

Optimal viewing conditions

1. List the ideal viewing conditions for conventional processed radiographic film.

2. How can light surrounding the film on a viewing box be limited?

3. How can fine detail interpretation on the radiographic image be improved?

4. Why should a radiographic viewing box be clean?

5. List the ideal viewing conditions for digital radiographs.

6. What is the main advantage of digital image interpretation over conventional radiographic film?

Radiographic anatomy of the teeth and supporting structures

1. List the hard tissue components of a tooth.

2. Which of these tissues has the highest density and, therefore, absorbs the most X-ray photons during a radiation exposure?

3. Does the term radiopaque describe white or black shadows on a radiographic image?

4. Does the term radiolucent describe white or black shadows on a radiographic image?

5. Is enamel more or less radiopaque than dentine?

6. Is pulp tissue more or less radiopaque than enamel?

7. Is pulp tissue more or less radiopaque than dentine?

8. Is cementum generally well visualised on a dental radiograph?

9. Name the supporting structures of the teeth as seen on a dental radiograph.

10. What supporting structure is positioned between the tooth root and the lamina dura? What density is this structure on the radiographic image?

11. What is the lamina dura?

12. Is the lamina dura radiopaque or radiolucent?

13. What supporting structure lies between the cortical plates in both jaws and is composed of thin radiopaque plates surrounding many small radiolucent pockets of marrow?

14. What supporting structure is at the gingival margin of the alveolar process that surrounds the teeth? What density is this healthy structure on the radiographic image?

15. What are the radiological features of the median palatine suture on a periapical or upper occlusal radiograph?

16. Where is the anterior nasal spine demonstrated on a periapical radiograph? What is its shape and density?

17. What are the radiological features of a normal incisive foramen?

18. The maxillary antral space may be visualised on an intra-oral or extra-oral radiographic image. Is a healthy antral space radiopaque or radiolucent?

19. What does a normal maxillary floor look like on a radiographic image?

20. In which jaw is the inferior dental nerve canal located?

21. What radiographs can demonstrate the inferior dental nerve canal?

22. Is the inferior dental nerve canal radiolucent or radiopaque?

23. Name the labelled anatomical landmarks on the periapical radiograph shown in Figure 5.33.

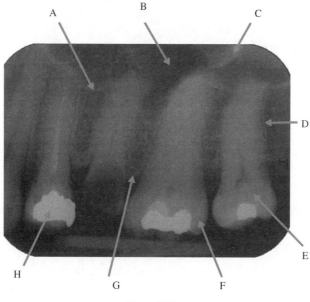

Figure 5.33

24. Name the labelled anatomical landmarks on the upper standard occlusal radiograph shown in Figure 5.34.

25. Name the labelled anatomical landmarks on the dental panoramic radiograph shown in Figure 5.35.

Dental caries

1. Are extra-oral or intra-oral radiographs optimal for caries assessment?

2. What is the radiographic technique of choice for caries assessment of a dentate child or adult in the posterior dentition?

3. What type of caries may be better demonstrated on a panoramic radiograph than a bitewing radiograph?

4. Which is generally considered higher dose, a panoramic radiograph or a set of bitewing radiographs?

5. Other than demonstrating a new carious lesion on a radiograph, what other diagnostic information may the clinician require with respect to the coronal aspects of the teeth?

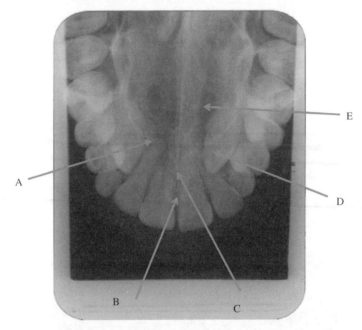

Figure 5.34

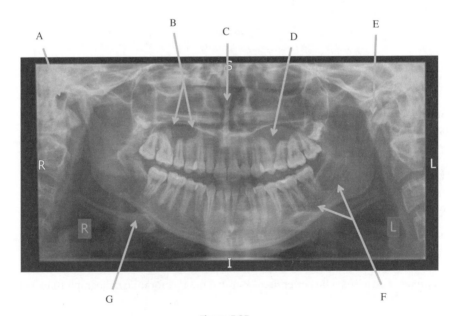

Figure 5.35

6. What is the suggested time frame between bitewing radiographs for an adult patient with a high caries risk?

7. What is the suggested time frame between bitewing radiographs for an adult patient with a moderate caries risk?

8. What is the suggested time frame between bitewing radiographs for an adult patient with a low caries risk?

9. Does dental caries appear radiolucent or radiopaque compared to the enamel and dentine.

10. Does an amalgam restoration appear radiolucent or radiopaque compared to the enamel and dentine.

11. Is a higher or lower kV better for caries assessment?

12. Approximately how much tooth tissue demineralisation is required for a carious lesion to be visible on a radiograph?

13. Does a radiograph tend to overestimate or underestimate the size of a carious lesion?

14. What technical fault during a bitewing radiograph can lead to poor diagnostic quality for the assessment of inter-proximal caries?

15. How may existing tooth restorations obscure caries in the tooth?

16. Name the artefactual radiographic shadow at the cervical region of the teeth that can mimic caries.

17. How is this artefactual radiographic shadow produced?

18. How can this artefactual radiographic shadow be distinguished from caries?

Periapical tissues and periapical disease

1. Where is the periodontal ligament space?

2. What are the radiological features of the periodontal ligament space?

3. Where is the lamina dura?

4. What are the radiological features of the lamina dura?

5. What is the other name for **trabecular bone**?

6. Where in the jaws is the trabecular bone found?

7. What is the most common radiograph used to assess the periapical tissues of the teeth?

8. What other radiographs demonstrate the roots and supporting structures of the teeth?

9. Normal radiolucent shadows may become superimposed on the apical tissues in a radiographic image; an example would be the maxillary antrum. What effect may this superimposed shadow have on the appearance of the healthy apical tissues?

10. Name a radiopaque shadow that can be superimposed over the apical tooth tissues.

11. What effect can this radiopaque superimposition have on the assessment of the periapical tissues?

12. Which dental panoramic positioning error can compromise the assessment of the periapical tissue of the maxillary teeth?

13. In dental health how would you expect the periapical tissue to appear radiologically?

14. What radiological features would you expect to see in an early acute apical periodontitis?

15. What radiological features would you expect to see in the development of a periapical abscess?

16. With long-standing chronic apical infection of a tooth, what would you expect to see radiologically?

17. In symptomatic apical pathology of the teeth, endodontic treatment or extractions are generally the first line treatment options. Which UK guidelines provide recommendations regarding imaging of the periapical tissues during endodontic treatment?

18. Which type of periapical technique should be employed during endodontic assessment and why?

19. Should a pre-operative radiograph be taken prior to starting endodontic treatment?

20. Is a radiograph required to confirm working length(s) of the root canal?

21. Should a radiograph be taken at the end of endodontic treatment?

22. Is cone beam CT considered a standard imaging technique for the assessment of teeth prior to endodontic treatment?

Periodontal tissues and periodontal disease

1. Are radiographs the primary method of diagnosis in periodontal disease?

2. What are the main indications for imaging the periodontal tissues?

3. Which UK guidelines provide recommendations regarding imaging of the periodontal tissue following a thorough clinical evaluation?

4. When do the guidelines suggest the use of horizontal bitewing radiographs for the assessment of the periodontal tissues?

5. When do the guidelines suggest the use of vertical bitewing radiographs for the assessment of the periodontal tissues?

6. What is the radiographic examination of choice to assess the periodontal tissues of the anterior teeth?

7. What radiograph is indicated if there is clinical suspicion of a perio-endo lesion?

8. Why are paralleling technique periapical radiographs favoured over the bisecting periapical technique in the assessment of the periodontal tissues?

9. What are the limitations of a dental panoramic radiograph in the assessment of the periodontal tissues?

10. When may a dental panoramic radiograph be considered to aid in the assessment of the periodontal tissues?

11. Is cone beam CT considered a standard technique for the assessment of periodontal bone support?

12. In film-based techniques to assess for caries, the film should be well exposed to show good contrast between enamel and caries. In the assessment of periodontal bone levels, should the film be overexposed or underexposed? Discuss your answer.

13. What are the radiological features of healthy periodontium?

14. Is bone loss seen on a radiograph a sign of active periodontal disease?

15. What types of periodontal bone loss pattern can be described from a radiographic image?

16. List four radiological features of chronic periodontitis.

17. List four secondary local factors that can be seen radiologically that can complicate and predispose to periodontal disease.

18. Which teeth are classically involved in aggressive juvenile periodontitis?

19. In advanced periodontal bone loss, what radiological features may be seen?

20. List three limitations of radiographic assessment of the periodontal tissues.

Localisation of un-erupted teeth

1. Which tooth in the dentition is most likely to require localisation due to un-eruption and ectopic position?

2. What reasons may a tooth fail to erupt?

3. What is **parallax**?

4. How is parallax used in dental radiography to localise an un-erupted canine?

5. Describe the **SLOB** rule.

6. If an un-erupted canine tooth lies within the dental arch which way will the tooth move with respect to the tubehead when applying parallax?

7. Parallax can be either performed in the horizontal or vertical plane. Give an example of two radiographic projections that may be used to localise an upper ectopic canine tooth in the horizontal plane.

8. Give an example of two radiographic projections that may be used to localise an upper ectopic canine tooth in the vertical plane.

9. What 3D form of imaging is now more widely used in the localisation of canine teeth that are closely approximated to the incisor teeth?

SECTION I Answers: Radiation physics

Atomic structure

1. An **atom** is a particle of matter, which is the smallest component of an element. It consists of a dense central nucleus made up of nuclear particles called protons and neutrons. Clouds of electrons in specific orbits or shells surround the nucleus. The particles are held together by electric and nuclear forces.

2. **Protons** have a positive (+ve) charge, **neutrons** have no charge and **electrons** have a negative (−ve) charge.

3. K and L shells.

4. 2 (K) and 8 (L).

5. **Atomic number** (Z) is the number of protons in the nucleus of the atom. (Z = no of protons). Z defines the element and determines its chemical properties and behaviour.

6. **Atomic mass number** (A) is the total number of protons and neutrons within the nucleus of the atom (A = no. of protons + no. of neutrons).

7. **Isotopes** are atoms with the same atomic number but with a different atomic mass number as a result of different number of neutrons.

8. A **radioisotope** is an isotope that is radioactive. Radioisotopes emit radiation during their decay to a stable form and have uses in medical diagnosis and treatment.

9. **Neutrons** and **protons** have almost the same mass (neutrons are slightly heavier), both are found in the nucleus of the atom. They both contribute to the atomic mass number (A) of the atom.

10. Electrons have a negative charge, whereas protons have a positive charge. Electrons are much smaller than protons, they are 1/1840 the mass of a proton. Protons reside in the nucleus of an atom, whereas electrons orbit the nucleus.

11. A **neutral atom** occurs when the number of orbiting electrons is equal to the number of protons in the nucleus. The atom is electrically neutral as the number of positive charges balances out the number of negative charges.

12. An **ion** is an atom or molecule in which the number of electrons does not equal the number of protons, resulting in an atom with a net positive or negative electrical charge.

13. Ionisation.

14. Excitation.

15. **Electron binding energy** is a measure of the energy required to remove electrons from their orbiting shells. The binding energy is higher the closer the shell is to the nucleus of the atom. This is because the attraction forces are stronger.

Properties of X-rays

1. Wilhelm Conrad Roentgen discovered X-rays by chance in 1895. He was awarded the Nobel Prize in Physics in 1901 for this ground-breaking discovery.

2. Roentgen called them X-rays after the mathematical symbol **X** for unknown.

3. Otto Walkoff. He is reported to have placed small glass photographic plates, wrapped in rubber dam, in his own mouth and exposed them for 25 minutes.

4. An **X-ray** is a type of electromagnetic radiation and forms part of the electromagnetic spectrum. An X-ray beam is made up of wave packets of energy, which are called **photons**. X-rays are very high-frequency waves and carry a lot of energy.

5. The electromagnetic spectrum.

6. The ionising components of the electromagnetic spectrum include the following:
   - Gamma radiation
   - **X-rays**
   - Ultraviolet radiation (higher frequency ultraviolet radiation begin to have enough energy to break chemical bonds)

   The non-ionising components of the electromagnetic spectrum include the following:

- Ultraviolet radiation
- Visible light
- Infrared radiation
- Microwaves
- Radio waves

The spectrum ranges from high-energy (short wavelength) gamma and X-rays to low-energy (long wavelength) radio waves.

7. The main difference between **ionising** and **non-ionising** radiation is in the amount of energy that the radiation carries. Ionising radiation carries more energy than non-ionising radiation. The ionising form of radiation has the power to create charged ions by displacing electrons in atoms. Non-ionising radiation, on the other hand, has the capacity to change the position of atoms but not to alter their structure, composition and properties. Ionising radiation includes X-rays, gamma rays, radiation from radioactive sources and sources of naturally occurring radiation, such as radon gas. Non-ionising radiation includes visible light, infrared radiation and electromagnetic fields.

8. The main properties of X-rays are as follows:
   - X-rays are wave packets of energy called photons. The X-ray beam used in diagnostic radiography comprises millions of photons of varying energies.
   - They have a short wavelength.
   - They are invisible and cannot be detected by human senses.
   - They have no mass or weight or charge.
   - X-rays travel at the speed of light in a vacuum.
   - They travel in a straight line.
   - X-rays obey the inverse square law.
   - They cannot be reflected by a mirror or fluids or deviated by a magnet.
   - They have penetrating power and are attenuated (absorbed or scattered) by matter.
   - X-rays cause ionisation of matter, hence the term ionising radiation.
   - They can cause chemical and biological damage to living tissue.
   - They can cause certain substances to fluoresce and emit light.
   - X-rays cause chemical changes to occur on radiographic and photographic films.

9. No.

10. **Diagnostic**: The detection, for example, of a bony injury or caries in a tooth.
    Therapeutic: The treatment of cancers.

11. Ionising radiation sources are used in the following industries:
    - Nuclear power
    - Manufacturing
    - Construction
    - Engineering
    - Oil and gas production
    - Medical and dental sectors
    - Education and research organisations

12. Ionising radiation is attenuated by distance, it obeys the **inverse square law: intensity is proportional to $1/d^2$**

This means that the intensity of the X-ray beam is reduced by a quarter when the distance from the X-ray source is doubled. This is, therefore, an important concept in radiation protection.

Dental X-ray generating equipment

X-ray tubehead

1. A tubehead, positioning arms and a control panel.

2. The main components of the X-ray tubehead are as follows:
   - Evacuated glass X-ray tube
   - Step-up transformer
   - Step-down transformer
   - Surrounding lead casing
   - Oil bath
   - Aluminium filtration
   - Collimator
   - Spacer cone/beam indicating device

3. The **step-up transformer** increases the mains voltage of 240 V to the high kilovoltage, of 60–90 kV, required across the glass X-ray tube.

4. The **step-down transformer** adjusts the 240 mains voltage down to the low current (7–10 V) needed to heat the cathode filament.

5. The outer **lead casing** prevents X-ray leakage from the tubehead. Lead is an important material used in radiation protection because of its high molecular density.

6. Yes, the equipment must not be used until it has been checked and repaired as required, as there is potential for radiation leakage.

7. Oil. Both copper and oil are thermo conductors and therefore facilitate the removal of the heat created during X-ray production.

8. The **aluminium filter** is a device to remove or filter out low-energy X-rays, so they are not part of the X-ray beam. Low-energy soft X-rays (less than 30 keV) contribute little to the radiographic image as they are so heavily absorbed by the patient's soft tissues, and thus would result in an increased patient dose.

9. Rectangular, the same shape and size as an intra-oral image receptor.

10. No, the collimator shapes the X-ray beam.

11. 200 mm.

X-ray tube

1. Figure 5.36
   A diagrammatic representation of the basic components of the X-ray tube (Figure 5.36).

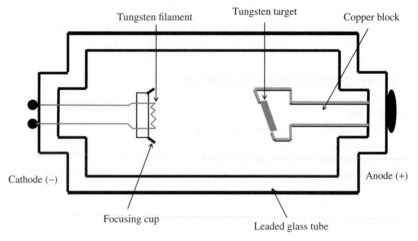

Figure 5.36

2. Tungsten.

3. The tungsten target is embedded in a copper block. Both copper and the oil surrounding the tube are good thermo conductors and aid in the removal of heat following X-ray production.

4. Tungsten (chemical symbol W) is a robust, hard metal and has the highest melting point of all the elements (3370 °C). It can therefore keep its shape at high temperatures. It has a high atomic number of 74, is strong, malleable and ductile and can be pulled into wire to make the filament for the cathode.

5. No.

6. The **leaded glass housing** creates a vacuum within the tube. The lead casing absorbs unwanted X-rays from escaping as the X-rays are emitted in all directions at the focal spot.

7. The basic function of the **cathode** is to create and expel the electrons from the electrical circuit and focus them in a well-defined beam aimed towards the anode. In a process known as thermionic emission, heat is used to drive the electrons from the cathode.

8. The **focusing cup** aims the stream of electrons towards the focal spot on the anode target.

9. The **anode** has two primary functions: firstly to convert electronic energy into X-rays and secondly to remove the heat created in the process of X-ray production.

10. Kilovoltage (kV).

11. The kilovoltage (kV) determines the amount of energy carried by each electron. For each kilovoltage, each electron has 1 keV of energy. By altering the kilovoltage, the operator actually assigns a specific amount of energy to each electron.

12. Milliamperage (mA).

Production of X-rays

1. **Kilovoltage (kV)** is the voltage applied across the tube. **Milliamperage (mA)** is the electrical current that flows through the tube. **Time (s)** is the duration of the exposure time.

2. Heating of the tungsten filament.

3. The high voltage (kV).

4. The focusing cup at the cathode.

5. Heat-producing collisions.

6. Approximately 99% heat production and 1% X-ray production.

7. Bremsstrahlung or braking radiation.
   The incoming electron penetrates and passes between the outer electron shells and approaches the tungsten atom nucleus whereby it is slowed down (hence the term braking radiation) and deflected by the nucleus resulting in a loss of energy in the form of X-rays. The degree of electron deflection and the extent of braking determine the amount of energy that the electron loses and, therefore, correlates with the energy of the X-ray photon produced. In this method of X-ray production, a wide range of photon energies is therefore possible.

8. Low-energy photons predominate in the continuous X-ray spectrum, as small deflections of the electrons are more common.

9. The potential difference (kV) across the X-ray tube.

10. Characteristic radiation.
    The incoming electron displaces an inner shell electron from the tungsten atom causing either excitation or ionisation of the atom. The orbiting electrons reposition themselves to form a ground state atom by jumping from one energy level to another with the resultant creation of an X-ray photon with a specific (characteristic) energy. The photons emitted are characteristic for the tungsten atom.

11. 69.5 keV.

12. Yes, the 85 kV exceeds the critical voltage of 69.5 kV.

13. No.

14. The continuous spectrum.

15. **The combined spectrum** is the total spectrum of the useful X-ray beam by combining the continuous and characteristic spectra in dental X-ray equipment using 69.5 kV and above.

16. The **quality** describes the average energy of the X-ray photons, which determines the penetrating power of the X-ray beam. Low-energy photons have little penetration power and as such may have an effect on patient dose but not on the diagnostic quality of the image.

17. The kilovoltage (kV).

18. The **intensity** is the total energy contained in the X-ray beam (product of the quality and quantity of X-ray photons) per unit area per unit time.

19. Decreases contrast resulting in a longer grey scale.

20. Decreases dose.

21. Darkening of the image.

22. Increases dose.

23. Darkening of the image.

24. Increases dose.

25. Approximately 240 V.

26. The mains supply is altered in two ways:
    - The step-down transformer in the X-ray tubehead reduces the voltage to allow a low-current voltage (7–10 V) to heat the tungsten filament for electron production.
    - The step-up transformer in the X-ray tubehead increases the voltage to generate a high potential difference (60–90 kV) to accelerate the electrons across the X-ray tube vacuum.

27. The positive half of the cycle. This allows the electrons to be drawn towards the target. To eliminate the negative half of the cycle, a process termed rectification is used. This converts the alternating current to a direct positive current using a diode that allows current to flow in only one direction.

28. DC units. They keep the kilovoltage at peak/optimum output throughout any exposure ensuring X-ray production is more efficient. There are more high-energy and less low-energy photons produced per exposure, and shorter exposure times can be used when compared to AC equipment.

The control panel and circuitry

1. The main components are as follows:
   - The mains on/off switch
   - Exposure button
   - Warning light and audible sound when X-rays are being generated
   - Timer (electronic or impulse)
   - Exposure time selector

   Control panels may also have the following:
   - Film speed selector
   - Patient size selector
   - Kilovoltage selector
   - Milliamperage switch

- Exposure adjustment for long or short focus to skin distance

2. The milliamperage (mA).

3. The exposure time can be numerical, the time is selected in seconds or anatomical whereby the area of the dentition to be imaged can be selected and an automatic time adjustment is made.

4. No.

5. Yes, but only under direct supervision of the trained operator.

6. The operator should act quickly to turn the equipment off at the mains. The mains switch should be positioned outside of the controlled area. As the X-ray set has displayed a fault, it must be re-examined prior to further clinical use. The operator should inform the RPS or employer of the incident, and also the patient. The Health and Safety Executive needs to be notified when an employer suspects or has been informed that a person, while undergoing a medical exposure, was exposed to ionising radiation at least 20 times the intended dose.

Interactions of X-rays with matter

1. X-ray photons on interacting with patient tissues may be
   - Transmitted unchanged
   - Absorbed with total loss of energy
   - Scattered with no loss of energy
   - Scattered with some absorption and some loss of energy

2. **Attenuation** is the reduction in intensity of an X-ray beam as it passes through an object due to the absorption and scattering of photons.

3. **Scatter** is a physical process whereby the X-ray photons are forced to deviate with or without loss of energy.

4. **Absorption** is the transfer of energy from the X-ray photon to the absorbing material.

5. The **photoelectric effect** and the **Compton effect**.

6. Photoelectric effect.

7. Compton effect.

8. Compton effect.

9. Photoelectric effect.

10. Photoelectric effect.

11. Compton effect.

12. Compton effect.

13. Yes, as the density (atomic number) of matter increases so does the number of inner shell electrons on the atoms and as a result the probability of the photoelectric effect occurring increases.

14. Lead has a high atomic number of 82 and, therefore, is a good absorber of X-rays through the photoelectric effect.

15. Both the photoelectric and Compton effects.

16. Photoelectric effect.

SECTION II Answers: Radiation dose and the biological risks associated with X-rays

Dosimetry

1. Radiation-absorbed dose (D) is the concentration of energy deposited in tissue as a result of an exposure to ionising radiation. In this case, it means the energy absorbed by human tissue.

2. Gray, the subunits of which are termed the milligray (mGy) or microgray (μGy).

3. Equivalent dose (H_T) is an amount that takes the damaging properties of different types of radiation into account. Not all radiation is alike. Equivalent dose addresses the impact that the type of radiation has on tissue. As all radiation used in diagnostic medicine has the same low-harm potential (radiation-weighting factor of 1), the absorbed dose and the equivalent dose are numerically the same. Only the units are different.

$$\text{Equivalent dose } (H_T) = \text{Radiation-absorbed dose } (D)$$
$$\times \text{Radiation weighting factor } (W_R) \text{ in a particular tissue}$$

4. Sievert, the subunits of which are termed the millisievert (mSv) and microsievert (μSv).

5. Effective dose (E) is a calculated value that takes three factors into account:
- The absorbed dose to all organs of the body
- The relative harm level of the radiation
- The sensitivities of each organ to radiation

Some parts of the body are more sensitive to radiation than others, and the effective dose allows investigations of different parts of the body to be compared by changing all doses to an equivalent whole body dose. The International Commission of Radiation Protection (ICRP) has allocated each tissue a numerical value termed the **tissue-weighting factor** (W_T). The more radiosensitive a tissue is, the higher the tissue-weighting factor.

$$\text{Effective dose } (E) = \sum \text{Equivalent dose } (H_T) \text{ in each tissue}$$
$$\times \text{relevant tissue-weighting factor } (W_T)$$

6. Sievert, the subunits of which are termed the millisievert (mSv) and microsievert (µSv).

7. **Collective dose** is the sum of the individual doses received in a given time period by a specified population from exposure to a specified source of radiation. The collective dose is measured in man-sieverts (man-Sv)

$$\text{Collective dose} = \text{Effective dose }(E) \times \text{population}$$

8. The effective dose.

Sources of radiation

1. **Radiation** is the energy that comes from a source and travels through space or through material. It can be ionising or non-ionising.

2. **Background radiation** is the ionising radiation that humans are exposed to from the environment. Background radiation includes radiation from natural and artificial sources.

3. Everyone is exposed to some form of radiation from the environment in which we live. These natural sources include the following:
   • **Radon** – a naturally occurring radioactive gas.
   • **Cosmic rays** – are a source of radiation that reaches the Earth from space.
   • **The earth** – rocks and soils contain various radioactive materials present since the earth was formed.
   • **Living things** – plants absorb radioactive materials from the soil that pass up the food chain. Examples of foods include bananas, nuts and potatoes.

4. Human activity has added to background radiation by creating and using artificial sources of radiation. These include radioactive waste from nuclear power stations, radioactive fallout from nuclear weapons testing and medical X-rays.

5. Approximately 2.7 mSv per annum.

6. Approximately 84% background radiation versus approximately 16% artificial radiation.

7. Medical and dental diagnostic radiation.

Biological effects of ionising radiation

1. **Tissue reactions (deterministic effects)** are the damaging effects to the body that will definitely result from a specific large dose of radiation. A threshold dose exists, and the severity of the biological effect is proportional to the dose.

2. It is now understood that some biological effects of radiation do not occur at the time of irradiation but can arise a period of time after the exposure. As a result, the ICRP has subdivided the tissue reactions into early and late tissue reactions. Early tissue reactions are seen shortly

after irradiation, and examples would include skin redness or oral mucositis. Late tissue reactions can occur possibly years after exposure, an example would be osteoradionecrosis of the mandible following tooth extraction.

3. The **stochastic** effect is a random chance effect, and it is suggested that there is no threshold dose. As such any exposure to ionising radiation carries a chance of a stochastic effect occurring. The size of the exposure to ionising radiation does not affect the severity of the damage induced, but only affect the probability of it occurring. An example would be a cancer such as leukaemia.

4. Cancer induction.

5. The **heritable (genetic)** effect is a random chance effect, and it is suggested that there is no threshold dose. Radiation to the reproductive organs carries a risk of damage to the DNA of the sperm or egg cells. This could produce a congenital abnormality in the child of the person irradiated. Dental radiography procedures should not be irradiating the reproductive organs.

6. Stochastic effects, namely, cancer induction. This is a chance effect of damage and may occur at low radiation doses such as those produced in dental radiography. The International Commission on Radiological Protection suggest a 1:20,000 risk of a fatal malignancy developing for every 1 mSv of effective dose.

7. Skin erythema, oral soreness, ulcers, dry mouth and a higher risk of tooth decay.

8. No. Doses in dental radiography are very small and should not reach a threshold dose in which a tissue reaction would result.

9. Conceivably yes, there is no known safe dose.

X-ray damage and risk in dental radiography

1. Direct and indirect damage.

2. **Direct damage** – An X-ray photon or an ejected high-energy electron directly hits the chromosomal RNA or DNA in the nucleus of a cell and breaks the bonds between the nucleic acids. Damage may be temporary with subsequent repair but could lead to cell death, abnormal replication or failure of the cell to pass on information.
   Indirect damage – When a cell is exposed to ionising radiation, the radiation can interact with the water in a cell (about 75% of each cell consists of water). This is a process of ionisation of water molecules that results in the production of ions and free radicals that can recombine to damage DNA. These free radicals can recombine to form hydrogen peroxide (H_2O_2) and hydroperoxyl radicals that are both toxic to a cell and cause biological damage. Again damage may be temporary with subsequent repair but could lead to cell death, abnormal replication or failure of the cell to pass on information.

3. Factors include the following:
   • The number and type of damaged nucleic acid bonds.
   • The type of radiation and the intensity of the exposure.

- The time span between exposures.
- The ability of the cell to repair.
- The stage of the cells maturity when exposed to radiation.

4. Yes risk is age dependent. When given equal radiation doses, the risks for children and adolescents are greater than for adults. Children grow quickly and their cells are more sensitive to radiation. Since effects of radiation take years to develop, their youth extends the time for any potential effects from ionising radiation to occur.

5. Approximately 1 in 1,000,000.

6. Approximately 1 in 10,000,000.

7. The former, 70 kV, circular collimation and D speed film.

8. About 1–5 days of background radiation equates to the effective dose of a dental panoramic radiograph.

9. Yes, it can be a reassuring tool when a patient is concerned about the risks from a medical exposure. For example, if they understand that the dose from a dental panoramic radiograph is approximately equivalent to the dose of radiation they receive naturally over a 1–5 days period in the United Kingdom, then it puts the level of dose into context.

Annual dose limits and dose monitoring

1. Radiation **dose limits** are legal limits, and to exceed them is to commit an offence. They should however only be seen as representing an upper boundary and not values that are be expected to be reached. Different annual dose limit values are fixed for different groups of people. Dose limits are defined in the UK legislation and can be found in the Ionising Radiations Regulations 1999.

2. Dose limits are set to protect workers and members of the public from the effects of ionising radiation. They are set at a level that balances the risk from exposure with the benefits that the use of ionising radiation brings.

3. It is an offence under the Ionising Radiations Regulations 1999 to exceed a dose limit.

4. The Ionising Radiation Regulations (IRR 99).

5. Yes, there are different dose limits for different groups of people, which are as follows:
   - Adult employees 18 years and older
   - Trainees aged 16–18 years
   - Any other person, for example, a member of the public
   - Women of reproductive capacity and those who are pregnant or who are breast-feeding

6. There are no set dose limits for patients.

7. 1 mSv.

8. Classified and non-classified workers.

9. The whole body dose limit for any employee over the age of 18 is 20 mSv per annum. There is no separate dose limit for classified and non-classified persons. The limit is the same for both. If the individual is likely to get 3/10 or more of that limit (6 mSv per annum), then that person must be termed a classified worker. A classified worker must be 18 years or above. Under the age of 18 years, then the annual dose limit is 6 mSv.

10. The International Commission on Radiological Protection (ICRP).

11. Non-classified worker.

12. No, classified workers require both as compulsory as they can receive high levels of radiation in their work. In the non-classified group, personal monitoring is recommended if a risk assessment suggests that an individual may exceed 1 mSv of radiation per annum. In practice, this may be considered for staff taking 100 intra-oral or 50 dental panoramic radiographs per week.

13. There are four main types:
    - Film badges
    - Thermoluminescent dosemeters (TLD)
    - Optically stimulated luminescence dosimeters (OSLD)
    - Personal electronic dosimeters (PED).

14. Film badges.

15. It is in the interests of both the employee and developing foetus to inform the employer as soon as pregnancy is known. The employer needs to know this so they can perform a risk assessment and make any necessary changes to protection measures and apply the additional dose limits. It is not a legal requirement to inform the employer; however, if the employer is unaware they may not be able to take any further action.

16. The Health and Safety Executive (HSE).

SECTION III Answers: Radiation protection

Legislation

Ionising radiation regulations 1999

1. IRR 99 principally relates to the protection of workers and the public. It also addresses the equipment aspects of patient protection.

2. The Health and Safety Executive (HSE).

3. **Radiation Protection Adviser**.

4. A Radiation Protection Adviser (RPA) is an individual or body that provides advice to employers on compliance with the Ionising Radiations Regulations 1999.

5. Yes, it is mandatory. An RPA must be appointed in writing and consulted to give advice on IRR 99.

6. No. An RPA is an expert in radiation protection, usually a medical physics expert (MPE). A dental nurse can be a Radiation Protection Supervisor (RPS) within their organisation as long as they receive the relevant training.

7. An RPA advises on all aspects of radiation protection, this will include the following:
   - Controlled areas
   - Installation of equipment
   - Modification and testing of equipment
   - Risk assessment and contingency plans
   - Staff training
   - Dose assessment
   - Quality assurance programmes

8. **Radiation Protection Supervisor.**

9. Yes. Usually a dentist, hygienist or senior dental nurse is appointed as the RPS as long as they have the relevant qualifications and training.

10. Yes.

11. The employer.

12. Information that must be included is as follows:
    - The name of the Radiation Protection Supervisor (RPS) and the Radiation Protection Advisor (RPA).
    - The identification and description of the controlled area and a summary of the arrangements to restrict access.
    - Summary of working instructions.
    - Summary of contingency plans in the event of an accident.
    - The dose investigation level (a dose level of no higher than 1 mSv per annum is generally recommended for staff working in dental radiography).

    It is also recommended that the local rules include the following:
    - The name of the legally responsible person for the use of dental X-ray equipment
    - Name and contact details of the RPA
    - Arrangements of personal dosimetry
    - Arrangements for pregnant staff
    - A reminder to employees of their legal responsibilities under IRR 99

IR(ME)R 2000

1. The Ionising Radiation Medical Exposure Regulations 2000.

2. IR(ME)R 2000 principally relates to patient safety and protection.

3. The positions of responsibility are defined as follows:
   The employer
   The employer is the legal person or body corporate with overriding legal responsibility for a radiological installation. The employer is responsible for overall safety of the process and

ensuring that the staff and procedures abide by the regulations. The employer must provide a document of **written procedures** for medical exposures within the practice or organisation, and this should be kept with the **local rules** in a **radiation protection file**.

The referrer

The referrer is a registered medical or dental professional or other health professional (e.g. a hygienist) who is allowed to refer patients for a medical exposure. A referrer is responsible for supplying the practitioner with the information required to justify an appropriate radiological examination.

The practitioner

The practitioner is a registered medical or dental professional or other health professional who may take responsibility for a medical exposure. The practitioner justifies the exposure and as such must be adequately trained.

The operator

The operator is the individual who is responsible for performing any practical aspect of a medical exposure. This includes identification of the patient, positioning of the patient and film, setting exposure parameters, processing films, clinical evaluation of the radiograph and exposing test objects as part of a quality assurance programme. Due to the range of responsibilities carried out by the operator, one exposure may involve a number of different operators performing different functions. It is essential that each operator is trained in their individual roles, and that these are clearly defined by the legal person.

4. Yes.

5. No, they cannot refer a patient for a medical exposure and cannot justify the examination.

6. Well this depends on who is reading the question. In dental practice, appropriately trained and qualified dental nurses and other DCP's can act as operators. The principal dentist within a practice may be the IR(ME)R employer, practitioner and referrer and also act as the operator.

7. For an exposure to be justified, the benefit to the patient from the diagnostic information obtained should outweigh the risk of the exposure to ionising radiation. The exposure would normally be expected to provide new information to aid in diagnosis and treatment planning.

8. The IR(ME)R practitioner.

9. No, the 2013 FGDP Dental Radiography Selection Criteria Guidelines state that there is 'no possible justification for routine radiography of new patients prior to clinical examination'. A history and clinical examination is required to determine if radiographs are necessary and if so which examination is most appropriate.

10. Yes, on the whole if the radiographic procedure is not repeated, or an alternative examination performed (depending on circumstances and patient tolerance), then it would suggest that the exposure was not justified in the first place. The operator should assess why the radiograph was non-diagnostic and aim to repeat ensuring that the reasons behind the poor quality image are resolved.

11. Yes, an operator should attend an update course at least every 5 years, which covers the following:
    - Principles of radiation physics and risks of ionising radiation
    - Radiation dose and factors affecting dose with respect to dental radiography
    - Principles of radiation protection
    - Statutory requirements
    - Quality assurance

12. Yes, this may be appropriate in-house training that should take place on a regular basis.

Dose reduction in dental radiography

1. All doses should be kept **as low as reasonably practicable (ALARP)**.

2. **Justification**. Do the benefits of the radiation exposure outweigh the risks? Is the radiographic examination required to aid in diagnosis and management of the patient?

3. **Dose constraints** – The upper level of individual dose that should not be exceeded in a well-managed practice. Annual dose constraints are recommended as 1 mSv for employees directly involved with radiography (operators) and 0.3 mSv for employees not directly involved with radiography and for the general public.

4. **DRL** stands for **diagnostic reference levels**. Diagnostic reference levels are radiation dose levels for specific radiographic examinations for groups of standard-sized patients. These dose levels should not be exceeded for standard procedures when good practice regarding diagnostic and technical performance is applied.

5. The Radiation Protection Advisor (RPA) or medical physics expert.

6. Every 5 years.

Radiation protection of radiation workers and the general public

1. **General public** relates to all individuals who are not undergoing a medical exposure either as a patient or as a radiation worker. This will include people seated in the waiting area, persons passing by doorways or windows. This group may be at risk of radiation exposure if they are in line of the primary X-ray beam.

2. RPA guidance is required to protect the public, and considerations must include the following:
    - Appropriate siting of X-ray generating equipment in order that the primary beam does not penetrate into a communal space.
    - Appropriate thickness and materials of walls and windows.
    - Appropriate siting of equipment and the safe design of the controlled area.
    - Correct positioning of audible and visual warning signs.

3. Radiation dose may arise from faulty equipment such as damage to the tubehead leading to radiation leakage. It may result from poor positioning of the operator or other staff members for that matter. An example would be standing in the direct path of the X-ray beam or too close to the patient and thus receiving scattered radiation. A radiation dose may result from staying in the controlled area during an exposure while comforting the patient.

4. An operator can limit their exposure to radiation in the following ways:
   - Ensuring that adequate and update training in radiation protection is undertaken on a regular basis so that they understand the risks and how to work safely.
   - Remaining outside of the controlled area during a medical exposure.
   - Ensuring equipment is safe and well maintained and using the equipment following current guidance and good practice.
   - Abiding by the local rules.
   - Applying common sense.

5. The employer (legal person).

6. 5.

7. Not exceeding 5 years. A review should be brought forward sooner if there is new equipment, significant changes to working procedures or the introduction of new legislation.

8. It is retrospective.

9. No.

10. No limit is placed on the maximum number of radiographic exposures. IRR 1999 requires occupational exposures to be **as low as reasonably practicable (ALARP)**, and in some cases, personal dosimetry will be necessary to demonstrate what is happening. However, this is not usually necessary if the workload for each staff member is fewer than 100 intra-oral exposures per week. Below this workload, it is considered unlikely that any individual could exceed the 1 mSv annual dose limit for a member of the public. The Radiation Protection Supervisor should monitor radiographic workload levels.

11. The **controlled area** is a defined space where entry, activities, and exit are controlled to help ensure radiation protection. Warning lights or signs should be displayed. Only the patient (and if required a comforter/carer under special working agreement) should be in this designated space during a radiographic exposure. The controlled area only exists when X-rays are being generated.

12. The operator should be at least 1.5 m (preferably 2 m) from the source of ionising radiation with a 70 kV dental X-ray set. They should not be in the direct line of the X-ray beam, and they should be able to see the patient throughout the procedure.

13. Only the patient should be in this designated space during a radiographic exposure. A further person, namely, a comforter/carer, may need to stay with the patient, and in this instance they must wear appropriate lead protection to minimise their radiation dose.

14. In the case of an emergency, such as failure of termination of an exposure, the operator must be able to access the mains switch to turn it off without having to enter the controlled area.

15. The Radiation Protection Advisor (RPA).

16. No.

17. Normally, yes. It is extremely unusual for involvement in dental radiography to require a change in working practice during pregnancy. The employer is required to carry out a risk assessment to ensure that the dose to the foetus does not exceed 1 mSv during the declared term of pregnancy. Pregnant women should not hold patients during X-ray exposures.

18. No.

19. No.

20. Yes. A lead apron (with or without thyroid protection) should be provided and worn.

X-ray equipment and dose reduction to the patient

1. In direct current (DC) systems, X-ray production per unit time is more efficient. In each exposure, more high-energy photons (of diagnostic use) are produced and also shorter exposure times can be used. This method is therefore dose saving.

2. X-ray filters are used to selectively attenuate (block) low-energy X-rays from exiting the X-ray tubehead. Low-energy X-rays (less than 30 keV) contribute little to the image as they are so heavily absorbed by the patient's soft tissues, particularly the skin. This absorption would increase both patient's dose and subsequently the risk of a stochastic effect occurring.

3. Aluminium.

4. 1.5 mm.

5. 2.5 mm.

6. 200 mm.

7. A short fsd, less than the general requirement, would result in divergence of the X-ray beam with resultant magnification of the image.

8. About 60–70 kV.

9. About 60–90 kV.

10. 50 kV, low-kilovoltage X-ray sets result in higher absorption of X-rays into the patient's tissues due to the photoelectric effect, which you will recall, is a process of pure absorption. The photoelectric effect predominates with low-energy X-ray photons, and the probability of the photoelectric effect occurring is proportional to $1/kV^3$.

11. 50 kV, the lower the kV is, the more the photoelectric effect occurs. The photoelectric effect has a direct effect on contrast. Lower kV provides better contrast radiographs.

12. Rectangular, this shape just allows for coverage of the rectangular image receptor and measures maximally 40 × 50 mm. A circular collimator has a larger surface area, and the X-ray beam will extend outside the surface area of an intra-oral film or digital sensor.

13. F speed. F speed film is faster than E speed. The faster the film, the less exposure is required and the lower the radiation dose to the patient.

14. Solid-state digital sensor.

15. Paralleling technique and bisecting angle technique.

16. Paralleling technique.

17. There are many different types of holders in the market, essentially their use aids in accurate image receptor positioning and alignment of the tubehead and spacer cone in order that rectangular collimation can be used without coning off part of the image. By using a holder with fixed image receptor and X-ray tubehead position, the technique is reproducible. With an optimal reproducible technique, this limits the necessity for retakes and thus is dose optimising.

18. Phosphor materials are used in intensifying screens. Rare earth and calcium tungstate screens are examples. Film by itself can be used to detect X-rays, but it is relatively insensitive and, therefore, a lot of X-ray energy is required to produce a properly exposed X-ray film. To reduce the radiation dose to the patient, intensifying screens are used in extra-oral conventional dental radiography. When X-rays interact in the phosphor, visible or ultraviolet (UV) light is emitted. The intensifying screen acts as a radiographic transducer; it converts X-ray energy into light. It is the light given off by the screens that principally causes the film to be darkened. One X-ray photon will produce many light photons, thus the amount of radiation required to expose the film is reduced. Screen-film detectors are considered an indirect detector because the X-ray energy is first absorbed within the screen or screens, and then this pattern is conveyed to the film emulsion by the visible or UV light. This results in a two-step, indirect process.

19. The rare earth screens such as gadolinium and lanthanum are commonly used today in practice. They are reportedly five times faster than the calcium tungstate screens.

20. No, resolution is reduced.

21. Justification, does the examination need to be performed to aid in diagnosis and treatment planning? Do the net benefits of the radiation exposure outweigh the risks?

22. The following publications aid in selection criteria for dental radiography:
    - FGDP (UK) 2013, Selection Criteria for Dental Radiography, 3rd Edition. Faculty of General Dental Practice (UK) of the Royal College of Surgeons of England.
    - British Orthodontic Society 2008, Guidelines for the Use of Radiographs in Clinical Orthodontics, 3rd Edition, London.
    - Sedentex CT Guidelines – EC 2012, Guidelines on Cone Beam CT for Dental and Maxillofacial Radiology. European Commission of Radiation Protection.

23. The dentist may not have known that the lady has had a recent radiograph in the area of interest. This image may be all that is required to assess the tooth prior to extraction. You should discuss justification of this X-ray with the dentist before proceeding.

24. You should postpone the examination until the hiccups cease, the examination takes 15–18 seconds and there is a high risk that the boy will hiccup and move during the procedure, which can result in movement artefact. This will compromise image quality and possibly make the radiograph diagnostically unacceptable (grade 3).

25. Good operator technique is essential, poor radiographic positioning, for example, leads to repeat radiographs and increased dose to the patient. If you are not confident with a procedure, then you should ask for help; it is in the patient's best interests.

26. Evidence has shown that a lead apron does not reduce the dose to patients undergoing a dental X-ray exposure (neither intra-oral nor panoramic). A lead apron should, therefore, not be offered routinely to patients, even for their peace of mind, as this can perpetuate bad practice.

27. Yes. Enquiries about whether a patient is pregnant are only necessary in radiography where the primary beam is directed at the abdomen. The risk from other dental X-rays to the foetus is effectively zero. The important consideration here is justification of the radiograph. For example, a lady who is 3 months pregnant attends the practice in severe pain from a carious infected wisdom tooth that requires extraction. She has a temperature, has not eaten for 2 days and is in pain. The benefits of assessing this tooth radiologically to aid management outweigh the risks. Conversely a pregnant lady attends for a routine check-up and bitewing radiographs are due, in this case deferring the examination until after the birth is a reasonable option.

28. No, the radiation beam is not directed at the abdomen.

29. Protective aprons, having a lead equivalence of not less than 0.25 mm, should be provided for any adult who provides assistance by supporting a patient.

30. Lead aprons should be placed over a hanger and not folded as this may lead to cracking of the lead. If a lead apron cracks, radiation may pass through the apron thus compromising its radiation protection qualities. The aprons should be regularly inspected for damage.

31. No, but it is good practice to fit the patient with a thyroid collar or thyroid shield if the X-ray beam is directed at the thyroid gland, an example would be in maxillary occlusal radiography.

SECTION IV Answers: Image receptors and processing

Direct action film

1. X-ray photons.

2. The direct action films are sensitive to X-ray photons, and direct exposure of X-ray onto the film produces the invisible latent image that is subsequently processed to create the visible radiographic image.

3. Direct action film is used in the following:
   - Bitewing radiographs
   - Periapical radiographs
   - Occlusal radiographs

4. The components of the direct action intra-oral film packet are as follows:
   - The **outer plastic wrapper** is sealed and used to prevent ingress of moisture and light. There is a raised dot on the white plastic side for correct film orientation. The opposing side, which is placed opposite to the tube, is the side that opens and is dual coloured. The colours depend on film speed/manufacturer.
   - The **lead foil** is thin and embossed with a pattern. The lead foil shields the film from backscatter, which may fog the film and reduce image quality. Lead also absorbs some of the residual X-ray beam, thus preventing the photons from continuing into the patient's tissues. It is therefore dose reducing.
   - A sheet of **black paper** is positioned either side of the film, and its purpose is to protect the film from damage during opening and from the ingress of light and saliva.

5. The raised dot that is positioned one corner of the white surface of the film packet. The side of the film with the raised dot is always placed to face the X-ray beam.

6. The lead foil in the film packet has an embossed pattern. If the lead foil were positioned in front of the film with respect to the X-ray beam (the wrong way round), then this pattern would show on the resultant image and the image would be reversed. In addition, the image would be pale due to the lead absorbing some of the X-rays photons resulting in fewer X-ray photons reaching the film.

7. The radiographic film comprises four components:
   - Centrally is a **clear plastic base** that acts as a support structure for the film emulsion.
   - **Adhesive** coats both sides of the plastic base and fixes the emulsion to the plastic layer.
   - **Emulsion** is fixed to each side of the base and is composed of silver halide crystals embedded in a gelatin matrix. The halide crystals are sensitised by the X-ray photons that strike the film. During processing, the sensitised halide crystals are converted to metallic black silver to produce the visible radiographic image.
   - A **protective layer** of clear gelatin coats both sides of emulsion and acts as a protective barrier.

8. The **latent image** is an invisible image produced in a film emulsion by X-rays or visible light that can be converted into a visible image by development.

9. Silver bromide.

10. Film speed is related to the size of the silver halide crystals in the emulsion or to the thickness of the silver halide layer. X-rays are more likely to interact with a large crystal or the increased number of crystals in a thicker layer. Fast films (high speed) have larger crystals or thicker layers. Slow films have smaller crystals or thinner layers.

11. The image detail is inversely related to the speed. Faster speed film will result in poorer image quality.

12. The faster the film, the less exposure required and therefore the lower the dose to the patient.

13. The film speed will be labelled on the plastic outer film packet. Each film type has a full white coloured side; the side positioned away from the X-ray tube generally has two colours that distinguish the different film speed types. Colours may vary between brands.

14. F speed film.

15. ~20%.

16. Approximately 10 lp/mm.

17. A barrier wrap.

Indirect action film

1. Light photons.

2. Indirect action films are film/screen combinations. This type of film is sensitive to light photons that are emitted from the intensifying screens in response to X-ray photon interaction. The latent image is formed indirectly via the use of intensifying screens.

3. Indirect action film is used commonly in the dental primary care setting for the following examinations:
   - Panoramic radiographs
   - Cephalometric radiographs
   - Some practices also acquire oblique lateral radiographs
   Within the hospital setting other extra-oral images such as PA jaws, lateral skull, occipito-mental, reverse townes and submento-vertex (SMV) radiographs may be acquired by indirect action film.

4. The image receptor comprises the cassette, the film and intensifying screens. Two intensifying screens are used one in front of the film and the other at the back.

5. Indirect action films do not have a raised dot as seen in direct action film, instead they have identification such as metal letters **L** (left) or **R** (right) placed on the outside of the cassette during an exposure.

6. An **intensifying screen** is a device consisting of fluorescent material, which is placed in contact with the film in a radiographic cassette. Radiation interacts with the fluorescent phosphor, releasing light photons. These photons expose the film with greater efficiency than would the radiation alone.

7. The screen has a plastic supportive base that is covered by a reflective titanium dioxide layer. The reflective layer redirects the light to the film. On top of this is the rare earth phosphor layer that is lined by a protective coating. The protective coating is light transparent and is resistant to abrasion and damage from handling. The protective surface should be cleaned following manufacturers' advice.

8. There are two main types of phosphor materials used in intensifying screens: firstly there are **rare earth phosphors** such as gadolinium and lanthanum, and secondly **calcium tungstate**.

9. Rare earth phosphors are used more commonly as they are faster (approximately 5× faster) than calcium tungstate screens. Less radiation is required in rare earth screens.

10. An intensifying screen is placed in a cassette on either side of the film in close contact. The intensifying screen absorbs the transmitted X-ray beam, which is then converted into light photons. The front screen absorbs low-energy photons and the back screen absorbs the higher energy photons. One X-ray photon will produce a large number of light photons that then interact with the film emulsion.

11. The photoelectric effect.

12. Decrease dose.

13. Decrease resolution.

14. Approximately 5–7 line pairs per millimetre (lp/mm).

15. Direct action film.

16. The silver halide emulsion in indirect film is primarily sensitive to light, and the emulsion in direct action film is primarily sensitive to X-ray photons.

17. There are differing film emulsions that are sensitive to specific colours of light. The film emulsion needs to be sensitive to the light colour emitted by the intensifying screen for a radiographic image to be produced.

18. Poor film/screen contact will result in an area of the image appearing unsharp, cloudy or blurry. The result will be degradation of the image.

19. Screen speed is the amount of time it takes for the screen to emit light following exposure to X-rays.

20. The thickness and size of the phosphor crystals affects the screen speed. Larger crystals in thicker layers attain maximum speed.

21. Dose is reduced, the higher the screen speed.

22. Fine image detail is reduced, the higher the screen speed.

23. No, it will degrade the final image.

24. The cassette should not be used until it is either repaired or replaced. A fault in the closing mechanism can lead to light ingress onto the film and degradation of the final image.

Digital image receptors

1. Digital dental radiography comes in two forms:
   - Direct, such as charge-coupled devices. The sensors connect directly to the computer, usually via a cable, and provide instantaneous images.
   - Indirect, such as photostimulable phosphor plates. These plates are exposed to radiation and then digitally scanned. Therefore, in this digital image acquisition, a second process is required.

2. Charge – coupled device (CCD).

3. The images produced by solid-state sensors once exposed to X-rays provide an almost instantaneous digital image on the computer monitor. Phosphor plate sensors have to be processed. They are placed into a reader and scanned by a laser beam that subsequently leads to a digital image on the computer monitor.

4. The solid-state sensors are made up of tiny silicon chip-based pixels that are arranged in rows and columns (termed a matrix). A scintillation layer, which is made of material similar to rare earth intensifying screens, lies above the silicon layer. These, along with associated electronics, are housed within a rectangular plastic casing. A cable generally runs from the sensor to a docking station. Essentially, a solid – state is a computer chip that is encased in hard plastic.

5. X-ray photons interact with the scintillation layer of the solid-state sensor and are converted to light. The light then interacts with the silicon to create an electric charge for each specific pixel. The total charge developed and stored by the pixel is proportional to the light or X-ray energy incident on the pixel. After exposure of the solid-state sensor to radiation, the charges stored by each pixel are removed electronically (the image is read by transferring each row of pixel charges from one row to the next). At the end of a row, the charge is transferred to an amplifier creating an analogue output signal that is transmitted down the cable to the computer's analogue-to-digital converter. Subsequently, the digital image is produced.

6. The phosphor plates have a plastic flexible support base, on top of which there is a conductive and then a reflective layer. A phosphor layer at the top is covered with a protective coating.

7. Barium fluorohalide phosphor.

8. No, image production is not instantaneous. Phosphor plates have to be processed and scanned by a laser beam for a digital image to be acquired.

9. X-rays that interact with the phosphor layer of the phosphor plate are absorbed. The image plate is then manually placed into a reader where it is scanned by a laser. The stored X-ray energy in the phosphor layer is converted into light. The photomultiplier tube detects the light that is then converted into voltage and sent to the computer to be transformed into a digital image.

10. The plate has to be erased before re-use. In modern equipment, this is done at the end of the reading process by exposing the plate to white light.

11. Both phosphor plates and solid-state sensors are used in intra-oral radiography. Solid-state sensors are not readily available in occlusal sensor size due to the expense of manufacture.

12. Phosphor plates.

13. Phosphor plates.

14. Smaller.

15. Solid-state sensors.

16. X-rays that reach the sensor are converted to light by an intensifying or scintillation screen.

17. The connecting cable can make it difficult to position the sensor in the patients' mouth. The cable can get twisted and damaged.

18. Phosphor plates.

19. Yes, the solid-state sensors generally vary in thickness from approximately 5–7 mm. Phosphor plates are of a similar thickness to conventional film packets.

20. Solid-state sensors.

21. Solid-state sensors, as they are the most expensive to replace.

22. Phosphor plates, as they are comparable in size to conventional intra-oral film. In addition, there is no attached cable.

23. No.

24. No.

25. Sensors are covered in a protective plastic barrier envelope for cross-infection control purposes. The sensors cannot be autoclaved before re-use.

26. No.

Conventional versus digital imaging

1. Digital radiography.

2. The intensifying screens in conventional extra-oral radiography are used as a means of dose reduction. Intensifying screens are not used in intra-oral radiography.

3. No.

4. Both methods produce a 2D grey-scale representation of a 3D object.

5. No.

6. Yes, phosphor plates can be used in conventional film holders, and there are holders on the market that can be purchased specifically for solid-state sensors. Film holders should be used as best practice for bitewing and periapical radiography.

7. Yes, if ionising radiation is being used, a quality assurance programme is a mandatory requirement.

8. Advantages of digital imaging include the following:
   - Lower dose particularly with intra-oral radiography.
   - Instant image with solid-state sensors, therefore, time saving.
   - No need for chemical processing and the hazards associated with handling and disposing of the chemical solutions.
   - Easy storage of images and inclusion into patient records.
   - Image transfer electronically.
   - Ability to manipulate images.

9. Disadvantages of digital imaging include the following:
   - Expense, solid-state sensors are expensive to replace and are relatively fragile.
   - Intra-oral solid-state sensors have relatively smaller image gathering surface than film, and therefore more images may be required to cover the area of interest.
   - Image manipulation can be time consuming and possibly fraudulent in the wrong hands.
   - Need for back-up images and digital image security for the purposes of data protection.
   - Computer failure means that images may not be able to be acquired or viewed.
   - Need for a monitor to view the digital image. Conventional PC screens reduce or limit image quality, therefore diagnostic image quality monitors are necessary.
   - Need company technical back-up.
   - Needs to be compatible with practice management software.
   - There may be loss of image quality and resolution on hard copy prints.

Image processing

Chemical processing

1. Image processing is a systematic process of events aimed at converting the invisible latent image into the visible radiographic film or digital image.

2. The **latent image** is an invisible image, produced on a sensitised emulsion or in the digital sensors by exposure to X-rays or light, which will emerge in development.

3. No.

4. Manual or wet processing is still used in practice, but the most common method of chemical processing is automatic processing.

5. Self-developing films.

6. There are five stages as follows:
   - Development
   - Washing (this stage is eliminated in automatic processing)
   - Fixation
   - Washing
   - Drying

7. Two, developer and fixer.

8. Fixation.

9. Fixation.

10. Development.

11. Two washes, but note that in an automatic processor, the rollers squeeze off any excess developer solution before passing the film to the fixer solution. This eliminates the need for a water wash at this stage.

12. The first film wash removes any residual developer solution (rollers remove the excess developer in the automatic processor), the second film wash removes residual fixer solution.

13. The second wash to remove excess fixer in a manual processing system should be for a minimum of 10 minutes.

14. Light ingress can fog the film and as a result compromise image quality.

15. A daylight loading facility and hood.

16. Ventilation is essential in a darkroom. Chemicals, especially fixer, give off strong fumes that can be unpleasant and can aggravate respiratory problems. The processing chemicals are extremely unhealthy in an enclosed non-ventilated space.

17. The safelight wattage should not exceed 25 W, and the safelights should be positioned approximately 4 ft from the work surfaces. Safe light filters should be compatible with the colour sensitivity of the film being used. Any filter damage increases fogging risk, and therefore damaged or scratched filters should be replaced.

18. The **coin test** measures overall safety of the safelights, essentially it assesses the fogging effect of the safelights on film.

19. Yes.

20. Approximately 5 minutes.

21. 20 °C.

22. Approximately 8–10 minutes.

23. The clearing time relates to the amount of time required to remove the unsensitised silver halide crystals during the fixing process.

24. Phenidone and hydroquinone.

25. Ammonium thiosulphate.

26. Sodium sulphide.

27. Alkaline (pH ~ 10.5).

28. Acidic (pH ~ 4.5).

29. Solutions should be changed when the step wedge phantom or control radiograph demonstrates deterioration in image quality. Solutions should be replaced at least every 14 days irrespective of the number of films that have been chemically processed.

30. Developer is oxidised by air, so over a period of time the function of the chemicals is reduced and the quality of the processed images will deteriorate.

31. The image will be too dark.

32. The image will be too pale.

33. Increased temperature speeds up the action of the developer, and therefore the resultant image will be too dark.

34. The image will be too pale.

35. Fixer is acid. Developer is alkaline. The acid in fixer will neutralise at least some of the alkali in the developer, causing the developer to slow down or stop working altogether. The image would either be underdeveloped (pale) or not developed at all.

36. If fixer has contaminated your developer, you should discard the solution, clean the tank and mix up fresh solutions before developing your film.

37. The chemical solutions should be made up following the manufacturers' guidance.

38. Immediately the films may appear milky due to residual emulsion, and over time the film may become browner in colour. This will have a detrimental effect on the image quality.

39. The advantages of automatic processing over manual processing may be considered as follows:
    - The process is faster. A visible radiographic image is usually ready in about 5 minutes.
    - Some machines automatically replenish solutions.
    - There is a daylight hood, so a darkroom space is not required.
    - A thermostat can control the temperature.
    - The process is under better control and is fairly standardised.

40. The disadvantages of automatic processing over manual processing may be considered as follows:
- Initial expense.
- Yearly service costs and maintenance costs if faults detected.
- The processor may only be able to accommodate intra-oral film.
- Cleaning of the rollers and general maintenance is required.

41. This is an X-ray film that is in a packet along with developing and fixer solutions. The film is processed in its packet once it has been exposed to radiation removing the need for standard manual or automatic film processing.

42. Self-developing films produce the radiographic image quicker than manual or automatic processing. No other equipment is required. The chemical solutions are contained within the packet.

43. There are several disadvantages to self-developing films. Image quality tends to be poorer, and patient dose is higher as the packet does not contain lead foil. The packets are thin and flexible and are difficult to position into film holders. The image tends to deteriorate over time, and the films are more expensive than traditional film.

44. Self-developing films may be of benefit during a domiciliary visit when diagnostic information is required immediately to aid treatment. This tool may also be beneficial during a dental examination and treatment under general anaesthetic for a patient who is unable to tolerate a radiograph while conscious. A further use for this type of image receptor would be in remote areas where processing facilities are not available such as conflict zones or research work/missionary trips in Third World countries. For each of these scenarios, X-ray generating equipment is required. There are hand-held portable X-ray sets on the market.

45. Yes, a double film packet that contains two films and produces two identical images from one exposure can be used. Of course, a second option would be to obtain one image and then copy it digitally either with a scanner/digital camera or using duplicate film.

46. Yes, the operator may take a technically perfect radiograph only for poor processing to render it a grade 3, non-diagnostic film. Processing is a critical part of the process of acquiring a conventional X-ray image and as such is an important part of quality control within a quality assurance programme.

Digital processing

1. The word **pixel** means a picture element. Every radiograph, in digital form, is made up of pixels. They are the smallest unit of information that makes up an image. Pixels are typically arranged in tiny squares in a 2D grid termed a matrix.

2. Each pixel measures the total amount of X-ray absorption throughout the whole voxel.

3. 0–255.

4. Black. For a pixel to be assigned the number 0 it will have received maximum voltage because there was no x-ray attenuation in the patient.

5. White. For a pixel to be assigned the number 255 it will have received no voltage because there was total x-ray attenuation in the patient.

6. 256.

7. 20–70 µm.

8. Pixel size affects resolution, the smaller the pixel dimension the more pixels will be within the matrix and the better the resolution of the final image.

9. This is dependent on the type of digital sensor used and has an approximate resolution between 7 and 25 line pairs per millimetre (lp/mm).

10. Solid-state sensors.

11. Phosphor plates.

12. Digital images can be enhanced in several ways, these include the following:
    - Brightness
    - Contrast
    - Edge enhancement
    - Inversion (image reversal)
    - Magnification/zooming
    - Measurements
    - Pseudocolourisation

13. Brightness and contrast.

14. The image becomes lighter.

15. Increasing brightness is achieved by increasing the numerical value of each pixel in the image. By increasing the number of the pixel, it is given a lighter shade of grey.

16. The total image would be white.

17. The image will have less shades of grey, and the difference between black and white is increased.

18. Increasing contrast is achieved by reducing the pixel numbers in the darker half of the grey scale and increasing pixel numbers in the lighter half of the grey scale.

19. The image would be purely black and white with no shades of grey.

20. Blooming is a digital image fault caused by overexposure and overloading of the solid-state sensor. In the region where the sensor is overloaded or flooded, the image will appear black.

21. Blooming affects solid-state sensors.

22. No.

23. The internal electronics are seen if the sensor is incorrectly positioned front to back.

24. The magnet.

25. Scratches on the phosphor plate results in opaque artefact that relate to the areas of damage.

26. Debris on the phosphor plate results in opaque artefact on the digital image.

27. The image will be light fogged; exposure to light can partially erase the latent image prior to the scanning process.

28. The image quality is inferior to that of the digital image viewed on the monitor. This is due to the limitations of the printer, which is unable to copy 256 shades of grey.

29. Computed tomography, in particular cone beam computed tomography (CBCT).

SECTION V Answers: Image quality and quality assurance

The radiographic image

1. It is difficult with a 2D representation to understand or appreciate the overall true shape of the object. There will be superimposition of structures, making it difficult to interpret the exact site of certain shapes or structures within the image.

2. The **radiopaque shadows** on an image are the dense structures within the object that have stopped the X-ray beam and prevented X-rays passing to the image detector.

3. The **radiolucent shadows** on an image represent the areas where the X-ray beam has not been stopped and has passed through the object onto the image detector.

4. Teeth (enamel and dentine), bone and dental restorations are radiopaque.

5. Air and the pulp cavity of a tooth are radiolucent.

6. Density of the image is affected by the following:
  • The constituents of the object – for example, human tissue will include structures of varying densities such as bone, teeth, fat, muscle and blood.
  • The shape of the object.
  • The energy of the X-ray beam.
  • The geometric proportions of the object to the X-ray beam and image receptor.
  • The type of image receptor.

7. Image **contrast** is the difference between adjacent densities. The adjacent densities can range from white to black and various shades of grey in between. High-contrast images have few shades of grey, whereas low-contrast images have many shades of grey.

8. It decreases contrast producing more shades of grey within the image.

9. The object and image receptor should be as close together as possible being parallel to one another. The X-ray beam should be angled at right angles to the object and the image receptor.

10. It decreases subject contrast. The amount of scattered radiation is generally proportional to the total mass of tissue within the X-ray beam, so with a larger patient size there will be increased scatter leading to decreased contrast.

11. **Image sharpness** relates to how well an image can define an edge or border.

12. Loss of image sharpness may result from the following:
    - Patient movement.
    - The penumbra effect. It is a fuzzy, unclear area that surrounds a radiographic image and is affected by focal spot size that ideally should be a point source.
    - The object shape, an example would be cervical burnout at the cervical constriction of a tooth.
    - Use of intensifying screens.

13. **Image resolution** is a measure of the image receptors' capacity to resolve two points that are close together.

14. It is measured in line pairs per millimetre (lp/mm).

15. Resolution may be affected by image receptor type and speed, image sharpness and contrast.

16. Radiographic image quality will be influenced practically by the following:
    - The operator technique including the exposure parameters selected.
    - The equipment used (X-ray equipment and image receptor type).
    - The patient, factors to consider would include patient size, co-operation and the local anatomy.
    - The processing technique (film-captured radiograph).

17. An ideal radiographic image demonstrates the image to be the same size and shape as the object, therefore it is geometrically accurate without distortion. The image has good detail, density and contrast, thus providing the clinician with optimal information.

Film-based radiographic faults

1. Causes of a pale film would include the following:
   - Underexposure caused by inaccurate (too low) exposure time setting by the operator or a fault in the timer.
   - Underdevelopment caused by insufficient development, developer solution being exhausted, too cold or too diluted. This may result from developer contamination with fixer.
   - If a direct action film is reversed in the mouth, then the lead will absorb much of the X-ray beam resulting in a pale image.
   - Excessive tissue thickness of the patient.

2. Causes of a dark film would include the following:
   - Overexposure caused by inaccurate (too high) exposure time setting by the operator or a fault in the timer.
   - Overdevelopment (too long in the developer solution) or developer being too hot or too concentrated.
   - Light fogging from an extraneous source, this may be due to operator error, faulty safe-lights or damage to the automatic processor lid, poor film storage, expired films or faulty extra-oral cassettes.
   - Thin tissue thickness of the patient.

3. Causes of a marked film would include the following:
   - Careless handling by the operator resulting in bending of the film, finger nail or finger print marks.
   - Bite marks on films. This can occur on occlusal radiographs if the patient is not instructed properly and bites down too hard on the film.
   - Processing errors such as fixer splash, roller marks, films stuck together.
   - Static electricity.
   - Dirt/debris on intensifying screens.
   - Scratches can readily occur on phosphor plates if they are not handled with care.

4. Causes of low contrast would include the following:
   - Underdeveloped film
   - Overdeveloped film
   - Direct action film positioned the wrong way round
   - Processing errors such as inadequate fixer time or exhausted/diluted fixer chemicals
   - Film fogging
   - Patient size

5. Causes of a blurred or unsharp image would include the following:
   - Poor patient positioning, particularly in dental panoramic tomography.
   - Patient movement.
   - Double exposure.
   - Distortion of a film through bending.
   - Film type and speed, fast intensifying screens result in loss of detail.
   - Poor film/screen contact in intensifying screens.

6. **Coning off** is an error in taking a radiograph where the X-ray beam is incorrectly aligned with the image receptor. This results in a blank area on the image that may have either a straight or curved outline (dependent on collimator shape). Correct and accurate use of film holders and beam indicating devices for intra-oral radiography should prevent the coning off of an image.

7. A dark area.

8. Geometric distortion is seen in the following:
   - Poor positioning of the object with respect to the image receptor and X-ray beam. This is seen in the bisecting angle periapical technique when incorrect beam angulation may lead to elongation or foreshortening of the image. If the patient holds the image receptor in place, it may be bent leading to distortion of the image.

- Dental panoramic radiography; there is an element of distortion in a panoramic radiograph due to the method of image acquisition.

9. Yes, as the technical processes are the same.

10. Cervical burnout is a radiolucent area on the mesial and distal aspects of the teeth in the cervical regions that extends from the cemento-enamel junction (CEJ) to the crest of the alveolar ridge and can be mistaken for caries. It is caused by the normal anatomy of the teeth; the tissue is thin in the area of interest resulting in less attenuation of the X-ray beam. It is commonly seen in the premolar region on bitewing radiographs.

11. There is coning off at the base of the image. This can be corrected by ensuring that the film is placed correctly in a film holder in the patient's mouth with careful alignment of the film holder, spacer cone and collimator. The patient's teeth are not biting together, and the image is blurred due to movement. Careful instruction to the patient prior to the radiographic exposure can prevent movement and ensure the teeth contact the bite block.

12. There is coning off at the top of the image. This can be corrected by ensuring that the film is placed correctly in the holder with careful alignment of the film holder and spacer cone. The right premolar region and lower right first molar teeth are not seen due to a fogged (blackened) film. This is because half of the film has been exposed to light prior to processing. Light exposure to a film may be as a result of operator carelessness but also can occur if there is light ingress into a darkroom or damage to the daylight hood of an automatic film processor.

13. The film has been exposed twice during separate radiographic examinations. There is a periapical image superimposed over a bitewing radiograph with a resultant double, dark image. Care must be taken to ensure that when a film has been exposed to X-rays that it is either processed immediately or placed to one side (preferably labelled) so that it cannot be re-used while further exposures are performed.

14. There are markings on the upper part of the film consistent with the dimples on the lead foil and a black strip at the base. The film has been placed back to front in the patient's mouth and as a result is pale. There is also coning off of the image.

15. There is a black line running across the film consistent with a bend that may have occurred when the film packet was placed in the film holder. Careful film packet handling and appropriate storage of film will reduce the chance of this damage and resultant artefact.

16. An orthodontic appliance with metal components has been left *in situ*, which is superimposed over the apical tissues of the incisor teeth. Dentures and orthodontic appliances, along with any relevant piercings and jewellery, should be removed prior to dental radiography.

17. The teeth are distorted and curved due to excessive bending of the film packet during the exposure. This periapical radiograph was taken using the bisecting angle technique, and the film was bent by excessive finger pressure from the patient. Careful handling of film packets and the use of film holders and the paralleling technique reduce the chance of film bending. If the patient cannot tolerate film holders, then it is important to instruct the patient how to support the film packet appropriately or use another method of stabilisation.

18. Large hoop earrings have not been removed, and as a result there is ghost shadow artefact from this jewellery on both sides, which is superimposed over the posterior teeth and jaws. The occlusal plane has a slightly smiley appearance, suggesting that the patient's chin is too low. Jewellery, piercings and intra-oral appliances must be removed during this imaging and careful positioning using the light markers is essential.

19. The film is marked due to dirt on the roller mechanism in the automatic film processor. The image is also pale. This may be the result of too low an exposure setting or faulty timer. The cause may be due to a processing error such as over diluted or exhausted developer, inadequate development time, too low a temperature or contamination of the developer with fixer. The other cause for a pale film is excessive patient tissues.

20. The image is dark. This may be the result of too high an exposure setting or faulty timer. The cause may be due to over concentrated developer solution, too high a temperature of the developer or too long a developing time. The other cause for a dark film is thin patient tissues.

Quality assurance

1. **Quality control** is a process to review the quality of all factors involved in production; in radiography these are the specific measures for ensuring and verifying the quality of the radiographs produced.

2. **Quality assurance** is any systematic process of checking to see whether a product or service being developed is meeting specified requirements. Quality assurance ensures that the quality control procedures are effective and if there are problems that they are recognised quickly and corrected promptly.

3. The **quality assurance programme** aims are to produce radiographic images of sufficiently high quality that ensure consistently adequate diagnostic information at the lowest possible cost and lowest radiation dose to the patient.

4. Yes, a quality assurance programme is mandatory if ionising radiation is being used in an organisation.

5. Yes, see the above-mentioned answer 4.

6. The responsibility and implementation of a quality assurance programme requires a named person, this is often a senior partner but could be a dental nurse with the relevant training. Overall responsibility lies with the employer.

7. Yes, all necessary procedures must be laid down in writing.

8. Essential quality control procedures in dental radiography include the following:
   - Image quality
   - Patient dose and X-ray equipment
   - Darkroom, films and processing (unless digital)
   - Training
   - Audit

9. Regular inspection of the digital sensors should be undertaken.
   - With respect to solid-state sensors, regular checks should be made for cracks or damage to the cables and sensor casing. There should be assessment for non-uniformity of the receptor.
   - With phosphor plates, regular visual checks for scratches and dirt should be made and the plates should be passed through the reader to detect for scratches on a daily basis. Regular cleaning of the plates should be undertaken following the manufacturer's advice. Again there should be assessment for non-uniformity of the receptor.
   - Monitors require cleaning on a regular basis and calibration checks that can be performed using specific test patterns designed for this purpose.

10. Guidance Notes for Dental Practitioners on the Safe Use of X-Ray Generating Equipment – Department of Health, June 2001.

11. A Grade 1 film is of excellent diagnostic quality with no errors of patient preparation, exposure, positioning, processing or film handling.

12. A Grade 2 film is diagnostically acceptable. There may be some errors in patient preparation, exposure, positioning, processing or film handling, but the radiograph is a useful aid to diagnosis and treatment management.

13. A Grade 3 film is diagnostically unacceptable. Errors of patient preparation, exposure, positioning, processing or film handling create a film of no diagnostic use.

14. No.

15. No.

16. Yes, if a Grade 3 film is not repeated (allowing for extenuating circumstances), the question should be raised as to whether it was justified in the first place.

17. Yes, but as digital images can be manipulated, there is a possibility that image quality can be enhanced unlike film-captured images. In addition, chemical processing is not used. A 1–3 rating system is suggested in Radiography and Radiology for Dental Care Professionals, 3rd Edition, Whaites E and Drage N 2013, p. 201. The authors consider a similar rating system (grade 1, 2 and 3) to film-captured images, but take into consideration the differences between digital- and film-based techniques.

18. It is important to consider the indications for the examination. The image may be, for example, of poor quality throughout but may actually give the clinician adequate diagnostic information in the area of interest to help in the management of the patient.

19. Not less than 70%.

20. No greater than 20%.

21. No greater than 10%.

22. 3 years.

23. Audit. A common radiography audit is to either retrospectively or prospectively analyse a number of radiographs by giving them a quality rating of 1, 2 or 3. The results can be compared to the standard targets and if targets are not being met consider and confirm reasons for this, implement change and re-audit.

24. This is a simple method of identifying all rejected images (grade 3) and to document the faults and sources of error. This will help to identify errors early so that the problems can be addressed and resolved quickly. As a result of this analysis, an equipment fault may be identified or it may be concluded that improvements in radiographic technique or further staff training are required.
    The following data should be recorded:
    - Date.
    - Nature of fault.
    - The known or suspected cause of the fault.
    - Number of repeat radiographs required.
    - It is also useful to name the operator if there is more than one in the dental practice.

25. Reasons for film rejection may include the following:
    - Patient movement resulting in blurring of the image.
    - Poor film positioning leading to coning off, magnification or loss of detail.
    - Geometric distortion.
    - Incorrect anatomy imaged.
    - Film too pale or too dark as a result or incorrect exposure factors or processing error.
    - Poor contrast.
    - Double exposure.
    - Artefact such as light fogging, fixer splash, nail marks, bite marks.

26. Image quality can be assessed daily by comparing each radiograph taken to a high-quality standard reference film.

27. **A**s **L**ow **A**s **R**easonably **P**racticable.

28. A **critical examination** is a test carried out on all new X-ray equipment prior to its routine use.

29. The installer.

30. An **acceptance test** is carried out by the RPA/medical physicist before equipment is used clinically. This test provides baseline values, including patient dose, against which subsequent routine tests can be compared.

31. The legal person.

32. At least every 3 years.

33. If there has been repair, modification or relocation of X-ray-generating equipment.

34. Yes, this must be kept in a radiation protection file as part of the quality assurance programme.

35. Daily checks may include the following:
- Correct function of safety devices
- Assessment of warning lights and audible alarms
- Counterbalance assessment to confirm satisfactory, maintainable positioning of the tubehead

36. For each piece of X-ray equipment, there should be details of the manufacturer, model and serial number, year of manufacture and installation.

37. General cleanliness of surfaces and film hangers, this should be checked daily.
Light tightness, this should be checked yearly.
Safelights adhere to the appropriate filters, wattage (no more than 25 W) and distance (no more than 4 ft away) from the work surfaces in order to prevent film fogging.

38. Light causes fogging of a film; this darkens the film in the region of light exposure.

39. The coin test.

40. A simple check is to load a cassette with an unexposed film and place it on a windowsill in full light for several minutes. The film should then be processed, and any ingress of light will appear as fogging (darkening) of the film.

41. Film/screen contact test. A piece of graph paper is placed into the cassette between the film and intensifying screen. The film is then exposed to a very low dose of X-rays (approximately 0.01 s exposure time) and then developed. If film/screen contact is good, sharp lines from the graph paper will be projected onto the film. If film screen contact is poor, the lines will be blurred in the area of inadequate contact. This can be undertaken in dental practice.

42. Information should include the manufacturer's instructions including special precautions on using the chemicals and the correct temperatures required for optimal processing. There should be details on changing or replenishing solutions, how often they are changed and how they are monitored for deterioration.

43. Chemical processing solutions should be changed approximately every 2 weeks, this should however be guided by the manufacturer's instructions or if the step wedge or control radiograph demonstrate deterioration of image quality sooner.

44. Daily, ideally each morning.

45. At least fortnightly.

46. It is a test object. This is a purpose-built step wedge phantom constructed using pieces of lead foil from intra-oral film taped to a wooden tongue spatula. Manufactured step wedges can be bought, but this example can be made simply and cheaply within the dental practice setting. It is used to monitor deterioration in chemical processing solutions. The step wedge is X-rayed using known and recorded exposure factors. The film is initially processed in new chemical solutions to produce a standard film of reference. This exact process is repeated each day using the same exposure factors. Each daily film is compared visually with the reference film to assess for a decrease in contrast that would suggest deterioration of processing solutions.

47. Yearly, unless a problem occurs in the interim period.

48. X-ray film should be stored in a dry, clean and cool environment away from ionising radiation. The X-rays should be handled carefully and packed in a way that does not cause pressure mark artefact. Expiry dates should be checked. Manufacturers will detail ideal storage conditions of their products, and this information should be followed.

49. Digital sensors should be stored in a dry, clean and cool environment away from ionising radiation. The sensors should be handled carefully, not dropped and packed in a way that does not cause scratches, bending or damage. Solid-state sensors may break if dropped, and therefore common sense would suggest that they are not stored in difficult to reach areas.

50. Screens are easily damaged. Their fluorescent emission will be affected if the active surface is soiled even slightly. Screens therefore must be kept clean, otherwise light photons will be prevented from reaching the film and creating an image, and the film in that area will appear clear. Dirt will also create 'high' spots that will create wear. Screens are best cleaned following the manufacturer's guidance. The screen should be dry before closing the cassette otherwise the gelatin on the surface of the screens may stick together. A cassette should not be left open, as it will accumulate dirt and dust on the screen.

51. The information is the name of the staff member and their responsibility and role. The document should also state the date and type of training each staff member has obtained and a recommended date for reassessing training needs.

52. It is a legal requirement.

53. Every 5 years.

54. Yes.

55. Clinical audit is a process that measures the quality of services, patient care and outcomes against a benchmark or set standard. If an audit shows failure to reach the standards, then reasons for the failings should be addressed and the appropriate changes made. In dental radiography, a quality assurance programme is in place to highlight problems early so that they can be corrected and thus audits are an important tool in this process.

56. Common audits in dental radiography include the following:
- clinical evaluation (image quality rating) of radiographs;
- justification of radiographs;
- Assessment of written report of radiographs in patient records.

57. The working procedures include the following:
- Local rules as required in the United Kingdom under the Ionising Radiation Regulations 1999.
- Employers written procedures as required in the United Kingdom under IR(ME)R 2000.
- Operational procedures or systems of work.
- Procedures log.

SECTION VI Answers: Patient care

Patient care during dental radiography

1. Patients can be anxious about having a radiation exposure, as they may be concerned about the potential health risks. They may be in pain and therefore worried that the procedure may bring additional discomfort. The equipment itself may be frightening, and this may in particular concern young patients and those with special needs.

2. Young children may find the procedure very frightening particularly if they have not had an X-ray before. Extra support is often required also for those individuals with disabilities, learning difficulties and phobias.

3. Clear explanation, avoiding jargon, is very important. Patients need to be informed of the procedure and reassured. You can make them comfortable and do your upmost to ensure that the examination is carried out as comfortably, accurately and as quickly as possible avoiding the need for a repeat exposure.

4. Most importantly, the patient is required to stay still to avoid movement artefact and the possible necessity to repeat the examination. In a dental panoramic radiograph, patient positioning such as tongue to the roof of the mouth and closing the lips is required.

5. The patient should be watched throughout the entire exposure to check that they are not moving and are obeying instructions. If a patient is moving during a dental panoramic radiograph, it may be necessary for the operator to terminate the exposure before it has finished to avoid unnecessary radiation and a resultant grade 3 film.

6. It is a good practise to have the exposure variables set up in order that the procedure can be performed quickly once the patient, image receptor and tubehead have been positioned correctly. This will reduce the chance of patient movement and reduce discomfort in an intra-oral procedure by limiting the time that the patient has to hold the image receptor in their mouth.

7. Glasses, jewellery and hairpins may need to be removed along with any removable metal dentures, orthodontic appliances or oral piercings. Removal of the above will be dependent on the type of radiographic projection.

8. The X-ray beam may project a blurred shadow of the necklace onto the image receptor degrading the quality of the image.

9. Children generally require smaller intra-oral image receptors than adults due to the smaller size of the mouth and oral cavity.

10. Patients come in all shapes and sizes, so film size selection is important. An individual with a small mouth may struggle with the larger intra-oral image receptors. A large tongue can also inhibit image receptor placement. Other anatomic hurdles include a high arch or shallow palate, narrow dental arches, limited mouth opening and restricted neck movements. Obesity can also make image receptor and patient positioning more challenging. Patients who have a strong gag reflex may not be able to tolerate intra-oral radiography at all.

11. Cooperation may be a problem, and this is where good communication to both parent and child is essential. A child may find it difficult to remain still, particularly during a longer procedure such as a dental panoramic radiograph (approximately 15-second exposure time). A young child may find it uncomfortable having even a small image receptor placed in their mouth, so particular care and patience are required.

12. There may be learning and communication difficulties that make it difficult for the patient to understand the procedure and therefore cooperation may be poor. The head is a personal space, and some individuals may not cope well with having an image receptor put into their mouth. Individuals who are deaf or have compromised hearing may require slow speech for lip reading or even sign language. Other disabilities include uncontrolled movements such as tremor as seen in Parkinson's disease. Patients who have facial weakness, for example, from a stroke may not tolerate radiographs well. Spinal problems resulting in excessive curvature of the spine may mean that radiographic projections such as a lower occlusal radiograph or a dental panoramic radiograph cannot be performed.

13. This technique should not be performed if you feel that cooperation is poor and the resultant radiograph is likely to be non-diagnostic. Clear instructions need to be provided, and it may be useful to perform a trial run to assess whether the child can remain still. Be aware though that tolerance and attention span levels at this age may be low. The alternative is to discuss other methods of radiography with the dentist. This may include left and right oblique lateral radiographs that may provide the relevant diagnostic information.

14. Each case is individual and different, and it is important to have various strategies in place to help your patient cope with dental radiographs. In this case, the mother has offered you some important information. It would seem sensible to sit the girl on her mother's lap (the mother acts as carer and as such wears lead protection as detailed in the local rules) in order that she can support and calm her daughter by stroking her hair during the procedure.

15. It can be very difficult to obtain a radiograph in a patient who gags, performing endodontic treatment may be even more challenging. Anxiety of the procedure can make the gag reflex worse. An empathetic approach, good communication and instruction are paramount, allaying anxiety and relaxing the patient is the first step in the process. The patient is best seated upright. A form of distraction may work, for example, ask the patient to raise their left leg a couple of inches from the chair while the image receptor is positioned while breathing slowly through the nose. It may not be possible to obtain a good quality radiograph, and an alternative extra-oral technique may have to be considered although not ideal.

Control of infection

1. The Health and Safety at Work Act 1974.

2. A non-invasive procedure.

3. The main risk would be salivary contamination from one patient to another via contamination of equipment or work surfaces. Operators are at risk of salivary contamination via an unprotected skin wound or exposure to the eye.

4. To prevent the transmission of infections/microorganisms from one person to another by either direct or indirect means.

5. Hepatitis B.

6. The operator must perform the same cross-infection protocol on each patient. A patient with a known infection risk may not choose to disclose this information when asked by a health-care worker. It is safest to assume that all individuals may be an infection risk and thus should be treated identically. The exception to this would be those individuals with, or suspected to have, a transmissible spongiform encephalopathy such as Creutzfeldt–Jacob disease (CJD).

7. Prior to a radiographic procedure, the following should be disinfected:
   • Work surfaces that are to be used
   • The X-ray-generating equipment
   The operator must wear personal protective equipment (PPE), changing gloves as and when required and ensuring that if plain films are to be used they have not been previously exposed.

8. The operator must wear the correct personal protective equipment (PPE), this as a minimum should be gloves and eye protection. Removing and re-gloving should be undertaken as required. The work surfaces should be zoned so that only the specific area that has been disinfected is used.

9. The radiographic film packet must be disinfected prior to processing unless a barrier-wrapped film is used, in this case the wrapping is removed with gloved hands and the film is placed onto a clean surface. The work surfaces, chair and X-ray-generating equipment must be disinfected. Film holders and dental panoramic bite pegs must be sterilised. Gloves must be changed and disposed of correctly.

10. After every use or if it is thought that cross-infection measures have not been carried out.

11. After every use or if it is thought that cross-infection measures have not been carried out.

12. There is no need to disinfect the X-ray film packet as the barrier would be removed prior to processing and disposed of in the clinical waste.

13. No.

Waste disposal

1. Clinical.

2. Domestic.

3. In an identified lead foil container. An authorised contractor will collect this on a regular contracted basis.

4. Spent chemical processing solutions should be poured into identified plastic containers that are clearly labelled. An authorised contractor will collect the solutions on a regular contracted basis.

   5. Special waste.

   6. Yes.

   7. Control of Substances Hazardous to Health.

   8. Clinical.

   9. Clinical.

   10. Clinical.

   11. The phosphor plate is not discarded and is reusable once it has been cleared (erased). A phosphor plate would only be discarded if it was damaged/faulty and was not producing images of adequate quality.

   12. Clinical.

SECTION VII Answers: Dental radiography

Bitewing radiography

   1. Intra-oral.

   2. A bitewing radiograph demonstrates the dental crowns and crestal bone levels of the upper and lower posterior dentition on one side. It may not show all of the premolar and molars.

   3. The main indication for this radiographic technique is for caries assessment. This will include identifying disease following clinical examination but may be indicated to monitor or assess disease progression and existing restorations.

   4. Yes, but in teeth with pocket depths of more than 6 mm, vertical bitewings or periapical radiographs are indicated. Please note that radiographic periodontal assessment is an adjunct to the clinical assessment and should not be used as the sole method for diagnosis.

   5. Horizontal bitewings.

   6. In the horizontal bitewing technique, the image receptor is positioned with the long axis horizontally; conversely the long axis is vertical for a vertical bitewing.

   7. Vertical bitewings are generally more informative than horizontal bitewings in detecting moderate-to-severe periodontal disease. The selection criteria guidelines (3rd edition, October 2013), when considering periodontal assessment, suggest that for uniform pocketing less than 4–5 mm with little or no recession then horizontal bitewing radiographs are indicated but for pocket depths of 6 mm or more then vertical bitewings plus or minus paralleling technique periapicals should be employed.

   8. The crowns of the premolar and first and second molar teeth.

9. No.

10. Bitewing image receptors are held between the teeth and the lateral aspect of the tongue while the patient bites together. Historically, a wing/tab was attached to the film (hence the phrase bitewing), but they have now generally been replaced with holders. Holders allow for ease of positioning of the X-ray tubehead and spacer cone with respect to the image receptor, resulting in accurate positioning that can prevent coning off and facilitate reproducible images.

11. The three components are as follows:
   - a device for holding the image receptor in a position that is parallel to the teeth;
   - a bite platform to stabilise the holder between the patient's teeth;
   - an X-ray beam-aiming device.

12. The posterior teeth should be as close to the image receptor as possible, preferably in contact, and the long axis of the tooth and image receptor should be parallel.

13. Young children.

14. The patient should be seated upright with stable head support and the occlusal plane parallel to the floor.

15. Parallel.

16. The distal aspect of the lower canine tooth.

17. To the mesial aspect of the lower third molar.

18. The X-ray beam is angled at right angles (90°) to the teeth and image detector in the horizontal plane, with an approximate 5°–8° downward vertical angulation to compensate for the upward rise of the dental arches.

19. Coning off as well as overlapping of the contact areas of the teeth may result.

20. Distortion of the teeth as the buccal and lingual cusps of the teeth would not be superimposed.

21. If the X-ray beam does not pass between the contact points, then there will be superimposition of the inter-proximal surfaces of the teeth, and this will compromise caries assessment. If there is dental crowding, then preventing superimposition of contact points may not be achievable.

22. Young children do not tend to tolerate image receptor holders as well as adults and, therefore, the tab technique may have to be used. In addition, children have smaller mouths and generally require the smallest image receptor.

23. Advantages of using image receptor holders in bitewing radiography include the following:
   - The image receptor is held firmly in position and cannot be displaced by the tongue.
   - The beam-aiming device controls the direction of the X-ray tubehead both in the vertical and horizontal planes.

- Avoids coning off of the image.
- The images are considered more reproducible, but this will be operator dependent. Tab bitewings technique allows the operator to make educated, yet arbitrary assessment of the necessary horizontal and vertical positions of the X-ray tubehead.
- Can be used for film and digital image receptors.

24. Disadvantages of using image receptor holders in bitewing radiography include the following:
- The patient may find the positioning uncomfortable, particularly the larger solid-state sensors. Young children with small mouths may not tolerate holders.
- Expense.
- Some holders are disposable but most require autoclaving after use. Tabs are disposable.

25. Good contrast is required to differentiate the dental tissues from one another and to allow any demineralisation of the tissue to be demonstrated.

26. Underexposure reduces burn out of the thin alveolar crestal bone, allowing for optimal assessment of the bone levels.

27. Carious lesions are generally larger clinically than radiologically. Approximately 50% demineralisation of tooth tissue is required to demonstrate caries radiologically.

28. This is a grade 1 right bitewing of a young patient. The image has acceptable definition and contrast with no blurring or coning off. The image includes the mesial aspect of the first premolar teeth and the erupted molars. The bite platform is central to the image and horizontal. The alveolar crests are nicely seen, and there is no overlap of the approximal surfaces of the teeth.

29. This is slightly subjective, but given the indications this should technically be considered a grade 3 bitewing. The image has acceptable definition and contrast with no blurring or coning off, but there is superimposition of the approximal surfaces of the teeth due to incorrect horizontal angulation of the X-ray tubehead and this compromises caries assessment of the molar teeth. The image is marked and scratched due to poor handling.

Periapical radiography

1. Intra-oral.

2. A periapical radiograph demonstrates individual teeth including the crown and root morphology, the crestal bone and the associated periapical tissues.

3. The main indications for this radiographic technique include the following:
- Periodontal assessment
- Root morphology prior to extraction
- Root and pulpal canal morphology for the purposes of endodontic and surgical endodontic procedures
- Assessment of periapical disease

- Position, presence and status of un-erupted or ectopic teeth
- Assessment of bone quality and bone height prior to or after implant placement
- Dental trauma assessment
- Localisation of teeth using parallax

4. Yes, but bitewing radiographs would be optimal for caries diagnosis in the posterior dentition.

5. Periapical radiographs can image the incisor and canine teeth in full, whereas bitewing radiographs aim to include the premolar, first and second molars. Both techniques may encompass the third molar tooth if it is in a position whereby the patient can tolerate the intra-oral image receptor placement.

6. The image receptor should be positioned as close to the teeth as possible and ideally parallel. (In practice, achieving absolutely parallel positioning is seldom feasible).

7. Parallel.

8. The long axis should be vertical.

9. The long axis should be horizontal.

10. The X-ray beam should be at right angles (90^0) to the long axis of the tooth and image receptor.

11. The paralleling technique.

12. The paralleling technique.

13. The paralleling technique.

14. With the **bisecting angle technique**, the image receptor is placed as close to the tooth as possible (the image receptor is not positioned parallel to the long axis of the tooth), commonly this is by gentle finger support from the patient but specific receptor holders for the bisected angle technique are available. The operator mentally bisects the angle formed between the long axis of the tooth and the long axis of the image receptor and the X-ray beam is angled at 90° to this imaginary bisecting line. The X-ray beam is centred on the apical area of the tooth or teeth.

15. The vertical angulation is the angle formed by continuing the line of the central X-ray beam until it meets the horizontal occlusal plane. The angle will depend on the operator's perception of the imaginary bisecting line between the long axis of the tooth and the image receptor.

16. The image will either be elongated if the vertical angulation is too small or foreshortened if the vertical angulation is too large.

17. There will be overlapping and superimposition of the crowns and roots of the teeth.

18. In the **paralleling technique**, the image receptor is placed in an appropriate holder and positioned in the mouth parallel to the tooth in question. The holder is positioned so that the teeth to be imaged are touching the bite block. A cottonwool roll can be placed on the underside of the bite block to aid in correct positioning and patient comfort. The tooth and image receptor do not touch due to local anatomy. The X-ray tube is aimed at right angles, both vertically and horizontally to the tooth and image receptor. This technique has no guesswork because it utilises a holder with fixed image receptor and X-ray tubehead position.

19. The positioning device on the holder determines the tubehead angulation.

20. The three components are the same as for the bitewing holders and comprise the following:
    • A device for holding the image receptor rigid in a position that is parallel to the teeth.
    • A bite platform to stabilise the holder between the patient's teeth.
    • An X-ray beam-aiming device.

21. The patient should be seated upright with stable head support and the occlusal plane parallel to the floor.

22. Figure 5.15.

23. Due to the patient's palatal and dental anatomy, the use of holders in the paralleling technique means that the receptor and tooth are not as closely approximated, to the entire tooth, as in the bisecting angle technique.

24. Magnification of the image. Incorporating a long focal spot to skin distance of 200 mm or more reduces magnification. This results in a more parallel and less divergent X-ray beam.

25. The main advantages of the paralleling technique include the following:
    • Reproducible images can be produced at different clinical appointments and with different operators.
    • Geometrically accurate images with little magnification, foreshortening or elongation of the image. The holders automatically determine the horizontal and vertical angles of the X-ray tubehead.
    • Accurate demonstration of the teeth and periodontal bone levels.
    • No superimposition of the zygomatic buttress overlying the tooth apices.

26. The main disadvantages of the paralleling technique include the following:
    • Expense of image receptor holders
    • Autoclaving of the holders
    • Operator difficulty in positioning the holder
    • Patient tolerance
    • The patient's oral anatomy may inhibit the accurate positioning of an image receptor holder.

27. The main advantages of the bisecting technique include the following:
    • Cheap, this procedure can be done without holders.
    • Relatively easy to position the receptor in the patient's mouth.
    • Comfortable for the patient.
    • Commonly no autoclaving required.

28. The main disadvantages of the bisecting technique include the following:
- Non-reproducible images.
- Geometric inaccuracy if the imaginary bisecting line is miscalculated and the horizontal and vertical angulations are incorrect. Poor horizontal angulation will lead to overlapping of the dental crowns, and incorrect vertical angulation results in either elongation or foreshortening of the image.
- The buccal roots of the maxillary premolar and molar teeth are foreshortened.
- Bending of the image receptor by digit pressure will lead to image distortion.
- The periodontal bone levels are poorly demonstrated.
- Coning off of the image.
- Superimposition of the zygomatic buttress over the posterior maxillary tooth apices.

29. Four are generally required when the bone levels need to be assessed; it may be possible to use three when assessing the apical tissues. This is operator dependent.

30. 3.

31. 2.

32. 2.

33. 15, but this may vary because this is operator and patient dependent.

34. The orientation dot should be placed opposite the crowns of the tooth in order to aid film mounting and to ensure that the dot is not superimposed over the apical tissues.

35. Yes.

36. Yes, the plates can be used in the conventional film holders due to their comparable size and thickness to film packets.

37. Yes, but the solid-state sensors are thicker than film and phosphor plates and require custom-made holders.

38. Upper left and lower right premolar and molar teeth.

39. Left and right maxillary and mandibular incisors. The holder position demonstrated is also used for upper left and lower right canine teeth.

40. Upper right and lower left premolar and molar teeth.

41. Good practice during endodontic treatment is the use of a rubber dam, which is stabilised with rubber dam clamps. This makes it difficult for the operator to visualise the tooth of interest and to place the image receptor correctly. In addition, if there are instruments coming out of the tooth, standard holders cannot be used.

42. Conventional film holders cannot be used, but there are specific holders for endodontic cases whereby the holder has a basket in the bite block that contains the exposed instruments while still allowing the film and tooth to remain parallel.

43. The absence of teeth makes image receptor positioning difficult due to the lack of ridge height, resulting in a shallow palate or reduced lingual sulcus depth. In the edentulous patient, the bisecting angle technique is often the technique of choice.

44. The upper left premolar and molar crowns are not fully imaged and the teeth are elongated (stretched). The distortion is a result of too small a vertical angulation between the X-ray beam and the occlusal plane. This periapical image was obtained with the bisecting angle technique. In addition, there is coning off in the canine region.

45. The upper left premolar and molar teeth are foreshortened (stubby). This is as a result of too large a vertical angulation between the X-ray beam and occlusal plane. This periapical image was obtained with the bisecting angle technique.

46. The radiopaque circle superimposed over the apices of the lower left incisor teeth represents the magnet on a Digora phosphor plate that is seen because the plate has been placed back to front in the patient's mouth.

Occlusal radiography

1. Intra-oral.

2. Holders are not required as the image receptor is placed onto the occlusal surfaces of the teeth and held in place by the patient gently biting together.

3. The vertex occlusal radiograph was previously used to assess the bucco-palatal position of the upper canine teeth. The X-ray beam was aimed downwards through the vertex of the skull and through the long axis of the teeth. There was direct radiation to the pituitary gland, and the lens of the eye and the reproductive organs were quite possibly in the line of the X-ray beam as well making it an undesirable X-ray projection when other forms of dental imaging at lower dose could provide the relevant information.

4. 5.7 × 7.6 cm.

5. The upper standard occlusal shows the anterior maxillary teeth and the anterior maxilla.

6. The main indications for this radiographic technique include the following:
- The periapical assessment of the incisor teeth. This may be required in patients who are unable to tolerate periapical radiographs. It is useful following dento-alveolar trauma of the anterior dentition whereby film placement and position are generally more comfortable than periapical radiographs.
- Assessment and localisation of ectopic teeth such as canines or supernumerary teeth using parallax.
- Assessment of cysts or tumours in the anterior maxilla, an example would be a nasopalatine duct cyst.

7. The patient should be seated comfortably with the head supported and the occlusal plane parallel to the floor. A thyroid collar or thyroid shield should be provided, as the thyroid gland is likely to be in the direct line of the X-ray beam.

8. The white rough surface with the raised dot should face uppermost.

9. The long axis of the receptor should be placed between the left and right corners of the mouth, therefore, across the dental arch.

10. The long axis of the receptor should be placed antero-posteriorly with respect to the dental arch.

11. The patient is asked to bite together gently to hold the image receptor in place. A firm bite may cause marks on the image receptor and degrade image quality.

12. The tubehead is positioned above the patient in the midline aiming down through the nasal bridge.

13. Approximately 65°–70°.

14. The main indications for this radiographic technique include the following:
- The periapical assessment of the posterior teeth. This may be required in patients who are unable to tolerate periapical radiographs.
- Assessment of cysts, tumours or bony abnormalities in the posterior maxilla, an example would be an odontogenic tumour.
- Dento-alveolar trauma of the posterior maxilla.
- Assessment of the antral floor on one side.
- Assessment of retained or displaced roots, supernumerary teeth or odontomes.

15. The patient should be seated comfortably with the head supported and the occlusal plane parallel to the floor. A thyroid collar or thyroid shield should be provided, as the thyroid gland is likely to be in the direct line of the X-ray beam.

16. For an upper oblique occlusal radiograph, the image receptor is placed with the long axis antero-posteriorly onto the dental side of interest. In the upper standard occlusal projection, the long axis of the receptor should be placed between the left and right corners of the mouth, therefore, across the dental arch. This however will be dependent on the size and tolerance of the patient.

17. The X-ray tubehead is aimed downwards through the cheek onto the area under investigation.

18. Approximately 65°–70°.

19. Yes, this is best practice and is a method of dose optimisation as the thyroid gland may be in the direct line of the X-ray beam.

20. There is no indication for the use of thyroid collar protection in a lower occlusal examination as the X-ray beam is directed upwards and the thyroid gland is not in the direct line of the X-ray beam.

21. True occlusal.

22. The lower 90° occlusal radiograph shows a view of the tooth-bearing portion of the mandible and the floor of the mouth.

23. The main indications for this radiographic technique include the following:
    - Assessment of the bucco-lingual position of the teeth and bucco-lingual bone anatomy in the case of cysts or tumours with related bony expansion.
    - Mandibular trauma, for example, assessing displaced mandibular fractures of the anterior mandible in the horizontal plane.
    - Detection of submandibular gland calculi in the region of the main duct.

24. The white side of the film is placed downwards in the patient's mouth, so the dual-coloured side faces upwards.

25. The patient's head should be tipped backwards as far as they are comfortable with the back of their head supported.

26. The X-ray tubehead is positioned below the patient's chin in the midline focused on an imaginary line that joins the first molar teeth at 90° to the image receptor.

27. 90°.

28. Yes, by turning the long axis of the film. As it is positioned antero-posteriorly to the relevant side of the mandible, the X-ray tubehead can be centred over the area of interest still at 90° to the image receptor.

29. Lower standard occlusal.

30. The lower 45° occlusal radiograph shows the lower anterior teeth and the anterior part of the mandible. The resultant image is similar to a bisected angle periapical radiograph of the anterior teeth, but in the occlusal image the lower border of the mandible is demonstrated.

31. The main indications for this radiographic technique include the following:
    - The periapical assessment of the anterior teeth. This may be required in patients who are unable to tolerate periapical radiographs in the floor of the mouth.
    - Assessment of cysts, tumours or bony abnormalities in the anterior mandible.
    - Dento-alveolar trauma or a displaced mandibular fracture in the vertical plane.

32. The white side of the film is placed downwards in the patient's mouth, so the dual-coloured side faces upwards.

33. The patient should be seated comfortably with the head supported and the occlusal plane parallel to the floor.

34. The X-ray tubehead is positioned in the midline aiming upwards centred on the chin.

35. 45°.

36. The lower oblique occlusal radiograph shows the region of the main submandibular gland on the side of interest. As the image is oblique, the anatomy is distorted.

37. The main indications for this radiographic technique include the following:
- Detection of submandibular gland calculi in the region of the main gland
- Assessment of cysts, tumours or bony abnormalities in the angle of the mandible.

38. The white side of the film is placed downwards in the patient's mouth, so the dual-coloured side faces upwards.

39. The long axis of the receptor should be placed antero-posteriorly with respect to the dental arch on the side of interest.

40. The patient should be seated comfortably with the head supported, the chin raised and the head rotated away from the side of interest.

41. The X-ray tubehead is aimed upwards and anteriorly towards the image receptor from below and behind the angle of the mandible. The tubehead should be parallel to the lingual surface of the mandible.

42. A specific angle is not measured, and positioning will be dependent on the anatomy of the patient and the judgement of the operator.

43. The lower 90° or true occlusal. In this examination, the patient has to tip their head backwards with the back of their head supported.

44. Lower 90° (true) occlusal.

45. Upper standard occlusal.

Panoramic radiography (PR)

1. Extra-oral.

2. A full panoramic radiograph demonstrates all of the teeth and their supporting structures.

3. The main indications for this radiographic technique in dental practice include the following:
- Assessment of a bony lesion or tooth whose size and/or position precludes its complete demonstration on intra-oral radiographs such as third molars.
- Prior to surgery under a general anaesthetic.
- Prior to a dental clearance or multiple dental extractions where the state of the dentition would make intra-oral radiography very difficult.
- As part of an orthodontic assessment to determine the condition, presence and position of teeth.
- As an adjunct to periodontal assessment where pocketing is greater than 6 mm and intra-oral radiography is either not tolerated by the patient or unavailable.
- History of trauma to the lower jaw to assess for mandibular fracture.
- Assessment in the vertical plane for implants at multiple sites.
- TMJ dysfunction, this is only indicated if there is a history of trauma preceding onset or recent evidence of progressive pathology.
- Patients who have trismus or are unable to tolerate an intra-oral film.

4. No, there is no justification for screening panoramic radiographs.

5. Other terms for the panoramic radiograph are as follows:
- Panoral
- Pantomogram
- Orthopantomogram
- OPT
- OPG
- DPT
- DPR
- PR
- PAN

6. Tomography is a technique for displaying a representation of a cross section through a human body or other solid object. In conventional medical X-ray tomography, a sectional image through a body can be created. This is achieved by moving an X-ray source and the film in opposite directions during the exposure. Consequently, structures in the focal plane appear sharper, while structures in other planes appear blurred.

7. A **tomograph** is the radiographic equipment used in tomography.

8. A **tomogram** is a radiographic image produced by tomography.

9. Dental panoramic tomography uses rotational narrow beam tomography.

10. The **focal trough** is a 3D curved zone in which structures, namely the jaws, are reasonably well demonstrated on a panoramic radiograph. A panoramic image largely consists of the anatomy located within the focal trough, structures outside of the focal trough are blurred, magnified or minified and are not clearly demonstrated.

11. The dental arches are not circular but are curved, and there are variations in jaw size, jaw relationship and curvature between individuals. A horseshoe-shaped focal trough is necessary to allow for the patient's arches (area of interest) to be positioned within the 3D space. The equipment employs narrow beam rotational tomography using two or more centres of rotation.

12. The shape and height of the X-ray beam and the size of the image receptor determine the vertical height of the focal trough.

13. No, only half of the image receptor will have been exposed. As with other forms of narrow beam tomography, a different part of the focal trough is imaged throughout the exposure. The image is created in stages as the equipment orbits around the patient's head.

14. X-ray production is continuous. Throughout the cycle, the centres of rotation required to produce the elliptical horseshoe-shaped focal trough are automatically adjusted.

15. There are four main components, namely an X-ray tubehead, a control panel, an image receptor (plus or minus carriage) and patient positioning equipment, including light beam markers and chin and head supports.

16. The operator can adjust field size and select a range of field limitation options. They can choose from a range of arch sizes and shapes dependent on patient size and can adjust the height of the equipment and also the antero-posterior position of the bite peg. In addition they can select the appropriate mA and kV.

17. Upwards.

18. Approximately 6°–8°.

19. Approximately 18 seconds.

20. Approximately 15 seconds.

21. 60–90 kV.

22. Traditional equipment uses indirect action film with intensifying screens in an extra-oral cassette. Newer image receptors include the removable phosphor plates, the removable flat solid-state sensors that fit into existing equipment (they are the same size as a cassette) and fixed solid-state sensors that are integrated within the equipment.

23. The operator must ask the patient to remove any earrings, necklaces, facial piercings, glasses, metal hairpins and removable orthodontic appliances or dentures that may cause artefact and degradation of the resultant image.

24. No.

25. The operator should explain the procedure to the patient in order to reassure them. Relevant information to relay will include the way the equipment moves and the need to remain still throughout the entire exposure.

26. The operator must position the patient accurately using the head supports, bite peg and the light beam-positioning guides.

27. Accurate positioning is critical to ensure that the teeth lie within the focal trough. If the patient is placed asymmetrically, too far forward, or too far back with respect to the image receptor, then the areas of interest may lie outside of the focal trough and hence will not be crisply displayed.

28. The tongue must be placed up to the roof of the mouth, so it contacts the palate during the full exposure time. If the tongue does not contact the palate, there will be a resultant air shadow space that will be superimposed over the apices of the maxillary teeth. This will hinder optimal assessment of that area.

29. The lips should be gently closed to prevent an air shadow space being superimposed over the incisor teeth.

30. No, the lead can cause artefact to the resultant image.

31. No, the lead can cause artefact to the resultant image.

32. A **ghost shadow** is an artefactual shadow produced by the tomographic movement and created by objects positioned between the X-ray source and the centre of rotation.

33. The right. A ghost shadow is cast on the opposite side to the real image.

34. Magnified.

35. Higher due to the upward projection of the X-ray beam.

36. Blurred.

37. The hard tissue structures that result in ghost shadows include the palate, cervical spine and posterior mandible.

38. The dental panoramic image has lower resolution than intra-oral radiography. The image represents a section of the patient, structures out of the focal trough may not be visualised or will be blurred and the clinician needs to recognise this limitation. As patients come in different shapes and sizes, certain jaws will not conform to the boundaries of the focal trough and some structures will be out of focus or distorted. There is distortion and magnification of the image as a result of tomographic movement and the distance between the image receptor and the focal trough.

Air, soft tissue and ghost shadows are superimposed over the tissues causing possible interpretation difficulties. The length of the procedure carries a risk of patient movement that can have a detrimental effect on the image. A panoramic radiograph may not be suitable for certain patients, for example, children under the age of 6 and people with certain disabilities, which may make their positioning and ability to remain still difficult.

39. The film should have integral left (L) and right (R) markings to enable accurate orientation.

40. Intra-oral radiographs.

41. A positioning error. This is however dependent on both the operator and the equipment.

42. Positioning the patient correctly is critical, the operator may compromise image quality by failing to achieve the following:
- position the patient in an upright position;
- ensure edge-to-edge incisor position on the bite peg;
- correctly align the light beam markers in the vertical or horizontal plane, thus not positioning the jaws correctly in the focal trough;
- instruct the patient to place the tongue up to the roof of the mouth and close the lips;
- instruct the patient to remain still throughout the duration of the exposure.

43. The operator must watch the patient throughout the entire X-ray exposure.

44. The anterior teeth are narrowed and are not in focus.

45. The anterior teeth are magnified in width and are not in focus. A useful phrase to remember is **too far in teeth thin, too far out teeth stout**.

46. The posterior teeth and ramus will be enlarged on one side of the image and reduced on the other. An example: if the patient's head is turned so that the left mandible is farther from the image receptor and the right side is closer, then there will be magnification of the posterior teeth and mandible on the left.

47. The image will have a 'smiley' occlusal plane with the condyles demonstrated at the upper aspect, or even excluded from the image, and the anterior teeth out of focus as they are out of the focal trough.

48. The image will have a flatter-distorted occlusal plane (opposite of the smiley appearance), splayed condyles and loss of sharpness of the maxillary incisors as they are positioned outside of the focal trough.

49. The patient is positioned too close to the image receptor, the canine line is posteriorly placed, and it should lie between the upper left lateral incisor and canine teeth. As a result, the anterior teeth will appear narrowed and not in focus.

50. The patient is positioned with chin up. The Frankfort plane is incorrect. As a result, there will be a flatter-distorted occlusal plane (opposite of the smiley appearance), splayed condyles and loss of sharpness of the maxillary incisors as they are positioned outside of the focal trough.

51. There is blurring of the right molar teeth suggesting subtle horizontal movement. In addition, the right molar teeth and mandibular ramus are magnified, which is indicative of rotation of the patient with the right mandibular ramus further away from the image receptor. The lower incisor teeth are out of focus.

52. The occlusal plane has a smiley appearance, and the right condyle is incompletely imaged at the upper aspect of the image. The chin is too low. The anterior teeth are out of focus as they are out of the focal trough.

53. There is blooming artefact of the image overlying the left and right angles of mandible. Blooming is a digital image fault caused by overexposure and overloading of the solid-state sensor. In the region where the sensor is overloaded or flooded, the image will appear black.

54. Field limitation techniques can be utilised. The clinician requires information relating to the posterior dentition, but there is no indication or justification to image the anterior maxilla and mandible. The operator can preselect parts of the patient that are to be exposed on the control panel, therefore removing unnecessary radiation dose.

55. No, there are two issues here. Firstly, the image is likely to result in movement artefact due to the patient's involuntary muscle movements, but more importantly, a panoramic radiograph is not the optimal examination for the indications provided. A paralleling periapical radiograph would be the examination of choice.

Oblique lateral radiography

1. Extra-oral.

2. An oblique lateral radiograph demonstrates the posterior maxillary and mandibular teeth and their supporting structures.

3. The main indications for this radiographic technique include the following:
   - assessment of the status of the posterior teeth;
   - assessment of the presence and position of the posterior teeth;
   - detection of mandibular fractures;
   - assessment of cysts, tumours or bony abnormalities in the posterior maxilla, an example would be an odontogenic tumour;
   - assessment of the salivary gland region;
   - use in patients that cannot tolerate intra-oral or dental panoramic radiographs.

4. Oblique lateral radiograph. It is a very useful technique to use for assessment of the posterior dentition in a young child or individual who cannot tolerate or cooperate with a panoramic radiographic exposure of 15–18 seconds.

5. Parallel.

6. Perpendicular.

7. In an oblique lateral radiograph, the sagittal plane of the patient and the image receptor are not parallel as with the true lateral projection. In both techniques, the X-ray beam is aimed perpendicular to the image receptor, but in the oblique lateral view the X-ray beam is oblique to the sagittal plane of the patient.

8. The equipment required includes the following:
   - a dental X-ray set;
   - an extra-oral cassette containing film and intensifying screens or a phosphor plate as the image receptor.

9. The cassette is held by the patient (or a carer as required) against the side of the face overlying the area of the jaws that are under investigation.

10. The patient is seated as upright as possible in the dental chair. The head is rotated to the side of interest and the chin is raised. This head positioning is required to posture the contralateral ramus forwards and to increase the space between the neck and shoulder and between the posterior ramus and the cervical spine.

11. The **radiographic keyhole** is an anatomical space between the posterior ramus and the cervical spine, the more the patient raises their chin the larger the space becomes. The X-ray beam is aimed through this space for certain oblique lateral projections.

12. Opposite side.

13. Aiming the X-ray beam through the radiographic keyhole behind the ramus means that the beam will not pass directly between the contact areas of the posterior teeth.

14. Aiming the X-ray beam beneath the lower border of the mandible will create distortion in the vertical plane as the X-ray beam is angled upwards.

15. Aiming the X-ray beam beneath the lower border of the mandible.

16. Aiming the X-ray beam through the radiographic keyhole.

17. The area of interest.

18. The operator must be informed of the area of the jaws under investigation, as this will affect the position of the cassette, the position of the patient's head and the position of the X-ray tubehead.

19. The young child may need to be seated on a carer's lap, if so they can be rotated 90° so that the cassette and their head can be supported on the adult's chest. Alternatively, the child can be rotated 90° on the chair and the backrest can support both the cassette and head in a stable position.

20. The cassette is positioned on the left side of the patient and the X-ray tubehead directed through the right radiographic keyhole to image the left posterior maxillary and mandibular teeth.

Cephalometric radiography

1. Extra-oral.

2. The lateral cephalometric radiograph demonstrates the facial soft tissue profile, the teeth, jaws and the rest of the facial skeleton including the cranial base. The upper cervical spine will be in part imaged.

3. An orthodontist.

4. The main indications for this radiographic technique include the following:
   • Orthodontics. This may include initial diagnosis, treatment planning, monitoring of treatment and then appraising treatment.
   • Orthognathic surgery. This may include preoperative assessment of the teeth, soft tissue and skeletal patterns, treatment planning and post-operative appraisal.

5. British Orthodontic Society 2008 Guidelines for the Use of Radiographs in Clinical Orthodontics. 3rd Edition. London.

6. The lateral cephalometric radiograph provides a standardised and reproducible image, whereas the lateral skull radiograph does not. This reproducibility is essential for the management of the patient during orthodontic treatment.

7. The equipment required to produce this radiograph is as follows:
   • Cephalostat – This is apparatus to stabilise the patient's head to ensure a reproducible patient position. There is a cassette holder possibly an anti-scatter grid.
   • Cassette.
   • Aluminium wedge filter.
   • X-ray generating equipment.
   • Processing equipment (if film-captured image).

8. Yes, the phosphor plate can be positioned into the cassette.

9. It can be a stand-alone unit but can be incorporated into dental panoramic equipment and cone beam computed tomography units.

10. Ear rods within the cephalostat stabilise the patient's head. Less commonly infra-orbital guide rods may be used.

11. An anti-scatter grid prevents the scattered X-ray photons from within the patient reaching the film and subsequently degrading the image.

12. An aluminium wedge filter attenuates the X-ray beam in the region of the facial tissues in order that the soft tissue profile can be demonstrated.

13. Triangular shape.

14. Computer software enhances the patient's soft tissue profile on the radiographic image.

15. Approximately 1.5–1.8 m.

16. Parallel.

17. Perpendicular.

18. Perpendicular.

19. The **Frankfort plane** is a cephalometric plane that passes through the inferior border of the bony orbit and the upper margin of the auditory meatus.

20. Parallel.

21. Perpendicular.

22. The ear rods are inserted into the external auditory meati.

23. The X-ray beam will be centred on the ear rods.

24. Cephalometric tracing provides a diagrammatic representation of anatomical points on the lateral radiograph, which can be manually or digitally recorded. It is the landmarks traced that aid the clinician in obtaining the measurements required to aid in orthodontic or orthognathic surgery treatment planning.

25. This is the Frankfort plane as described earlier. Orbitale (Or) represents the lowest point on the infra-orbital margin, and Porion (Po) relates to the superior aspect of the bony external auditory meatus.

26. The teeth should be in intercuspation.

SECTION VIII Answers: Radiological interpretation

Dental terminology

1. **Radiology** is the science that deals with diagnostic, therapeutic and research applications of high-energy radiation.

2. **Dental radiology** is the science that deals with the use of radiation in the diagnosis of dental disease.

3. **Dental radiography** is the method of producing an image or picture for intra-oral and extra-oral structures on an image receptor using X-ray.

Image interpretation

1. Dental radiographs enable the clinician to assess for the presence or absence of disease and to gain information on the extent and possible nature of a disease process. The information from a radiographic image enables the clinician to formulate a differential diagnosis and create a suitable treatment plan in the best interests of the patient.

2. Yes of course, if the radiographic image is not viewed and interpreted, then it should not have been justified and performed in the first place.

3. All radiographs should be assessed, and an accompanying written report is mandatory under the IR(ME)R 2000 regulations.

4. There may be an incidental pathological finding that is of significance to the patient that is discrete from the specific site of interest.

5. The clinician who assesses the radiograph whether that is a dentist, doctor or a radiologist.

6. If the dental nurse has performed the radiograph, then they should provide a critical assessment of the image to assess technique, exposure factors and processing and to consider the image quality rating. The quality rating will influence whether a repeat radiograph is necessary.

7. The essential requirements may be considered as follows:
   - Optimal viewing conditions.
   - Access to any previous and relevant radiographs for comparison.
   - Understanding the black, white and grey image and its limitations as a 2D representation of a 3D object, namely the patient.
   - Knowledge of the types of radiographic projections in order that technique, geometric accuracy and film quality can be assessed.
   - Knowledge of the radiographic features of normal anatomy.
   - Knowledge of the radiographic features of different pathologies.
   - A systematic approach to assessment in order to describe specific findings in a logical sequence.

8. Ask, show the dentist the image and let them decide on whether you need to repeat the exposure or use a different projection. Repeating the exposure without this relevant conversation may only result in an unnecessary radiation dose to the patient.

Optimal viewing conditions

1. The dry radiographic film should be viewed on a clean and bright viewing box in a dimly lit and quiet room.

2. Placing an appropriately sized black cardboard mount around the film on the viewing box removes the extraneous light and optimises viewing conditions.

3. Fine detailed assessment can be improved with magnification tools if using a film-captured image or by computer manipulation if digitally based.

4. The viewing box should be free of dust and debris that may superimpose onto or damage the image thereby creating artefact that hinders optimal assessment.

5. Digital radiographs should be displayed on an appropriate high-resolution monitor and should be viewed in a dimly lit and quiet room. The quality of the monitor resolution should be part of the quality control checks within the quality assurance programme.

6. The digital image can be manipulated. Sharpness, contrast and brightness, for example, can be changed to improve viewing conditions and image quality.

Radiographic anatomy of the teeth and supporting structures

1. Enamel, dentine and cementum.

2. Enamel.

3. White.

4. Black.

5. Enamel is more radiopaque than dentine.

6. Enamel is radiopaque when compared to pulp, which is radiolucent.

7. Dentine is radiopaque when compared to pulp, which is radiolucent.

8. Cementum is a very thin layer on the root surface of the tooth, it is usually not particularly apparent radiologically unless the tooth has hypercementosis.

9. The supporting structures include the lamina dura, periodontal ligament space, alveolar crest and trabecular bone.

10. The periodontal ligament space. It is radiolucent.

11. The lamina dura is a thin layer of dense bone surrounding the periodontal ligament space and tooth socket.

12. Radiopaque.

13. The trabecular or cancellous bone.

14. The alveolar crest. It is radiopaque.

15. The median palatine suture extends from the alveolar crest between the central incisor teeth and continues posteriorly to the posterior aspect of the hard palate. It appears as a thin radiolucent line with a radiopaque border.

16. It can be seen on a periapical radiograph of the central incisor teeth in the midline usually about 1.5–2 cm above the alveolar crest. It is radiopaque as it is bone and is 'V' shaped.

17. The incisive or nasopalatine foramen is located in the anterior maxilla in the midline just behind the central incisor teeth. It is oval shaped and is generally less than 6 mm in maximum dimension. As it is a foramen (a hole), it is radiolucent.

18. The healthy antral space is filled with air and therefore will be radiolucent.

19. The maxillary antral floor is a thin radiopaque line that may be in close proximity to the roots of the posterior teeth.

20. The mandible.

21. The inferior dental nerve canal can be visualised on a lower posterior periapical, a dental panoramic radiograph and a lateral oblique radiograph. It will be superimposed on a lateral cephalometric radiograph and therefore is not well visualised in this projection.

22. The nerve canal is radiolucent; however, it has a thin radiopaque periphery. These are termed tramlines.

23. A. Floor of the left maxillary sinus
   B. Left maxillary sinus space
   C. Zygomatic buttress
   D. Lamina dura of the upper left second molar
   E. Dentine of the upper left second molar
   F. Enamel of the upper left first molar
   G. Alveolar crest
   H. Amalgam restoration

24. A. Lateral wall of the nasal fossa
   B. Median palatine suture
   C. Anterior nasal spine
   D. Upper left canine
   E. Nasal fossa

25. **A.** External auditory meatus
    B. Hard palate
    C. Nasal septum
    D. Left maxillary sinus space
    E. Left condyle
    F. Left inferior dental nerve canal
    G. Hyoid bone

Dental caries

1. Intra-oral radiographs, namely, bitewings or paralleling periapicals due to the superior resolution and fine detail when compared to extra-oral images.

2. Bitewing radiographs.

3. Occlusal caries.

4. The effective dose of a panoramic radiograph will be higher than bitewing radiographs using a rectangular collimation and F speed film.

5. The clinician may wish to monitor caries progression or assess existing restorations for marginal fit and secondary caries.

6. Six monthly bitewing radiographs.

7. Yearly bitewing radiographs.

8. Bitewing radiographs every 2 years.

9. Radiolucent.

10. Radiopaque.

11. The lower the kV, the better the contrast of the image. Good contrast is required for caries assessment and, therefore, a lower kV is preferred.

12. About 40–50% demineralisation is necessary for the defect to be evident.

13. Underestimate. A carious lesion tends to be larger clinically than radiologically.

14. Inaccurate horizontal beam angulation can cause superimposition of the inter-proximal tooth surfaces that can disguise small carious lesions. Inaccurate horizontal beam angulation may also make a carious lesion in enamel appear larger.

15. The restoration may be projected over the caries as a result of the beam angulation, thus obscuring the defect on the final image. The shape of the restoration may simply obscure the caries. The radiograph is 2D, and as a result this is a limitation for caries diagnosis.

16. Cervical burnout.

17. Cervical burnout occurs at the cervical region of the teeth where the dental tissue is thin, as such there is less attenuation of the X-ray beam in these areas and very little opaque shadow is demonstrated in the cervical region on the radiographic image. The cervical area therefore appears radiolucent or burnt out.

18. Cervical burnout is located at the cemento-enamel junction (CEJ) and has demarcated boundaries extending vertically from the CEJ or restoration to the alveolar crest. Caries does not have defined boundaries. Cervical burnout generally affects multiple teeth, particularly premolars, and it has a triangular shape, whereas caries tends to be more saucerised. Clinical assessment should be able to distinguish whether caries is in fact present.

Periapical tissues and periapical disease

1. The periodontal ligament is a part of the periodontium that provides the attachment of the teeth to the surrounding alveolar bone by way of the cementum. It surrounds the root of the tooth, lying between tooth and the socket outline, the lamina dura.

2. The normal periodontal ligament appears as the periodontal space of 0.4–1.5 mm on radiographs, a radiolucent area between the radiopaque lamina dura of the alveolar bone proper and the radiopaque root.

3. The lamina dura surrounds the tooth socket.

4. A healthy lamina dura appears as a thin continuous radiopaque line surrounding the radiolucent periodontal ligament space.

5. Cancellous or spongy bone.

6. The trabecular bone lies between the cortical bone in both the maxilla and mandible. It surrounds the socket outline of the teeth and extends into the furcation region of the premolar and molar teeth.

7. A periapical radiograph, paralleling technique.

8. The panoramic radiograph shows all of the teeth and their associated periapical and periodontal tissues. Oblique lateral, cephalometric and occlusal radiographs can demonstrate root morphology and the periapical tissues of specific teeth in the dentition. Cone beam CT is a newer technology that demonstrates the apical tissues three-dimensionally.

9. The effect of the antral shadow can reduce the amount of bone that would be projected on the radiographic image, thus making the lamina dura appear less obvious or even absent and by making the periodontal ligament space more radiolucent or prominent. The space should however remain intact and continuous.

10. Examples would include the zygomatic buttress in the maxilla and the external oblique ridge of the mandible.

11. The radiopaque shadows may completely obscure the detailed anatomy of the periapical tissues.

12. If the patient's tongue is not placed up to the palate during the exposure, then there will be an air space superimposed over the apices of the maxillary teeth. The size of the air space will depend on the gap between the dorsum of the tongue and the hard palate.

13. The periodontal ligament space and lamina dura would be of normal dimension being continuous around the roots of the tooth and intact throughout. The trabecular bone would extend up to the alveolar crest at the cemento-enamel junction of the tooth.

14. In initial acute inflammation, there may be no radiological change of the periapical tissues or there may be subtle widening of the periodontal ligament space.

15. Early features of a periapical abscess would be the loss of the lamina dura at the apex of the tooth. As the inflammation spreads further, an ill-defined area of radiolucency will develop at the tooth apex.

16. There may be development of a periapical granuloma or radicular cyst at the apex of the non-vital tooth. Both will be represented as a well defined and corticated unilocular radiolucency at the apex, which is generally surrounded by dense sclerotic bone termed a sclerosing osteitis. The bone remodels around the area of inflammation as a protective mechanism/barrier. If the chronic apical area becomes acutely infected, the radiolucency will lose its corticated outline and will become irregular at its periphery.

17. FGDP (UK) 2013 Selection Criteria for Dental Radiography, 3rd Edition. Faculty of General Dental Practice (UK) of the Royal College of Surgeons of England.

18. The paralleling technique should be used, as it is a reproducible and accurate technique allowing comparison between images.

19. Yes.

20. In theory yes, unless the clinician is confident in the use of an apex locator.

21. Yes, as this will assess the quality of the obturation and importantly will act as a baseline to which further radiographs may be compared.

22. No, it should not be used routinely for the purposes of endodontic work up but may be used in selected cases whereby a high-resolution, small-volume scan could be acquired.

Periodontal tissues and periodontal disease

1. No, radiographs are used to complement the clinical assessment. A radiograph cannot assess the periodontal pocketing depths, tooth mobility, bleeding or pus that may be seen at the gingival margins during a clinical examination. A radiograph will not inform as to whether disease is active or not.

2. The main indications would include the following:
- assessment of bone loss around a tooth and whether this extends into the furcation space;
- assessment of local factors such as overhanging restorations, calculus that may be a causative factor for the clinical presentation;
- assessment of the root morphology and length if, for example, endodontic treatment or tooth extraction is indicated;
- assisting in treatment planning;
- monitoring disease progression;
- evaluating treatment outcomes, an example of which would be following periodontal surgery and guided tissue regeneration.

3. FGDP (UK) 2013 Selection Criteria for Dental Radiography, 3rd Edition. Faculty of General Dental Practice (UK) of the Royal College of Surgeons of England.

4. When the clinical examination demonstrates generalised pocketing of less than 4–5 mm (BPE 3) and little or no gingival recession.

5. When the clinical examination demonstrates generalised pocketing of 6 mm or more (BPE 4). Additional periapical radiographs should be used in areas where the periodontal bone is not demonstrated on the bitewing images.

6. Paralleling technique periapical radiograph.

7. Paralleling technique periapical radiograph.

8. The paralleling technique is standardised and reproducible, further images can be taken for comparison such as monitoring or evaluation of treatment. They provide reproducible images that can be produced at different clinical appointments and with different operators. They are geometrically accurate images with little magnification, foreshortening or elongation of the image. The holders automatically determine the horizontal and vertical angles of the X-ray tubehead and spacer cone. Accurate demonstration of the teeth and periodontal bone levels is acquired, and there is no superimposition of the zygomatic buttress overlying the tooth apices.

9. The dental panoramic radiograph is not a dose-saving examination when compared to dose-optimising periapical or bitewing radiographs. The panoramic radiograph produces distortion of the periodontal bone levels due to the upward angulation of the X-ray beam as it travels behind the patient's head. The maxillary bone on this radiographic image can appear less than it actually is and the mandibular bone can be exaggerated. The bone support of the anterior teeth (particularly if they are proclined) can be poorly demonstrated due to the narrow focal trough. Ghost shadows and artefact can also degrade assessment of the tissues, and movement artefact can produce blurring of the image.

10. A dental panoramic radiograph may be indicated if the patient cannot tolerate the intra-oral radiographs and if there is severe trismus.

11. No. Cone beam CT should not be used routinely for the purposes of periodontal bone assessment but may be considered in selected cases of an infra-bony, or furcation defect where a 3D assessment would aid in treatment planning. A small-volume, high-resolution scan would be the technique of choice.

12. For the assessment of periodontal status, the film should be underexposed when compared to caries assessment exposure factors. This is necessary to avoid burnout of the inter-dental crestal bone.

13. The crestal bone should be within 2–3 mm of the cemento-enamel junction. With age however this distance will increase. The alveolar crestal bone should be smooth and corticated, being horizontal in the posterior dentition and more tapered to a point in the anterior region. The crestal bone cortication runs continuous with the lamina dura of the teeth, and the periodontal ligament space should be thin and relatively uniform.

14. No, this can only be assessed clinically. Bone loss may represent age-related changes or represent treated or stable disease.

15. Horizontal, vertical and furcation bone defects. The extent of the bone loss can be described in a radiographic report, detailing the sites and extent of bone loss, the pattern of loss and any causative factors that are evident.

16. Radiological features of chronic periodontitis include the following:
    - loss and irregular flattening of the defined and corticated inter-dental crestal bone;
    - widening of the periodontal ligament space at the crestal level within the furcation space and inter-dentally;
    - loss of bone support either locally or in a generalised pattern;
    - vertical and horizontal bone defects on the mesial or distal root surfaces or more complicated intra-bony defects;
    - furcation bone defects;
    - secondary local factors.

17. Secondary local and complicating factors can include the following:
    - primary or secondary caries;
    - calculus;
    - overhanging restorations;
    - poorly fitting restoration margins;
    - lack of contact points;
    - impacted or tilted teeth;
    - pin or post-perforations.

18. The incisor and first molar teeth.

19. In aggressive/advanced periodontal disease, there will be rapid bone destruction, there may be large vertical bone defects and teeth may even appear as if they are floating with no structural bone support. There may be signs of a perio-endo lesion. Teeth may appear tilted or drifted.

20. Limitations include the following:
    - The image is a 2D representation of a 3D object, and therefore, it is difficult to assess the buccal and lingual/palatal bone levels. Superimposition of structures can make accurate interpretation difficult.

- Intra-bony defects cannot be fully assessed two-dimensionally.
- Burnout of the crestal bone due to overexposure. This leads to poor definition of the anatomy, and manipulation in digital imaging can help to rectify this problem.
- Geometric inaccuracies can lead to distortion of the crestal bone, and this is why reproducible images are essential.
- There is no reliable information on the soft tissues of the periodontium.

Localisation of un-erupted teeth

1. Maxillary canine teeth.

2. A tooth may fail to erupt due to limited available space in a crowded arch. Canine teeth have a long path of eruption and may not follow the correct path. Supernumerary teeth and odontomes may inhibit the path of eruption of a tooth. An odontogenic cyst or odontogenic tumour may envelop the tooth crown and cause displacement and prevent eruption.

3. **Parallax** is the way an object's position or direction seems to change depending on the viewing angle. To experience parallax, simply cover one eye and focus on a static object. Then move the cover to the other eye. As each eye provides a different viewing angle, the object will appear to move when of course it has not.

4. In dental radiography, an un-erupted canine tooth can be imaged at two different angles. This is achieved by placing the X-ray tubehead in different positions, either horizontally or vertically. The movement of the canine tooth with respect to the beam angulation can help the clinician to clarify whether the tooth is buccal or palatal to the arch.

5. **SLOB** stands for **S**ame **L**ingual **O**pposite **B**uccal. If the tooth of interest is palatally positioned, it will appear to have moved in the same direction as the X-ray tubehead. If the tooth is buccal to the arch it will appear to move in the opposite direction to the tubehead.

6. The tooth will not appear to have moved.

7. Two periapical radiographs may be used with a shift in the horizontal angulation of the X-ray tubehead. An upper standard occlusal radiograph and a periapical at different horizontal tubehead angles would also achieve horizontal parallax.

8. A dental panoramic radiograph with the tubehead angled upwards at 6°–8° and an upper standard occlusal radiograph with the tubehead angled downwards at about 65° can achieve vertical parallax.

9. Cone beam CT is often used when there are two questions. Firstly, where is the canine with respect to the arch; secondly, has this tooth caused resorption of the adjacent teeth?

Bibliography

FGDP (UK) 2013 Selection Criteria for Dental Radiography, 3rd Edition. Faculty of General Dental Practice (UK) of the Royal College of Surgeons of England.

Isaacson KG, Thom AR, Horner K, Whaites E 2008 Guidelines for the Use of Radiographs in Clinical Orthodontics, 3rd Edition. British Orthodontic Society, London.

NRPB/DH 2001 Guidance Notes for Dental Practitioners on the Safe Use of X-ray Equipment. National Radiological Protection Board/Department of Health, London.

Sedentex CT Guidelines – EC 2012. Guidelines on Cone Beam CT for Dental and Maxillofacial Radiology. European Commission of Radiation Protection.

Whaites E, Drage N 2013a Essentials of Dental Radiography and Radiology, 5th Edition. Churchill Livingston Elsevier.

Whaites E, Drage N 2013b Radiography and Radiology for Dental Care Professionals, 3rd Edition. Churchill Livingston Elsevier.

CHAPTER 6
Orthodontic dental nursing

SECTION I Questions: Anatomy useful to orthodontics

LEARNING OUTCOMES

At the end of this section, you should be able to identify any gaps in your knowledge associated with the following:

- Recognise anatomical structures useful in orthodontics
- State anatomical structures within orthodontics

Post Registration Qualifications for Dental Care Professionals: Questions and Answers, First Edition.
Nicola Rogers, Rebecca Davies, Wendy Lee, Dominic O'Sullivan and Frances Marriott.
© 2016 John Wiley & Sons, Ltd. Published 2016 by John Wiley & Sons, Ltd.
Companion Website: www.wiley.com/go/rogers/post-registration-dental-care-questions

1. Patients often like to eat and drink with their orthodontic appliances *in situ*. Name four muscles of mastication the patient would use.

2. To be able to insert an orthodontic retainer at night. Which muscles are involved in mouth opening?

3. The patient will need to close their mouth for a wax bite. Which muscles are involved in mouth closure?

4. Which nerve supplies the muscles of mastication?

5. Often when placing a photographic mirror into the patient's mouth, to take a photograph of the lower arch, we require the patient to lift their tongue behind the mirror. What is the attachment called at the floor of the mouth which joins the tongue?

6. You need a good impression of these when an upper removable appliance is required. What are the ridges on the palate called just behind the incisors?

7. When bonding a patient, it is important to have excellent moisture control. There are three salivary glands and ducts, what are they called?

Gland	Duct

8. If an orthodontic end of wire is inhaled, which lung is most likely to go into and what complication would it cause?

9. Fill in the chart on the eruption and exfoliation of the following teeth?

Primary teeth	Eruption	Exfoliation
A		
B		
C		
D		
E		

10. Fill in the chart on the formation and eruption of the following teeth?

Permanent teeth	Formation		Eruption	
	Upper	**Lower**	**Upper**	**Lower**
1				
2				
3				
4				
5				
6				
7				
8				

11. How long after eruption is the root on a permanent tooth fully formed?

12. What would be the dental age of a patient with the following teeth present?

(a) $\dfrac{6EDC21 \mid 12CDE6}{6ED321 \mid 123DE6}$

(b) $\dfrac{6E4C21 \mid 12C4E6}{6E4321 \mid 1234E6}$

(c) $\dfrac{654C21 \mid 12c456}{654321 \mid 123456}$

(d) $\dfrac{7654321 \mid 1234567}{7654321 \mid 1234567}$

SECTION II Questions: Classifications and terminology

LEARNING OUTCOMES

At the end of this section, you should be able to identify any gaps in your knowledge associated with the following:

- The causes of malocclusion
- Recognising orthodontic terminology
- Stating facts on orthodontics

1. What is Orthodontics?

2. What causes Malocclusion?

3. Write the definitions for the following molar relationships using Angles classification.
   (a) Class I
   (b) Class II
   (c) Class III

4. What is the definition to the following using the British Standard Institutes incisor classification.
    (a) Class 1
    (b) Class 2 division 1
    (c) Class 2 division 2
    (d) Class 3

5. Carl who is a 14-year-old male has attended today for an orthodontic assessment. It is noted that the lower second premolars are developmentally absent, what is the dental terminology for this?

6. List in order the most commonly missing teeth, not including the wisdom teeth.

7. Write the definitions to the following terminology
    (a) Overjet
    (b) Overbite
        (i) Complete overbite
        (ii) Incomplete overbite
    (c) Transposition
    (d) Crossbite
    (e) Scissor bite
    (f) Supernumerary.

8. Where in the mouth is the most likely place for a supernumerary to occur?

9. What is the difference between 'competent' and 'incompetent' lips?

10. How do you tell if a patient is forcing lip closure?

11. What are the typical clinical signs of a patient who sucks their thumb?

12. What is the minimum age if you classed a patient as having a prolonged habit?

13. It is important in some orthodontic treatment planning to know if the patient is about to start their pubertal growing. What age is the pubertal growth in:
    (a) Boys
    (b) Girls

14. What is anchorage?

15. Explain the different ways anchorage can be achieved.

16. Which type of tooth movement does an active removable orthodontic appliance do?

17. What do we mean by tip?

18. What do we mean by torque?

19. On average, how much root resorption will occur during each orthodontic treatment?

20. Explain how a tooth moves through bone when a light orthodontic force is placed onto the tooth through a fixed appliance.

21. How many grams of force are used for the following types of tooth movement?
   (a) Tipping
   (b) Bodily movement
   (c) Rotations
   (d) Extrusion
   (e) Intrusion.

22. What happens when too much force is placed onto a tooth?

SECTION III Questions: Records

LEARNING OUTCOMES

At the end of this section, you should be able to identify any gaps in your knowledge associated with the following:

- Identify clinical records and equipment associated with orthodontics
- State the relevant radiographs used in orthodontics
- Discuss different indices relevant to orthodontics
- Explain cephalometrics tracing and Eastman points
- List the risks and benefits in orthodontics

---

1. What clinical records do we take and why?

2. The Orthodontist goes through all the treatment options, treatment proposed, advantages/disadvantages, risks and benefits, cost, commitment, consequences of refusing treatment, unfinished treatment and long-term retention, what is this type of consent?

3. A patient has been asked if they are happy to have impressions and photographs taken for their dental notes for treatment planning. What type of consent is this?

4. A 35-year-old female had made an appointment to have orthodontic treatment, she has turned up for the appointment on time. What type of consent is this?

5. How are study models trimmed?

6. List two methods of storing orthodontic models.

7. What is a model called when it has had teeth moved on it and placed on with wax?

8. List and explain the equipment required for good clinical photographs.

9. List the relevant radiographs used in orthodontics and what they are used for.

10. Which radiographs are used for the following:
    (a) Vertical parallax
    (b) Horizontal parallax.

11. Write short notes on IOTN.

12. What is the IOTN of the following statements?
    (a) Severe contact point displacements greater than 4 mm
    (b) Defects of cleft lip and palate and other craniofacial anomalies
    (c) Increased overjet greater than 6 mm but less than or equal to 9 mm
    (d) Increased and complete overbite with gingival or palatal trauma
    (e) Increased overjet greater than 9 mm
    (f) Impeded eruption of teeth (except for third molars) due to crowding, displacement, the presence of supernumerary teeth, retained deciduous teeth and any pathological cause
    (g) Extensive hypodontia with restorative implications (more than 1 tooth missing in any quadrant) requiring pre-restorative orthodontics.

13. What can the orthodontic therapist do without the prescription of a dentist under direct access?

14. Write short notes on PAR.

15. With PAR scoring, what weighting is added to the following:
    (a) Overjet
    (b) Overbite
    (c) Centre line
    (d) Anterior segments
    (e) Buccal occlusion.

16. How is treatment success monitored?

17. What is required to do a cephalometric tracing by hand?

18. What is required to digitize a cephalometric radiograph?

19. Using the Eastman system for cephalometric tracing, what are the definitions for the following points?
    (a) A point
    (b) B point
    (c) N
    (d) S
    (e) Me
    (f) Pog
    (g) Po
    (h) Or
    (i) ANS

   (j) PNS
   (k) Go
   (l) Gn

20. A lateral cephalograph can be traced to identify the skeletal pattern. For the following, state what skeletal pattern would be using the following ANB angles.
   (a) 3°
   (b) 5°
   (c) 2°
   (d) −2°
   (e) 8°
   (f) 0°

21. What is the average MMPA using the Eastman analysis?

22. List the benefits of Orthodontic treatment.

23. Explain the risks to Orthodontic treatment.

SECTION IV Questions: Appliances

LEARNING OUTCOMES

At the end of this section, you should be able to identify any gaps in your knowledge associated with the following:

- Removable orthodontic appliances and their uses
- Functional orthodontic appliances and their uses
- Fixed orthodontic appliances and their uses
- EOT – headgear and their uses
- Retention and their uses
- TADs and their uses.

Removable appliances

1. What is the definition of a removable appliance?

2. What type of tooth movement does a removable orthodontic appliance produce?

3. List the advantages of an orthodontic removable appliance.

4. List the disadvantages of an orthodontic removable appliance.

5. What does the laboratory require to be able to fabricate an upper removable appliance?

6. List what is required for the fitting of an orthodontic removable appliance.

7. Name the component and describe what it does and the size of the wire used (Figure 6.1).

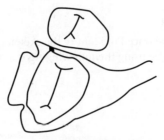

Figure 6.1

8. Name the component and describe what it does and the size of the wire used (Figure 6.2).

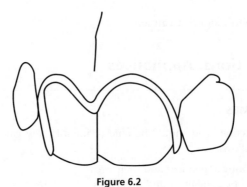

Figure 6.2

9. Name the component and describe what it does and the size of the wire used (Figure 6.3).

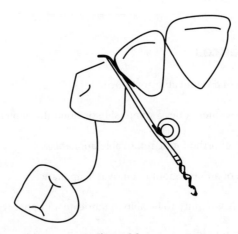

Figure 6.3

10. Name the component and describe what it does and the size of the wire used (Figure 6.4).

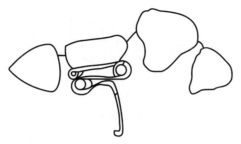

Figure 6.4

11. Name the component and describe what it does and the size of the wire used (Figure 6.5).

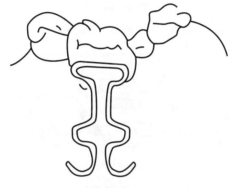

Figure 6.5

12. Name the component and describe what it does and the size of the wire used (Figure 6.6).

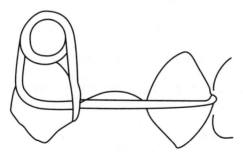

Figure 6.6

13. Name the component and describe what it does and the size of the wire used (Figure 6.7).

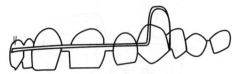

Figure 6.7

14. Name the component and describe what it does and the size of the wire used (Figure 6.8).

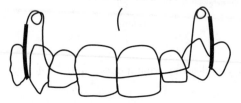

Figure 6.8

15. Name the component and describe what it does and the size of the wire used (Figure 6.9).

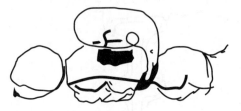

Figure 6.9

16. How does a Khloen bow get fitted to an upper removable appliance?

17. What acronym does the Orthodontist use to design a removable orthodontic appliance, and what do the letters stand for?

18. Why would an anterior bit plane be placed on an URA?

19. How would the Orthodontist know if the removable appliance is being worn?

20. How often should a patient attend with an active removable appliance *in situ*?

21. What instructions would be given to the patient once the appliance has been fitted?

Functional appliances

1. At what stage is a functional appliance fitted to produce the best dental changes?

2. What does a functional appliance do?

3. What effects can a functional appliance have on a growing patient?

4. List four removable functional appliances?

5. List two fixed functional appliances?

6. Name the two types of bites that need to be taken for a functional appliance.

7. Which measurements will the Orthodontist take at a review functional appointment.

8. For a compliant patient wearing their functional appliances, how long would you expect this phase of treatment to be?

9. What angle are the blocks on a Clarks Twin Block?

10. When the functional appliance phase has been completed, what would the Orthodontist expect to see posteriorly?

Fixed appliances

1. What is the definition of a fixed orthodontic appliance?

2. What are the advantages of a fixed orthodontic appliance?

3. What are the disadvantages of a fixed orthodontic appliance?

4. What materials can a bracket be made from?

5. Name the four component features of a straight wire bracket.

6. Name the three features that a bracket can do.

7. List three prescription types available on the market for a preadjusted edgewise bracket

8. Why does the Orthodontist invert the brackets on the upper lateral incisors?

9. What is the difference between passive and active self ligating brackets?

10. What are ceramic brackets made from?

11. What are the problems with ceramic brackets?

12. What are the stages of fixed appliance treatment.

13. Describe the shapes and materials that archwires are processed?

14. What size archwire is normally used for initial levelling and alignment of arches?

15. What are the properties of a NiTi archwire?

16. With heat activated archwires, what does TTR stand for?

17. What are the properties of a stainless steel archwire?

18. Name the following component and describe which instrument is used in conjunction with the placement onto a tooth (Figure 6.10).

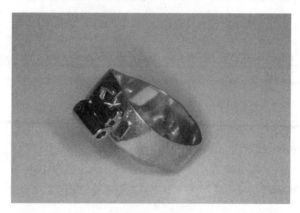

Figure 6.10

19. Name the following component and describe which instrument is used in conjunction with the placement onto a tooth (Figure 6.11).

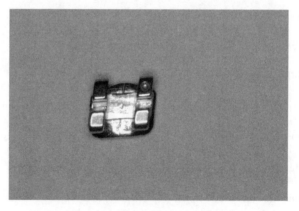

Figure 6.11

20. Name the following component and describe which instrument is used in conjunction with the placement of it (Figure 6.12).

21. Name the following component (Figure 6.13).

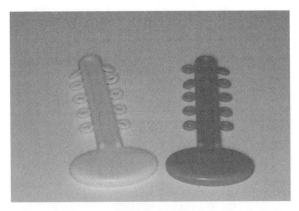

Figure 6.12

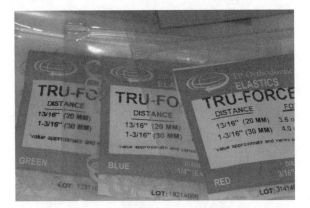

Figure 6.13

22. Name the following components and describe which instruments are used in conjunction with the placement (Figure 6.14).

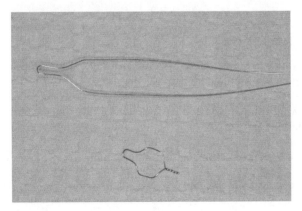

Figure 6.14

23. Name the following component and describe which instrument is used in conjunction with the placement (Figure 6.15).

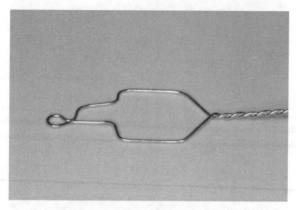

Figure 6.15

24. Name the following component, describe which instrument is used in conjunction with the placement and what the main purpose of this component is (Figure 6.16).

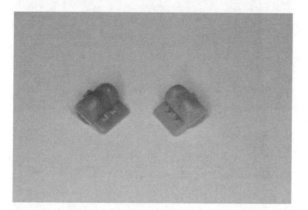

Figure 6.16

25. Name the following component, describe which instrument is used in conjunction with the placement and what the component does (Figure 6.17).

26. Name the following components and describe which instruments are used in conjunction with the placement (Figure 6.18).

27. What is the procedure in cementing an orthodontic band?

28. What instructions would you give to a patient after they have been fitted with a fixed appliance and an 0.014″ NiTi.

29. What is meant by finishing and detailing?

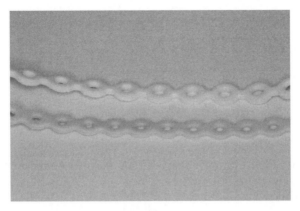

Figure 6.17

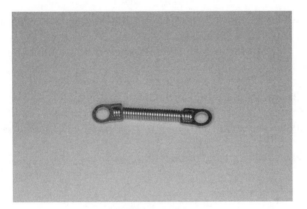

Figure 6.18

30. How are class II intra oral elastics worn?

31. How are class III intra oral elastics worn?

32. What is a box elastic?

33. What is a quadhelix used for?

34. What is a palatal arch used for?

35. What is a lingual arch used for?

Headgear – EOT

1. What is the definition of headgear?

2. What does EOA stand for?

3. What does EOT stand for?

4. How many hours a day should headgear be worn for EOA?

5. How many hours a day should headgear be worn for EOT?

6. How many grams of force does headgear require for EOT?

7. How many grams of force does headgear require for EOA?

8. What is the name of the instrument that measures the force on the modules for headgear?

9. What are the components for conventional EOT?

10. What are the three directions of pull a headgear can achieve?

11. What instructions would you give to a patient at the 'fitting' of a headgear.

12. What would you lay out for the orthodontist when they are fitting a headgear on a fixed appliance?

13. What does headgear reinforce during orthodontic treatment?

14. How many safety devices are recommended when the patient wears headgear?

15. How is a headgear fitted to a fixed orthodontic appliance?

Retention

1. What is the aim of retention and list the common types of retainers

2. When is retention planned for by the orthodontist?

3. How long is the retention period?

4. How is a vacuum-formed retainer constructed from debond to fit.

5. What instructions would you give to a patient who has just had removable retainers fitted.

6. What type of retention is commonly used to hold migrating teeth?

7. How is a bonded retainer attached to the upper 3-3?

8. Why is a Hawley-type retainer used rather than a vacuum formed retainer?

9. What is relapse?

10. What instructions would you give to a patient after they have been fitted with a bonded retainer?

TADs

1. What does TAD stand for?

2. What does it do?

3. How is a TAD placed?

4. What must the orthodontist take care about when placing the TAD?

SECTION V Questions: Interdisciplinary care

LEARNING OUTCOMES

At the end of this section, you should be able to identify any gaps in your knowledge associated with:

- Explain different interdisciplinary care treatment options.
- Explain the different advice given to patients.
- State the risks of surgery.

1. What do we mean by interdisciplinary care?

2. Which records are required for orthognathic planning?

3. What items are available to help the patient decide on treatment options and play a key role in informed consent?

4. What is the sequence of treatment for orthodontics and a surgical approach?

5. What are the objectives for combined orthodontics and orthognathic surgery?

6. List the risks of orthognathic surgery.

7. What advice would you give to a patient post operatively?

8. What is Genioplasty?

9. Name two common types of osteotomy.

10. Explain the difference between open and closed surgery for ectopic canines.

11. Which problems are likely to be seen on the orthodontic/restorative multidisciplinary clinic for assessment?

12. If upper laterals are missing what are the two options?

13. When a patient is going to have an implant what is important for the orthodontist to plan for?

14. What is important to look at if the patient has migrating teeth due to loss of periodontal support?

15. When the treatment for migrating teeth has been completed, what can the patient not like as much?

16. At what age would a baby with a cleft lip and palate have their lip repaired?

17. What is the prevalence of cleft lip and palate in Caucasians?

SECTION I Answers: Anatomy useful to orthodontics

1. **(a)** Masseter
   (b) Temporalis
   (c) Lateral pterygoid
   (d) Medial pterygoid.

2. Lateral pterygoid muscles (assisted by the digastric and mylohyoid muscles).

3. Contraction of masseter, temporalis and medial pterygoid muscles.

4. Mandibular division of the trigeminal nerve.

5. Lingual fraenum.

6. Rugae.

7.

Gland	Duct
Parotid	Stensons
Sub-mandibular	Whartons
Sub-lingual	Rivinus

8. Right lung as it is the straightest route. It could cause an infection/cyst on the lung and the patient would feel unwell.

9.

Primary teeth	Eruption	Exfoliation
A	6 months	6–7 years
B	9 months	7–8 years
C	12 months	9–12 years
D	18 months	9–11 years
E	24 months	10–12 years

10.

Permanent teeth	Formation		Eruption	
	Upper	Lower	Upper	Lower
1	3–4 months	3–4 months	7 ½ years	6 ½ years
2	10–12 months	3–4 months	8 ½ years	7 ½ years
3	4–5 months	4–5 months	11 ½ years	10 ½ years
4	1 ½ years	2 years	10–11 years	10–12 years
5	2 years	2 ½ years	10–12 years	11–12 years
6	Birth	Birth	6 years	6 years
7	3 years	3 years	12–13 years	12–13 years
8	8–10 years	8–10 years	17+ years	17+ years

11. 3 years

12. (a) 9 years
    (b) 10 years
    (c) 11 years
    (d) 12 years.

SECTION II Answers: Classifications and terminology

1. Orthodontics comes from the Greek word for straight teeth. It is the study of the variation of the development and growth of the structures of the face, jaws and teeth.

2. Genetic – missing teeth, growth or cleft
   Soft tissues – lips, cheeks and tongue
   Habits – digit habit
   Dental – crowding, early loss.

3. (a) Class I = The mesio-buccal cusp of the upper first molar occludes with the buccal groove of the lower first molar.
   (b) Class II = The mesio-buccal cusp of the upper first molar occludes anterior to the buccal groove of the lower first molar.
   (c) Class III = The mesio-buccal cusp of the upper first molar occludes posterior to the buccal groove of the lower first molar.

4. (a) Class 1 = The lower incisor tip lies on or immediately below the cingulum plateau of the upper central incisor.
   (b) Class 2 division 1 = The lower incisor tip lies posterior to the cingulum plateau of the upper central incisor. The upper central incisors are proclined or of average inclination. Therefore, the overjet is increased.
   (c) Class 2 division 2 = The lower incisor tip lies posterior to the cingulum plateau of the upper central incisor. The upper central incisors are retroclined. Therefore, the overbite is increased.

(d) Class 3 = The lower incisor tip lies anterior to the cingulum plateau of the upper central incisor. The upper central incisors bite edge to edge or the patient has a reverse overjet.

5. Hypodontia

6. Lower second premolars
   Upper lateral Incisors
   Upper second premolars
   Lower incisor.

7. **(a)** Overjet – the distance between the upper and lower incisors in the horizontal plane.
   (b) Overbite – vertical overlap of the upper and lower incisors when viewed anteriorly: one-third to one-half coverage of the lower incisors is normal.
   (i) Complete overbite – the lower incisors occlude with the upper incisors or palatal mucosa.
   (ii) Incomplete overbite – the lower incisors do not occlude with the opposing upper incisors or the palatal mucosa when the buccal segment teeth are in occlusion.
   (c) Transposition – the interchange in the position of two teeth.
   (d) Crossbite – a discrepancy in the buccolingual relationship of the upper and lower teeth. By convention, the transverse relationship of the arches is described in terms of the position of the lower teeth relative to the upper teeth.
   (e) Scissor bite – the buccal cusps of the lower teeth occlude lingual to the lingual cusps of the upper teeth (this can also be known as a lingual crossbite).
   (f) Supernumerary – a tooth which is one that is additional to the normal series.

8. In the midline of the palate near the central incisors.

9. Competent lips – when the lips are at rest, they come together easily and form an oral seal.
   Incompetent lips – when the lips are at rest they do not meet.

10. The chin looks like orange peel, and this is due to the mentalis muscle forcing closure.

11. Narrowing of maxillary arch and widening of mandibular arch
    Posterior crossbite
    Increased overjet
    Reduced overbite and asymmetrical anterior open bite
    Class II buccal segment.

12. 7 years

13. **(a)** Boys = 14 years (standard deviation 2 years)
    (b) Girls = 12 years (standard deviation 2 years).

14. Anchorage is the resistance to unwanted tooth movement – (Proffit).
    For every action there is an equal and opposite reaction (third law) – (Newton).

15. Simple – large tooth used against smaller

Compound – a number of teeth tied together and other structures usually acrylic base

Reciprocal – sets of teeth to move against or towards each other

Intermaxillary – teeth in one arch used for traction in other arch

Extra-oral – headgear

Absolute anchorage– Implants (TADS).

16. Mainly tilt teeth, but can also be used to intrude or extrude teeth.

17. Tip is the mesio–disto angulation of the tooth.

18. Torque is the labio-palatal angulation of the tooth by twisting the tooth around a centre of rotation.

19. 1–2 mm

20. 1–5 seconds – PDL is compressed on the pressure side and blood flow is altered.

Minutes – cell proliferation occurs within the periodontal ligament in areas of compression. Prostaglandins and cytokines are released, and osteoclasts migrate in from the surrounding blood vessels and resorb the bone.

Hours – changes occur and enzyme levels change.

2 days – tooth movement begins and fibroblasts and osteoblasts remodel the bone on the tension side where the PDL fibres have stretched.

Days – remodelling and reattachment of PDL fibres and calcification of osteoid into mature bone occurs

21. **(a)** 30–60 g
    (b) 100–150 g
    (c) 50–75 g
    (d) 50–75 g
    (e) 15–25 g

22. On the pressure side, the blood vessels are compressed which results in the death of the PDL:

Hyalinisation occurs and there is no tooth movement for 2–3 weeks

Undermining resorption occurs

Teeth become tender

Loss of vitality.

SECTION III Answers: Records

1. Notes – Written dental chart/examination – to have a reference point at the start of treatment. For medico legal – to cover treatment options/decisions.

Medical History – legal requirement, so that you can be prepared for a medical emergency and to see if there is any contraindication to treatment.

Previous orthodontic treatment – as they would have already had 1–2 mm of root resorption so this would need to be checked. Compliance with treatment and retention.

Previous trauma – the tooth would need to be moved slower as the pulp could die and the tooth changes colour.

Photographs – as a reference point and to show tooth shape and existing marks on the teeth.

Study models – assist in assessment and treatment planning, pre-treatment record.

Radiographs – to check presence, position and pathology of the patients dentition and surrounding structures.

All taken to assist with the high quality of patient care.

Can be used for research/audit and teaching.

2. Informed consent = it is good practice to get the patients to sign for this as well. If under the age of 16 to get both parties to sign, the patient and the parent.

3. Expressed consent.

4. Implied consent.

5. Gnatho statically trimmed.

6. Model box – either alphabetically or numerical
   Digital study model storage.

7. A Kesling set–up.

8. Digital camera with a macro lens and ring flash – to be able to take good close-up photos with minimal shadows so the photos are a good representation of the patient.

   Retractors – good retractors to be able to retract the soft tissues so that there is a good view of the teeth and supporting structures.

   Photographic mirrors – warmed in water to prevent condensation so that the biting surfaces and palatal/lingual surfaces plus soft tissues are clear and taken at 45° to the mirror.

9. DPT/OPG – shows the presence of primary and permanent teeth and in what stage of development they are. It confirms the absence of teeth. The position of the teeth and where the roots lie. The pathology is also clear as it will show apical condition, whether there are caries, any cysts and also supernumerary teeth. Shows the TMJ.

   Lateral cephalometrics – this is taken from the side of the head with the Frankfort plane horizontal to the floor. It is standardised so that it can be measured accurately. Used to trace or digitise from to plan Osteotomy surgery. Measurements can be taken to show the labial segment angulations, skeletal pattern, MMPA and facial proportions.

   Standard Anterior Occlusal (upper or lower)
   - Identification of abnormal pathology
   - Used to see any supernumerary teeth
   - Used in conjunction with an OPT as a parallax to see if a tooth may be buccal or palatal
   - To show presence of unerupted teeth (vertical parallax localisation either with an OPT or periapical film)
   - Bone in the palate (Cleft patients).

   Periapical
   - Assess root morphology
   - Check bone around a tooth – especially patients with periodontal problems

- Assess root resorption
- Assess apical pathology
- In combination with second periapical or standard occlusal to localise unerupted teeth by horizontal parallax.

Bitewings
- Used to check decayed molars or premolars

10. **(a)** DPT and Standard Occlusal
    (b) DPT and periapical or two periapicals.

11. It stands for the **Index of Orthodontic Treatment Need**
    It is divided into two components.
    1. **Dental Health Component** – This has five categories:
       (i) no need
       (ii) little need
       (iii) moderate need
       (iv) great need
       (v) very great need.
       The worst feature of the malocclusion is recorded, and this is decided from the acronym MOCDO:
    - Missing teeth
    - Overjets
    - Crossbites
    - Displacements (contact point)
    - Overbite
    - Buccal occlusion
       There is a ruler to help with assessment of the dental health component.
    2. **Aesthetic component** – This uses 10 colour photographs:
    - 1 – most attractive
    - 10 – least attractive.
       IOTN is used for acceptance for NHS treatment.
       Currently accepted – all 4's and 5's (DHC) and a 3 (DHC) with a 6 (AC)

12. **(a)** 4d
    (b) 5p
    (c) 4a
    (d) 4f
    (e) 5a
    (f) 5i
    (g) 5h

13. IOTN for the patient

14. Stands for Peer Assessment Rating.
    Used to check improvement from pre-treatment to post-treatment.
    Measurements should be done by a 'calibrated' person.
    Use study models to take measurements from.
    Scores are assigned to the various occlusal traits that make up the malocclusion.
    Some scores are weighted.

Individual scores are summed up to obtain a total that represents the degree, a case that deviates from the normal alignment and occlusion.

Score of zero indicates a good result and a higher score indicates increased levels of irregularity.

Score of change >70% is a greatly improved result.

Scores are made up by using a 'special PAR ruler' to measure the distance between contact points, and also doing other measurements by grading to specific scores, for example, antero-postero, vertical and overjet.

Used as an 'audit' tool.

15. (a) ×6
    (b) ×2
    (c) ×4
    (d) ×1
    (e) ×1

16. The outcome of orthodontic treatment can be monitored in terms of occlusal changes with PAR (Peer Assessment Rating). The pre- and post-treatment models should be assessed. A reduction of greater than 30% shows improved occlusal changes, or 22 points or greater.

17. Lateral cephalometric radiograph
    A lightbox
    Tracing paper
    Masking tape
    Sharp HB pencil
    Pencil sharpener
    Eraser
    Ruler
    Protractor
    Darkened room.

18. A digital cephalometric radiograph
    Software
    Computer
    Mouse.

19. (a) A point – point of deepest concavity on the anterior profile of the maxilla
    (b) B point – point of deepest concavity on the anterior surface of the mandible
    (c) Nasion – most anterior point of the frontal suture
    (d) Sella Turcica – midpoint of the sella turcica (Turkish saddle)
    (e) Menton – lowest point on the mandibular symphysis
    (f) Pogonion – most anterior point on the mandibular symphysis
    (g) Porion – upper and outermost point on the bony external auditory meatus
    (h) Orbital – most inferior anterior point of the margin of the orbit
    (i) Anterior Nasal Spine – the tip of the anterior process of the maxilla situated at the lower margin of the nasal aperture

(j) Posterior Nasal Spine – the tip of the posterior nasal spine of the maxilla
(k) Gonion – most posterior inferior point on the angle of the mandible
(l) Gnathion – most anterior and inferior point on the mandibular symphasis

20. (a) $3°$ = Class I
    (b) $5°$ = Class II
    (c) $2°$ = Class I
    (d) $-2°$ = Class III
    (e) $8°$ = Class II
    (f) $0°$ = Class III

21. 27^0 ±5

22. **Dental disease**: To reduce dental decay – with difficult areas to clean and a poor diet in susceptible children, improving their malocclusion may increase the potential for natural tooth cleansing and ease of cleaning, therefore reducing the risk of caries.

Periodontal disease: This disease – overcrowding, especially in the lower incisor region, may lead to teeth being squeezed lingually or buccally out of their investing bone, therefore reducing periodontal support. Traumatic occlusion within standing incisors can cause gingival recession.

Improve appearance/psychological benefit: Appearance of teeth – dento-facial anomalies have a negative effect on confidence and self-esteem. Therefore, treatment can be of huge benefit for the patient so they can stand taller and smile.

Restore position/function/distribute the forces of mastication evenly over all the teeth: Where teeth are out of alignment, treatment is designed to restore their position and function. Anterior openbites and those with large or reversed overjets may have difficulty incising food. Therefore, treatment is beneficial as this distributes the forces of mastication evenly over all the teeth.

Also where teeth are misaligned or unerupted the benefit of having all the teeth in the arch is that, for example, unerupted canines do not resorb the upper lateral roots.

Ease of cleaning: Cleaning of the teeth – crowding and displaced teeth can increase the risk of decay. However, research has shown than an individual's motivation has more impact than tooth alignment upon effective tooth brushing.

23. **Pain**: As teeth move, the patient may experience an ache. This can be for approximately 2–12 days. It will normally start about 4 hours after the patient has left the surgery.

Pulp damage: If the patient has had previous trauma to the tooth or the tooth is moved too quickly, then the pulp could die and cause pain and swelling. The tooth can discolour.

Decalcification: If patient neglects the need to keep their brace/teeth adequately clean, or have a high-sugar diet, they are at risk of developing decalcification and/or caries.

Periodontal problems: If a patient neglects to look after their appliance, teeth and surrounding gingivae, they are at risk of gum infections and possibly periodontal disease that is irreversible.

Enamel damage: Patients who have ceramic brackets on can wear the opposing teeth. On debond of ceramic brackets, enamel may fracture. Those with tongue piercing can wear a 'V' into the incisal tip.

Traumatic ulceration: It can occur if the appliance or archwire is rubbing the soft tissues constantly, especially the distal ends of archwires if they are left too long.

Allergic reaction: Patient could possibly have an adverse reaction on materials used in the dental practice such as nickel (e.g. in NiTi wires or brackets), latex (e.g. in tubing, gloves).

Root resorption: Root resorption is inevitable during orthodontic treatment. Usually 1–2 mm per course of treatment. However, a small proportion of patients will experience excessive root resorption that may compromise the life expectancy of a tooth. Factors associated with root resorption include the amount of root movement that takes place, long or narrow roots, atypically shaped roots, and the use of elastics and nail biting. Previous trauma to a tooth. If root resorption does occur during treatment, patients can be assured that it will stop and not progress once the appliances have been removed.

Exposure of canines: The canines could be ankylosed and therefore unable to be pulled into alignment of the arch.

Failure to complete treatment: This will leave the patient with incomplete treatment, which means the end result may not be stable.

Relapse: If patient does not follow retention instructions, then there is the risk of teeth relapsing.

SECTION IV Answers: Appliances

Removable appliances

1. An appliance that can be easily removed from the patient's mouth.

2. Tipping of the crowns of the teeth, overbite reduction, crossbite correction, extrusion and intrusion.

3. It can be put together in the laboratory, which makes it inexpensive.

   It is simple to adjust and therefore requires little clinical time.

   It is safe. If troublesome, it can be removed for short periods by the patient.

   It is removed for cleaning; therefore, oral hygiene is seldom a problem.

   It is removed for contact sports; therefore, damage to the patient (and appliance) is reduced to a minimum.

   If damaged, it can be repaired fairly easily, either in the Dental Surgery or in the Laboratory. Should it be beyond repair, the appliance may be adapted so that orthodontic progress is retained while a new appliance is constructed.

   Anchorage is increased by covering the palate with acrylic.

   Is used for overbite reduction in a growing child.

   Acrylic can be thickened to form anterior bite plane or buccal capping.

   Useful as a passive retainer or space maintainer.

   Is used in mixed dentition where mobile teeth may mean that a fixed appliance is not possible.

   Can be used in conjunction with a fixed appliance.

4. They tend to be bulky and take time to get accustom to.

   They are unsuitable for most treatment in the lower arch, as the shape of the lower molar teeth is quite bulbous and makes the appliance harder to retain, and also it is difficult to tolerate because of encroachment on tongue space.

Removable appliances push teeth, therefore only tilting movements possible.

Patients can remove the appliance and forget to place back.

A good technician is required.

The patient will lisp a while when they start to wear it.

The patient will produce more saliva when the appliance is fitted.

Intermaxillary traction is not practicable.

They are ineffective for multiple individual tooth movements.

5. It needs an alginate impression that includes all the upper teeth, sulcus and muscle attachments and a good impression of the palate showing all the anatomy including rugae.

    From this, they will cast up a working model from stone and fabricate the appliance from the design on the laboratory card.

    It is important to put the 'fit' date on the card so that it is ready for the date of the appointment.

6. Patients notes, models, X-rays

    Working model and appliance

    Mirror, Probe, Tweezers

    Stainless Steel Ruler

    Dividers

    Chinagraph Stick

    Adams Universal Pliers (No. 64) – to adjust molar clasps

    Adams Springforming Pliers (No. 65) – to adjust and modify springs

    Mauns Heavy Duty Wire Cutters – to shorten springs

    Articulating paper – if bite plane or teeth on appliance

    Straight handpiece and acrylic bur – to relieve acrylic to permit tooth movement

    Full face mirror – so that the patient can see how to remove and replace the appliance

    Photographs and examples of orthodontic appliances

    Instructions for the care of removable orthodontic appliances.

7. **Adams Crib**: A retaining clasp designed for molars, although sometimes found on premolars as well. It is used to grip a tooth to maintain the appliance. The crib is usually fabricated in hard 0.7 mm stainless steel wire and should engage about 1 mm of undercut. On primary molars, 0.6 mm stainless steel wire is used.

8. **Southend Clasp**: Is usually used around the upper anterior teeth. The Southend Clasp is used to retain the appliance in place or to maintain a space between posterior and anterior teeth. It is designed to utilize the undercut beneath the contact point between two incisors. It is usually fabricated in 0.7 mm or 0.8 mm hard stainless steel wire.

9. **Palatal Spring, Finger Spring or Cantilever Spring**: This is the commonest type of spring used for moving canines and premolars along the line of the arch either mesially or distally, usually used in conjunction with a labial bow to help guide the tooth around the arch, this prevents buccal flaring of the tooth. Made from 0.5 mm stainless steel wire. On a molar, 0.6 mm stainless steel wire is used, for example, on a nudger appliance.

10. **Z Spring**: The Z spring takes its name from the shape of the spring. It is used for moving instanding incisors forward into their correct position. It is a small double cantilever spring made from 0.5 mm stainless steel wire. The orthodontist can alter the direction of movement. They will activate the spring by 1–2 mm from the baseplate at an angle of 45 degrees in the direction of the desired movement. It is important that good anterior retention is required to resist the displacing effect of the spring.

11. **T Spring**: This spring also takes its name from its shape. It is used for buccal movement of a single premolar or molar. Good retention is required to resist the displacing effect of the spring. To activate, the orthodontist will pull the spring away from the acrylic at a 45 degree angle. It is made from 0.5 mm stainless steel wire.

12. **Buccal Spring Retractor**: This is a retractor, which is used when a canine needs to be moved palatally. The spring approaches the tooth from the buccal side to nudge the canine distally and palatally into the arch. Can be constructed with 0.5 mm tubed or 0.7 mm stainless steel wire.

13. **Labial Bow**: This is a wire running around the incisors, usually extending from the distal of the canines. It is useful for anterior retention. It will help guide tooth movement along the arch to prevent buccal flaring. It is used for retaining the appliance and can also be modified to retract the incisor teeth during later stages of treatment. The bow is made out of 0.7 mm or 0.8 mm stainless steel wire.

14. **Roberts Retractor**: This is used to retract proclined incisors. This spring is made from 0.5 mm stainless steel wire sheathed with tubing distal to the coils. It can be difficult to repair and requires an adequate depth of sulcus. To activate, the orthodontist bends the arms of the spring towards the incisors.

15. **Plint Clasp**: This clasp is used in conjunction with molar bands to engage under the tube assembly. It is made from 0.7 mm stainless steel wire. The orthodontist adjusts it by moving the clasp under the molar tubes.

16. Tubes are soldered onto the cribs for the Khloen bow, this is called an Adams crib with buccal tube.

17. A – Anchorage

    R – Retention

    A – Active

    B – Baseplate

18. To reduce the overbite by propping open the bite anteriorly, so that the molars and premolars can erupt more.

19. Wear facets on the bite plane.

    The acrylic looks dull.

    The cribs will be looser and require tightening.

    The overbite will be reducing or teeth will move over the bite.

Marks on the palate (post-dam).

Pt can speak in it.

Pt can insert and remove easily without a mirror.

20. Every 6–10 weeks

21. Wear as prescribed by the Orthodontist.
   OH
   - Clean teeth and appliance after eating – luke warm soapy water on appliance as toothpaste is abrasive.
   - Always rinse after food or drink.
   - Clean your palate as well.

   Diet
   - No sticky, hard or sugar foods. Definitely no chewing gum
   - No fizzy drinks
   - Fruit juices as meal times only
   - Limit snacks
   - Water or milk in between meals.

   Pain
   - It may ache for a few days – perseverance is the answer and whatever they take for a headache.

   Breakage
   - Remove for contact sports.
   - If not in mouth, keep in a rigid container.
   - Avoid 'clicking' the appliance in the mouth. Always remove and place as you have been directed.
   - If you cannot wear then come back earlier than next appointment.
   - Lost and damaged appliances may have a charge to replace or fix.

   May lisp for a few days – read out loud and your speech will improve quickly.

   Will produce more saliva for first few days – this is normal.

   Keep appointments.

   Dental 'check-ups' with GDP still recommended.

   Written instruction sheets to be handed to patient.

Functional appliances

1. At pubertal growth.

2. Uses the forces generated by the muscles of mastication, and other facial muscles, to achieve occlusal changes.

3. Maxillary restraint
   Accelerates mandibular growth
   Glenoid fossa remodelling
   Dento-alveolar effects.

4. Clarks Twin Block

Newport Twin Block

Andresen

Harvold

Frankel

Dynamax

Bionator

Monoblock

MOA – Medium Opening Activator.

5. Dynamax – lower part

Twin Block

Herbst

Advanc Sync.

6. Normal wax bite in centric occlusion

Postured wax bite.

7. Molar relationship

Overjet.

8. 6–9 months.

9. 70%.

10. Posterior Open Bite

Molars either Angles Class I or Class III.

Fixed appliances

1. An orthodontic appliance that is fixed to the teeth and cannot be removed by the patient.

2. Bodily tooth movement – this gives the orthodontist controlled movement in all three planes: in/out, tip and torque.

   Tooth movement that are not possible with removable appliances, for example, rotations.

   Worn all the time – patients should not be able to remove during treatment, therefore treatment can be completed quicker.

   They are less bulky than the acrylic on the palate of removable appliances, so they are easier to speak in.

   Easier for treatment in lower arch due to the brackets being attached to the teeth.

   Can move blocks of teeth at the same time.

   Better occlusal results are achievable, for example, with intra-oral elastics to help to inter-cuspate the occlusion together.

   During contact sports the fixed appliance can be used as a mouthguard, therefore reducing the chance of evulsion of a tooth.

? Greater stability of results – this is because the crowns and roots are placed into a better position than a removable appliance, because of bodily tooth movement, which gives a more stable result.

3. They are expensive and time consuming during construction.

If damaged the patient must come in straight way to get it repaired. Otherwise their teeth may move incorrectly.

Oral hygiene is difficult as there is a lot of parts to clean around. But it is possible.

Can look quite cumbersome to others, and therefore aesthetics can be a problem.

Cannot be removed by the patient even if in pain, so there is no release.

There is a greater risk of damage to teeth – decalcification from bad Oral Hygiene. Root shortening by 2 mm or more.

The clinic needs to carry a large inventory of stock and instruments.

Risk of inhalation/ingestion if bond failure occurs – will go through the system if ingested, if inhaled will go into right lung as this is a straighter root.

When adjusted, it will cause some pain initially.

Specialist Orthodontist treatment only.

4. Stainless Steel
Ceramic
Polycarbonate
Polyurethane

5. Identification marker, tie wing, archwire slot and bracket base.

6. First-order control – in/out
Second-order control – mesial/distal tip
Third-order control – crown inclination or torque.

7. MBT
Roth
Andrews
Damon

8. Used on palatally placed lateral incisors so that the prescription value reverses the torque in the bracket.

9. With passive gate on the bracket, the archwire has to go in easily without being pushed into the slot and therefore we have less friction. With an active bracket, the gate pushes the archwire into the slot.

10. Aluminium Oxide
   • Polycrystalline
   • Monocrystalline
   Zirconium Oxide
   • Polycrystalline

11. The tie wings can fracture during an archwire change.

    Tooth wear from the opposing bracket.

    The bracket can fracture on debond and bits of the bracket can fly across the room into eyes or can be inhaled by the patient and they are not radiopaque.

    The enamel on the tooth can fracture on debond.

12. Alignment and levelling

    Continued levelling and overbite reduction

    Space closure and molar relationship

    Finishing

    Retention

13. They are made from different materials, for example, NiTi, Stainless steel, beta titanium, Teflon coated.

    They came in various sizes. Round, for example, 0.014"; Square, for example, 0.020"×0.020"; or rectangular, for example, 0.019"×0.025".

    They arrive in straight lengths, on a coil or preformed.

    Some stainless steel wires are posted for auxiliaries.

    Some have preformed loops placed.

    Some have a reverse curve already placed, usually in rectangular NiTi. Also known as a 'rocker'.

    There are braided wires or multistrand – used for initial levelling and alignment or bonded retainers.

    Wires made for a patients treatment for each stage – as with incognito appliances.

14. Usually a round NiTi archwire is used to start with. It will depend on how irregular the teeth are. An 0.014" NiTi is a good start, in some cases a larger or smaller wire can be used. If a heat-activated wire is used, then a larger wire can be used.

15. Good springback

    Low friction

    Low stiffness

    Light continuous force

    Large range

    Non-toxic

    Poor biohost

    Cheap.

16. Temperature Transitional Range.

17. Low friction

    Low springback

    High stiffness

Good joinability

Non-toxic

Poor biohost

Cheap.

18. Upper left first molar band. It is sized on a study model and then tried into the mouth. It is placed over the first molar tooth, and a bite stick or band pusher is used to make sure it fits correctly. The band is then removed with posterior band-removing pliers. Glass Ionimer cement is placed inside the band covering all of the inside surface and the band is placed back onto the tooth as above. A damp cotton wool roll can be used to remove the excess cement from the tooth and instruments.

19. An Orthodontic bracket. This is a metal bracket for the upper left canine. The coloured marking is placed disto-gingival when bonding onto the tooth. A pair of bonding tweezers is used to hold the bracket, so composite (or GIC) can be placed onto the mess base and the clinician can place onto the LACC point of the tooth.

20. Elastomeric rings/Ormlast rings. These come in various colours and are placed onto the bracket tie wings to hold the archwire in place by mosquito forceps or a twirl on.

21. These are intra-oral elastics. They are placed by the patient and need to be changed daily or when they break. They come in a variety of sizes. Good instructions are required to give to the patient. An elastic placer can be given to the patient to aid placement/removal. In the surgery, mosquitoes can be used.

22. These are wire ligatures. They are used to hold a wire in place for less friction. Long ligatures can be used as a laceback to protect a thin archwire during alignment or to distalise a canine. Mathieu artery forceps are used to tie up the ligatures (these tie from instrument to bracket) or ligature locking pliers can be used for the long ligatures (these tie from bracket to instrument). Mosquitoes should never be used as it wrecks the beaks.

23. Kobiashi hook ligature. This can be used to hold the archwire in place on the bracket. It has a hook on it where the orthodontist can add inter-arch elastics or the patient can add intra-oral elastics. The Kobiashi quick ligatures can be placed with Mathieu artery forceps or the long ligatures with ligature locking pliers.

24. Rotation wedges. These are placed on the mesial or distal tie wings on a bracket underneath the archwire using a pair of mosquitoes. Their main purpose is to derotate a tooth.

25. Powerchain. This is used to close spaces on a stainless steel archwires. It is placed by using a pair of mosquitoes. The ends should be cut smooth, so they do not irritate the patient's soft tissues. Powerchain can also be used for buccal segment space closure by placing the chain from the hook on the molar to the hook on the archwire.

26. NiTi coil springs. Attached to fixed appliances and used to close spaces. They work throughout the 6 weeks in between appointments so that extraction site spaces close at a steady pace.

They can have ligature wire placed on one end to make the spring longer. Mosquitoes are used to place the spring or a pair of Mathieu if a ligature is attached to it.

27. The patient needs to attend to have a separator placed to make space. This is normally placed a week prior to the fitting of the band.

   The following week the separator is removed. The band is tried in for size and then cemented in place with glass ionomer cement. The orthodontist will need a band pusher or bite stick to place the band and a band remover to remove safety from the tooth during the trying-in stage.

28. **OH**
   - After any meal or snack, the appliance must be cleaned by brushing and rinsing.
   - Clean teeth, gums and braces well. This will take longer so allow time to do it, often a track of your favourite CD.
   - You must attend your GDP to have regular 'check-ups', so that fillings can be done and your general dental health is monitored.

   Diet
   - Sticky sweets and chewing gum must be avoided as it will damage the brace.
   - Hard or crusty bread must be cut up into bit size pieces so that it can be eaten easier.
   - No fizzy drinks. Sugary drinks/food can cause decalcification – white marks on your teeth around the brackets.
   - Do not chew pencils or hard objects as these can damage the brace.

   Pain
   - Appliances may cause some discomfort at first. If painful take what you normally take for a headache.
   - If the brace rubs and you get ulcers, dry the bracket with a tissue and place a piece of wax over it (container with wax given). This will alleviate the rubbing and the ulcer/sore bit will go. Do not worry if you swallow the wax, it is not harmful.

   Breakage
   - If the appliance breaks, then you should phone the department/practice to come in and have it repaired, else your teeth will move incorrectly or move back.
   - Wear a mouth guard for contact sport – one that can be adjusted in hot water, so it will fit as the teeth move.

   You will be expected to wear the appliance for 12–24 months if you look after the appliance and do not have any breakages.

   Discuss with patient and parent/guardian verbally with written information that can be used to refer back to if required.

29. Using a 0.019″×0.025″ stainless steel wire or a TMA wire, bends are placed to get the correct angulation and torque can also be placed to get the roots into the correct position.

30. From the hook distal from the upper lateral to the hook on the lower molar.

31. From the hook on the upper molar to the hook distal to the lower laterals.

32. It is an elastic that goes around in a 'square' or 'triangular' shape so that it reduces an open bite.

33. To expand the upper arch.

34. Used for anchorage to hold the molars where they are.

35. To hold the lower molars where they are. This can be used as a space maintainer and also as the lower part of a dynamax functional appliance.

Headgear – EOT

1. The applying forces to the teeth and or skeletal structures from an extra-oral source.

2. Extra-oral anchorage.

3. Extra-oral traction.

4. 10–12 hours.

5. 12–14 hours.

6. 450–500 grams.

7. 250–350 grams.

8. Correx gauge.

9. Headcap, Khloen bow (Nitom Safety Lock), Masel safety strap, either 'snap away' modules to headcap or extra-oral elastics (it depends on make).

10. High or Occipital pull
    Straight or Combi pull
    Low or Cervical pull.

11. Show patient how to fit the headgear:
    - Facebow – whisker
    - Head cap
    - Safety strap.

    Fixed appliance – facebow inserted into molar band tubes

    Removable appliance – facebow inserted into cribs tube

    Ensure all safety devices are worn correctly, to prevent injury to face and/or eyes. Patient/parent is competent, elastics removed first prior to removing facebow.

    If the headgear becomes loose, patient must ring dept and see orthodontist. Patient must not wear appliance until it has been checked by orthodontist.

    Must be worn for 10–14 hours a day, as instructed by orthodontist.

    Headgear to be worn at night-time only.

    OHI must be given.

    Written and verbal instructions given.

    If any injuries do happen. go to A&E dept **IMMEDIATELY**!

12. Patients notes

    Patients model box

    Mouth mirror

    Mauns heavy duty wire cutters

    Adams universal pliers

    Adams spring forming pliers

    Ruler

    Nitom Locking facebow (various sizes)

    Headcap with 'snap away' modules

    Chinagraph stick

    Sharps box

    Large hand mirror

    Patient information leaflet

    Chart for patient to record hours

    Written instructions.

13. Anchorage

14. 2

15. The Nitom Safety lock is fitted by locking the ends into the buccal tubes of the first molar bands and locked into place.

    The headcap is placed over the head.

    Holding onto the facebow, the 'snap away' modules are attached to the outer wings of the facebow one side and then the other side (or if elastics are used, e.g. with interlandi head-cap, then the elastics are joined to the facebow).

    If required, a Masel safety strap is attached to the facebow.

Retention

1. The aim of retention is to hold orthodontically treated teeth while the bone and fibres remodel around the teeth and prevent relapse due to previous orthodontic treatment or continued growth. Common types of retainers are as follows:
   • Vacuum-formed retainers (Essix)/thermo-formed retainers
   • Bonded retainers
   • Hawley retainers
   • Begg retainer.

2. At the start of treatment.

3. This varies between orthodontists but it is best practice to retain as long as possible because teeth will move all your life.

   The regime we use is: every night for the first year, then alternate nights for 6 months and then 2 nights a week for as long as possible.

4. Clinic

Impressions taken in alginate and then disinfected as per practice policy.

Laboratory card written up with prescription for lab for VFRs.

Laboratory

Impression cast in stone to make a working model.

Clear sheet placed over model and placed into vacuum machine.

Once the sheet has gone over all the teeth it is taken out and trimmed

The VFR is disinfected.

Clinic

VFR is fitted by the Orthodontist or Orthodontic Therapist.

Patient is shown how to insert/remove.

Instructions are given on the wear and care of appliance.

Written instructions are given to the patient. The EU medical directives sheet is given to the patient.

5. Clean your teeth with a small headed toothbrush and fluoride toothpaste, spit and do not rinse.

Take your retainers out of the pot and rinse them with water (not hot water).

Place them in firmly, so that they sit properly on your teeth.

You must not eat or drink with them in, only still water can be consumed.

In the morning you need to remove the retainer before breakfast, take it out of your mouth and clean it with a clean toothbrush with soap and water (tepid). Retainer Brite (or equivalent) can be used as directed.

Once cleaned, place it in your pot. Do not wrap in a tissue as retainer could be thrown away, and there will be a charge for a replacement.

If you pet chews the retainer or you lose the retainer then there is a cost to replace it.

If you break your retainer, then bring the bits back and there may or may not be a cost.

Remember to bring your retainers to your visits so they can be checked.

Keep regular 'check-up' appointments with your GDP, and remember to take your retainers with you in case you have any dental work done as they may need adjusting.

6. Bonded retainer – kept as close as possible to the incisal tip.

7. At the debond appointment, a fabricated bonded retainer wire is collected from the lab or made up in the surgery.

The palatal surface of the teeth is cleaned with pumice.

The patient has a rinse.

Cotton wool rolls are placed in the sulcus and a saliva ejector is placed.

The teeth are dried, and 37% phosphoric acid is placed on to the palatal surface of the teeth.

Then this is washed off and dried with air.

The cotton wool rolls are changed.

Bond is placed onto the palatal surface of the teeth.

This is dried.

The bonded wire is placed onto the teeth and held in place by elastics, floss or a jig.

Flowable composite is placed and then cured by the curing light.

The floss, elastics or jig is removed.

The occlusion is checked with articulating paper and adjusted if necessary with a tungsten carbide bur.

8. A Hawley is sometimes used instead of a vacuum-formed retainer so that vertical settling can occur for better interdigitization.

Hawley's are very useful for placing an artificial tooth until a permanent restorative replacement can be completed. Some Orthodontists will use a vacuum-formed retainer with a tooth for this.

9. Where there is a change in tooth position from the place, they were treated to.

10. **OH**
    - Clean teeth as normal with a toothbrush and toothpaste containing fluoride.
    - Use floss with a floss threader or superfloss to get around the bonded retainer being careful not to knock it off.
    - Can use TePe brushes or similar around the retainer again being careful not to knock it off.
    - A waterpik can be used to wash around the retainer.

    Diet
    - Do not bite into anything, cut food up into smaller pieces.
    - Do not have anything too hard or sticky.
    - Do not chew pens or finger nails.

    Breakage
    - If it should break, contact the surgery as soon as possible to have it repaired. Do not pull on it as it is easier to repair a small piece rather than the whole retainer coming off.
    - Use your vacuum-formed retainer to hold the teeth in position until you can be seen.
    - There may be a charge to repair the retainer.

TADs

1. It stands for Temporary Anchorage Device.

2. It reinforces anchorage.

3. A small amount of local anaesthetic is placed into the area to 'numb' the soft tissues. The TAD is then 'screwed' in between the roots of the teeth into the correct position.

4. Not to hit the PDL.

SECTION V Answers: Interdisciplinary care

1. It is where two or more specialities get together with a patient to decide on the best treatment options. For example, orthodontist and oral maxilla facial surgeon or orthodontist and restorative dentist.

2. Patients notes

   Study models

   DPT

   Lateral cephalometric

   Digitization and projection of how many mm to move hard tissues and the projection of soft tissues

   Intra- and extra-oral photographs

   Occasionally a cone beam will be required to check growth is complete.

3. BOS leaflet – Orthognathic surgery

   BOS – patient DVD about Orthognathic surgery

4. Planning

   Consent

   Extractions

   Fixed appliances – takes about 12–18 months
   - Alignment and levelling
   - Arch coordination – to make sure they will fit after surgery
   - Decompensation

   'snap' impressions and records

   Surgery planning finalised

   Wafers produced
   - Impressions
   - Facebow
   - Surgical hooks onto archwire

   Surgery

   Intermaxillary traction

   Complete any movement not undertaken pre surgery

   Fine detailing

   Debond 3–6 months after surgery

   Retention

   2-year post-operative review with records taken

   Data placed on BOS audit

5. Acceptable dental and facial aesthetics

   Good function

   Excellent oral health

   Stability

6. Swelling

   Bleeding

   Limited mouth opening

   Dietary changes and associated weight loss in the short term

Time off work and recovery

Changes in facial appearance

Changes in nerve sensation

Permanent damage to ID nerve

Need for re-operation

Infection

Need to remove plates

TMJ problems

Relapse

Problems swallowing

Tooth avulsion or other damage to periodontal support

Ophthalmic complications

Reduction in auditory capacity

Risk to GA – death.

7. Please use these items as you have been shown. It is important that you keep your mouth as clean as possible to reduce the risk of infection.
   - Corsodyl mouthwash – This should be used morning and evening for the next 2 weeks. When rinsing use 10 ml and swish around your mouth for 1 min. When you start to clean your teeth with toothpaste remember to rinse your mouth at a separate time.
   - 'Sponges on sticks' can be soaked in Corsodyl and rubbed around the teeth and braces gently twice a day for the first couple of days. This may need to be longer on areas you cannot clean with your toothbrush.
   - An oral B stages-1 brush which can be used from day 2 or 3. Start to clean your front teeth and gently move further back when you can.
   - An adult sensitive toothbrush can be introduced from day 5. Try and clean as much as possible.
   - Tepe brushes can be used to clean between your wire and teeth as soon as possible. Please be gentle especially around any operation areas as you may be sore or numb.
   - Vaseline can be used to make your lips feel softer and more comfortable after surgery. Use as required.
     REMEMBER A CLEAN MOUTH HEALS QUICKER THAN A DIRTY MOUTH
     Be reassured
     Your braces will be removed as soon as possible
     This is likely to be at least three months after your surgery

8. Movement of the chin

9. Maxillary procedures alone
     - Le Fort I
     - Le Fort II
     - Le Fort III
   Mandibular procedures
     - Sagittal split
     - Vertical Subsigmoid Osteotomy

Both arches
- Bimaxillary

10. Open: The canine is exposed and bone removed. A pack is placed over the exposure and removed 10 days later. The tooth is either left to erupt or a bond with chain can be bonded at day 10.

    Closed: The canine is exposed and bone removed, a caplin hook with chain (or something similar) is attached to the tooth and the palate is sutured back over with the chain showing so the tooth can have traction placed to aid eruption by pulling on the tooth.

11. Hypodontia – developmentally abscent

    Microdontia

    Post-trauma

    Missing teeth – from extractions

12. Option 1 – Close spaces. If the canines are a good colour and can be adapted to look like laterals or the patient does not want to pay for bridges/implants later.

    Option 2 – Open spaces. So that bridges/implants can be placed to artificially replace the laterals. This option has continuing upkeep costs for the patient.

13. Leave the roots parallel to the space and make sure there is enough space for the implant.

14. The periodontal disease must be stable prior to the commencement of orthodontic treatment.

15. Black triangles

16. 3 months

17. 1:700 live births